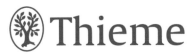

Top 3 Differentials in Pediatric Radiology

A Case Review

Rebecca Stein-Wexler, MD
Professor of Pediatric Radiology
Director, Radiology Residency Program
University of California Davis Medical Center and Children's Hospital
Sacramento, California

Series Editor

William T. O'Brien Sr., DO, FAOCR
Director, Pediatric Neuroradiology Fellowship
Cincinnati Children's Hospital Medical Center
Associate Professor of Radiology
University of Cincinnati College of Medicine
Cinncinnati, Ohio

Thieme
New York • Stuttgart • Delhi • Rio de Janeiro

Thieme Medical Publishers, Inc.
333 Seventh Avenue
New York, New York 10001

Executive Editor: William Lamsback
Managing Editors: J. Owen Zurhellen IV and Kenneth Schubach
Editorial Assistant: Conrad Kozlowski
Director, Editorial Services: Mary Jo Casey
Editorial Director: Sue Hodgson
Production Editor: Sean Woznicki
International Production Director: Andreas Schabert
International Marketing Director: Fiona Henderson
International Sales Director: Louisa Turrell
Director, Institutional Sales: Adam Bernacki
Senior Vice President and Chief Operating Officer: Sarah Vanderbilt
President: Brian D. Scanlan

Library of Congress Cataloging-in-Publication Data

Names: Stein-Wexler, Rebecca, editor.
Title: Top 3 differentials in pediatric radiology: a case review /
  [edited by] Rebecca Stein-Wexler
Other titles: Top three differentials in pediatric radiology
Description: Second edition. | New York : Thieme, [2018] | Includes
  bibliographical references and indexes.
Identifiers: (print) | (ebook)
  | ISBN 9781626233713 (E-book) | ISBN 9781626233706
  (paperback : alk. paper)
Subjects: | MESH: Radiography | Diagnosis, Differential |
  Case Reports
Classification: (ebook) | (print) |
LC record available at https://lccn.loc.gov/

The views expressed in this book are those of the author and contributors, and do not reflect the official policy or position of the United States Government, the Department of Defense, Department of the Army or the Department of the Air Force.

Copyright © 2019 by Thieme Medical Publishers, Inc.

Thieme Publishers New York
333 Seventh Avenue, New York, NY 10001 USA
+1 800 782 3488, customerservice@thieme.com

Thieme Publishers Stuttgart
Rüdigerstrasse 14, 70469 Stuttgart, Germany
+49 [0]711 8931 421, customerservice@thieme.de

Thieme Publishers Delhi
A-12, Second Floor, Sector-2, Noida-201301
Uttar Pradesh, India
+91 120 45 566 00, customerservice@thieme.in

Thieme Publishers Rio de Janeiro, Thieme Publicações Ltda.
Edifício Rodolpho de Paoli, 25º andar
Av. Nilo Peçanha, 50 – Sala 2508,
Rio de Janeiro 20020-906 Brasil
+55 21 3172-2297 / +55 21 3172-1896

ISBN 978-1-62623-370-6

Also available as an e-book:
eISBN 978-1-62623-371-3

Important note: Medicine is an ever-changing science undergoing continual development. Research and clinical experience are continually expanding our knowledge, in particular our knowledge of proper treatment and drug therapy. Insofar as this book mentions any dosage or application, readers may rest assured that the authors, editors, and publishers have made every effort to ensure that such references are in accordance with **the state of knowledge at the time of production of the book.**

Nevertheless, this does not involve, imply, or express any guarantee or responsibility on the part of the publishers in respect to any dosage instructions and forms of applications stated in the book. **Every user is requested to examine carefully** the manufacturers' leaflets accompanying each drug and to check, if necessary in consultation with a physician or specialist, whether the dosage schedules mentioned therein or the contraindications stated by the manufacturers differ from the statements made in the present book. Such examination is particularly important with drugs that are either rarely used or have been newly released on the market. Every dosage schedule or every form of application used is entirely at the user's own risk and responsibility. The authors and publishers request every user to report to the publishers any discrepancies or inaccuracies noticed. If errors in this work are found after publication, errata will be posted at www.thieme.com on the product description page.

Some of the product names, patents, and registered designs referred to in this book are in fact registered trademarks or proprietary names even though specific reference to this fact is not always made in the text. Therefore, the appearance of a name without designation as proprietary is not to be construed as a representation by the publisher that it is in the public domain.

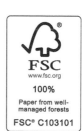

FSC
www.fsc.org
100%
Paper from well-managed forests
FSC® C103101

Dedicated to the memory of

Sandra L. Wootton-Gorges, **dear friend and colleague**

May all who read this book care for their patients with wisdom and compassion.

Contents

Series Foreword

The original "Top 3" concept was something engrained during my residency training in the military. From day 1, our program emphasized the importance of having gamut-based differentials as part of our daily readout sessions, as well as during didactic and clinical case-based conferences. The bulk of residency training was then centered around learning the key clinical and imaging manifestations of each entity on the list of differentials to be able to distinguish one from another, when possible. To avoid providing clinicians with a laundry list of differentials that would be of little value, we were encouraged to consider the "Top 3" differentials and any other important considerations based upon the specific clinical scenario or imaging finding(s) presented. I found that concept and approach to radiology so useful that I continue to utilize it to this day.

One thing I have learned throughout my radiology career, especially as a residency program director, is that not every individual learns or processes information in the same manner. Some individuals can read through a traditional textbook that is organized by pathology (i.e., developmental abnormalities, infectious processes, neoplasms, etc.) and readily recognize that the developmental abnormality in Chapter 1 is in the same differential for the infectious process in Chapter 2 and a few neoplasms in Chapter 3. Others, like me, best learn from gamut-based resources where content is organized based upon the key imaging findings, similar to how we practice radiology. If you are part of the latter group, then the "Top 3" approach may be the right fit for you. The intent of the series is to provide a comprehensive case-based alternative to traditional subspecialty textbooks where the focus remains on differential diagnoses. After all, when the dust settles and the core and certifying exams are nothing but distant (and hopefully pleasant) memories, this is what radiology is all about.

When it came time to recommend an author for the Pediatric Radiology subspecialty edition of the "Top 3" series, I immediately thought of Dr. Rebecca Stein-Wexler. Along with Dr. Sandra Wootton-Gorges, to whom this book is dedicated, Dr. Stein-Wexler taught me the intricacies of pediatric imaging during my residency training and was instrumental in my decision to pursue an academic career in pediatric neuroradiology. Her style and approach to working through even the most complicated cases at the viewing monitor is beautifully translated into the cases of this book. The result is perhaps one of the most practical resources available for learning or reviewing pediatric radiology.

Top 3 Differentials in Pediatric Radiology is organized into six sections: chest, cardiac, and airway imaging; gastrointestinal imaging; genitourinary imaging; musculoskeletal imaging; head and neck imaging; and brain and spine imaging. Each section begins with a series of differential-based cases and concludes with important "Roentgen Classics" – cases that have imaging findings characteristic of a single diagnosis. In this first edition, Dr. Stein-Wexler and colleagues have done an exceptional job in selecting common and important gamuts encountered in pediatric imaging practices with content suitable across a wide range of experience levels. The case discussions are centered on a key imaging finding (with a few exceptions that are centered on the patient presentation), which serves as the basis for the subsequent differential diagnoses. The didactic approach to the case discussions walks readers through the key clinical and imaging manifestations for each entity on the list of differentials, making this an incredibly high yield resource for board preparation and—even more importantly—clinical practice.

It is my sincere hope that you find this well thought out and expertly written book both enjoyable and educational.

William T. O'Brien Sr., DO, FAOCR

Foreword

Pediatric imaging is a discipline like no other subspecialty in Radiology. Not only does it encompass all imaging modalities and all parts of the body, but it also demands familiarity with manifestations of both normal and abnormal growth and development. It is no easy feat to create a comprehensive, yet manageable compilation of representative entities encountered when imaging children. Dr. Stein-Wexler, Professor of Pediatric Radiology and Director of the Radiology Residency Program at University of California Davis, has the depth of clinical knowledge and decades of experience instructing trainees and junior colleagues in the art and practice of Pediatric Radiology to successfully take on this challenge. Following her recently completed "tour de force" pediatric musculoskeletal textbook, Pediatric Orthopedic Imaging, Dr. Stein-Wexler has produced The Top 3 Differentials in Pediatric Radiology. In this current work, she has concisely distilled a large body of information into a format that is accessible for a wide-ranging audience, from students and residents who are just beginning their training to fellows and early career physicians, to more seasoned clinicians who wish to "brush up" on newer developments and concepts in the field. By its succinct yet systematic representation of a vast discipline, this book just may entice radiology residents to pursue a career in pediatric radiology!

Serving as both editor and author, Rebecca Stein-Wexler, has selected a talented group of contributors who have compiled 194 wonderfully illustrative sections that encompass a majority of the key clinical topics and imaging modalities. Each disease entity is conveniently organized by medical history, radiologic image(s), key findings, and top 3 differential diagnoses along with additional less likely diagnoses, the correct diagnosis, clinical pearls, and landmark references. This format makes this textbook a valuable review tool for certification examinations and for use as a basic general pediatric radiology primer, particularly for those of us who still enjoy the feel of paper in our hands! The Appendix facilitates these functions by summarizing the most common differential diagnoses for each disease entity. Finally, by listing each section and its content, the Index of Key Findings, can serve as a useful curriculum guide for trainees and educators alike.

Dr. Stein-Wexler is applauded for preparing this wide-ranging, yet manageable, summary of common radiologic findings in children. Anyone seeking a salient review of imaging features of common pediatric disorders will be well-served by this elegant textbook, and in turn, the knowledge imparted upon its readers will ultimately benefit the care of children. On behalf of the readers of your book and the children we serve, congratulations and thanks, Rebecca!

Tal Laor, MD
Professor of Radiology
Harvard Medical School
Academic Division Chief of Musculoskeletal Imaging
Boston Children's Hospital
Boston, Massachusetts

Preface

Top 3 Differentials in Pediatric Radiology: A Case Review is intended for the radiology residents and fellows who wish to learn what really matters during their initial exposure to pediatric imaging, as they prepare for exams and embark on their post-graduate career. It will also be useful to the practicing radiologist who seeks an easy-to-digest refresher. The book's 194 cases cover what is typically encountered in a busy practice. The chapters include the most relevant, useful, and important information for each diagnosis.

Children are not just little adults. And the range of pediatric imaging—normal and pathological—only partially overlaps that of adults. Normal anatomy changes with age. Some congenital anomalies are encountered only in the very young. Many common pediatric conditions are unheard of in older patients. And processes that are encountered across age groups—trauma, infection, some neoplasms—manifest differently in children.

This book emphasizes diseases that are unique to, or especially common in, children. It focuses on pathology that is encountered relatively often, but also includes unusual disorders and normal variants that may mimic disease. Radiographs and ultrasound constitute most of pediatric imaging, so many cases include examples of these modalities. Magnetic resonance, computed tomography, and nuclear medicine imaging are included where appropriate. Up-to-date references are provided for the reader who wants to probe more deeply.

Welcome to the fascinating world of pediatric radiology!

Acknowledgments

The gamuts in this book draw on insight from several brilliant pediatric radiologists. Local colleagues who provided invaluable advice include Thomas Sanchez, Anna Nidecker, and the late Sandra L. Wootton-Gorges of happy memory. Leslie L. Grissom and Jennifer L. Nicholas also helped a great deal with the initial planning stages of the book. In addition, Leslie Grissom, Jennifer Nicholas, Anna Nidecker, Matthew Bobinski, Jennifer Chang, Arzu Ozturk, and the late Sandra L. Wootton-Gorges provided thoughtful editorial suggestions after reading sections of the book.

I would like to thank my parents, Sherman and Hannah Stein, for inspiring me to write. And finally, I couldn't have done this without the encouragement and support of my husband, Tony, and unending distraction and comic relief from our adult children, Jason and Rachel.

Contributors

Karen Ayotte, MD
Pediatric Radiologist
The Permanente Medical Group
Walnut Creek, California

Duy Quang Bui, MD
Fellow, Neuroradiology
University of California Davis Medical Center
Sacramento, California

James S. Chalfant, MD
Resident, Radiology
University of California Davis Medical Center
Sacramento, California

Ellen Cheang, MD
Resident, Radiology
University of California Davis Medical Center
Sacramento, California

Michael Doherty, MD
Resident, Radiology
University of California Davis Medical Center
Sacramento, California

Leslie E. Grissom, MD
Clinical Professor, Radiology and Pediatrics
Nemours duPont Hospital for Children
Thomas Jefferson University
Wilmington, Delaware

Kriti Gwal, MD
Assistant Professor, Pediatric Radiology
UC Davis Medical Center and Children's Hospital
Sacramento, California

Stephen Henrichon, MD
Resident, Radiology
University of California Davis Medical Center
Sacramento, California

Ernst Joseph, MD
Resident, Radiology
Hospital of the State University of Haiti
Port-au-Prince, Haiti

Fabienne Joseph, MD
Chief Resident, Radiology
Hospital of the State University of Haiti
Port-au-Prince, Haiti

Wonsuk Kim, MD
Resident, Radiology
University of California Davis Medical Center
Sacramento, California

Aleksandar Kitich, MD
Resident, Radiology
University of California Davis Medical Center
Sacramento, California

John P. Lichtenberger III, MD
Associate Professor, Radiology and Radiological Sciences
Uniformed Services University
Bethesda, Maryland

Stephen Malutich, MD
Resident, Radiology and Nuclear Medicine
University of California Davis Medical Center
Sacramento, California

Myles Mitsunaga, MD
Resident, Radiology
University of California Davis Medical Center
Sacramento, California

Geoffrey D. McWilliams, MD
Chief Resident, Radiology
University of California Davis Medical Center
Sacramento, California

Ethan Neufeld, MD
Chief Resident, Radiology
University of California Davis Medical Center
Sacramento, California

Jennifer L. Nicholas, MD, MHA
Assistant Professor, Pediatric Radiology
Washington University School of Medicine
Mallinckrodt Institute of Radiology
Saint Louis, Missouri

Anna Nidecker, MD
Associate Professor, Neuroradiology
University of California Davis Medical Center
Sacramento, California

William T. O'Brien Sr., DO
Director, Pediatric Neuroradiology Fellowship
Cincinnati Children's Hospital Medical Center
Associate Professor of Radiology
University of Cincinnati College of Medicine
Cincinnati, Ohio

Aaron Potnick, MD
Assistant Clinical Professor, Pediatric Radiology
University of California Davis Medical Center
Sacramento, California

Shruthi Ram, MD
Resident, Radiology
University of California Davis Medical Center
Sacramento, California

Mike Evens Saint-Louis, MD
Chief Resident, Radiology
Hospital of the State University of Haiti
Port-au-Prince, Haiti

Patrick J. Sanchez, MD
Fellow, Neuroradiology
University of California Davis Medical Center
Sacramento, California

Thomas Ray Sanchez, MD
Associate Professor, Pediatric Radiology
Director of Pediatric Imaging
UC Davis Medical Center and Children's Hospital
Sacramento, California

Arvind Sonik, MD
Pediatric Radiologist
The Permanente Medical Group
Sacramento, California

Rebecca Stein-Wexler, MD
Professor of Pediatric Radiology
Director, Radiology Residency Program
University of California Davis Medical Center and
   Children's Hospital
Sacramento, California

Robert J. Wood
University of San Diego
San Diego, California

Sandra L. Wootton-Gorges[†]
Professor, Pediatric Radiology
Director of Pediatric Imaging
UC Davis Medical Center and Children's Hospital
Sacramento, California

Cathy Zhou, MD
Resident, Radiology and Nuclear Medicine
University of California Davis Medical Center
Sacramento, California

[†]Deceased.

Part 1

Airway, Cardiac, and Chest Imaging

1

Case 1

Karen M. Ayotte

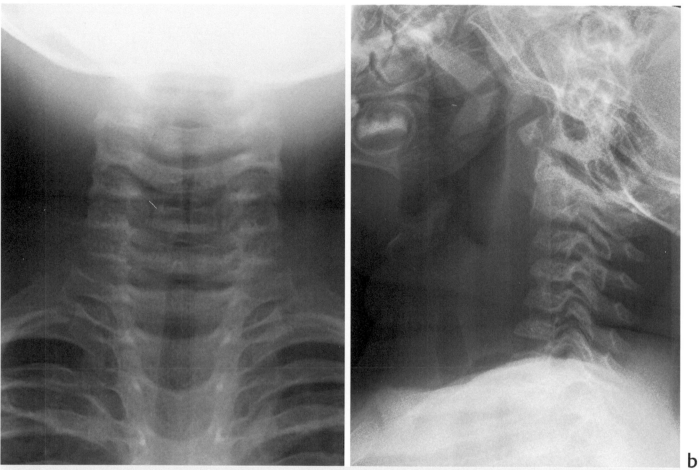

a ⬛ b

Fig. 1.1 Frontal view of the neck reveals subglottic tracheal narrowing with loss of normal shouldering of the airway, referred to as the "steeple sign" **(a)**. The lateral view demonstrates overdistention of the hypopharynx and subglottic narrowing; there is mild pseudothickening of prevertebral soft tissues and pseudosubluxation at C2–C3 **(b)**.

■ Clinical Presentation

A 15-month-old with stridor (▶ Fig. 1.1).

■ Key Imaging Finding

Narrowing of the airway.

■ Top Three Differential Diagnoses

• **Croup (laryngotracheobronchitis).** Croup is the most common cause of upper airway obstruction in children between 6 months and 3 years of age, with peak incidence around 1 year. The radiographic hallmark is symmetrical subglottic airway narrowing manifested by loss of normal shouldering of the upper airway on the frontal projection, referred to as the "steeple" sign. The lateral view commonly demonstrates overdistention of the hypopharynx, as well as narrowing of the subglottic airway.

• **Epiglottitis.** This potentially life-threatening disease affects older patients than those with croup. When the diagnosis is suspected, a provider capable of managing the child's airway should be immediately available during imaging. The radiographic hallmark is epiglottic enlargement (thumb sign) on the lateral view, as well as thick aryepiglottic folds. Epiglottitis may mimic croup on a frontal view.

• **Retropharyngeal abscess.** Space-occupying processes in the prevertebral and retropharyngeal soft tissues may exert mass effect on the airway, causing dyspnea and stridor. The differential diagnosis of widened prevertebral soft tissues includes abscess, hemorrhage, lymphadenopathy, and pseudothickening. If physiological pseudothickening is suspected, a repeat inspiratory exam with the neck fully extended or airway fluoroscopy may resolve the dilemma.

■ Additional Differential Diagnoses

• **Bacterial tracheitis.** Bacterial tracheitis is characterized by exudative plaques that adhere to the tracheal wall. Because of their flat, longitudinal configuration, they may be seen only on one view. Asymmetrical subglottic airway narrowing may resemble the radiographic appearance of croup. However, patients with bacterial tracheitis are typically older (6–10 years old) and more toxic. Adherent mucus in the airway mimics the plaques of bacterial tracheitis but should clear on repeat examination after coughing.

• **Aspirated foreign body.** Both aspirated and ingested foreign bodies may cause an abnormal airway contour on radiographs, and both may present with dyspnea and stridor. It is easy to determine the location of disk-shaped radiopaque foreign bodies (such as coins) on a frontal neck radiograph. Those in the trachea align in the sagittal plane, since the cartilaginous rings of the trachea are incomplete posteriorly, whereas those in the esophagus align in the coronal plane. Radiographic diagnosis of the more common radiolucent foreign bodies is problematic. Direct visualization is the next step in evaluation.

• **Hemangioma.** Hemangiomas tend to cause variably asymmetrical airway narrowing and are commonly detected before the age of 1 year. When subglottic, the patient's symptoms may mimic other more common etiologies of stridor. Radiographs show asymmetrical mass effect narrowing the airway.

■ Diagnosis

Croup.

✓ Pearls

• Croup is most common in children under 3 years of age; the "steeple" sign is seen on frontal radiographs.
• Lateral X-ray of epiglottitis shows epiglottic thickening (thumb sign) and thickened aryepiglottic folds.

• Retropharyngeal abscess demonstrates prevertebral soft-tissue swelling.
• Foreign body aspiration must always be considered in a child with stridor.

Suggested Readings

John SD, Swischuk LE. Stridor and upper airway obstruction in infants and children. Radiographics. 1992; 12(4):625–643, discussion 644

Yedururi S, Guillerman RP, Chung T, et al. Multimodality imaging of tracheobronchial disorders in children. Radiographics. 2008; 28(3):e29

Case 2

Rebecca Stein-Wexler

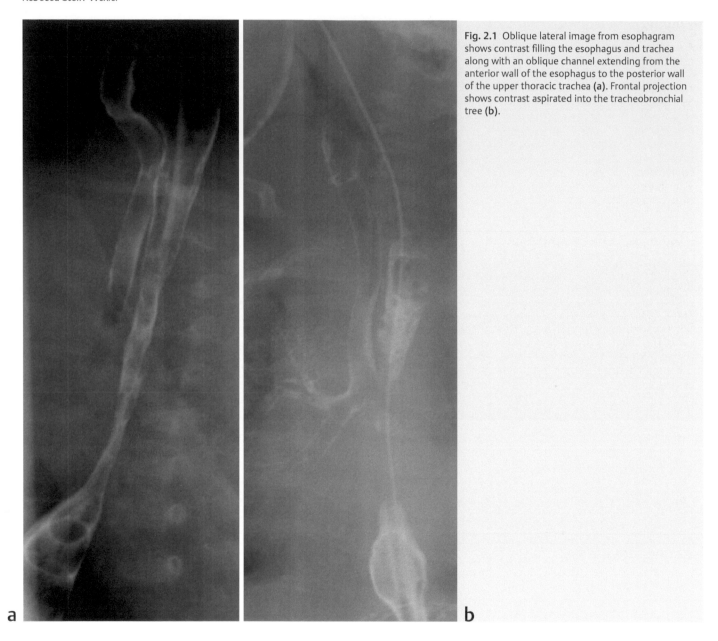

Fig. 2.1 Oblique lateral image from esophagram shows contrast filling the esophagus and trachea along with an oblique channel extending from the anterior wall of the esophagus to the posterior wall of the upper thoracic trachea **(a)**. Frontal projection shows contrast aspirated into the tracheobronchial tree **(b)**.

a

b

■ Clinical Presentation

A 4-year-old child who coughs while feeding (▶Fig. 2.1).

■ Key Imaging Finding

Contrast material in the trachea.

■ Top Three Differential Diagnoses

- **Aspiration.** Oropharyngeal coordination is critical and if disrupted may lead to aspiration in apparently normal children as well as in those with a history of prematurity, neurological impairment, and craniofacial malformations. Patients may be asymptomatic or present with poor feeding, apnea, cough, wheezing, reactive airway disease, and lower respiratory tract infections. If aspiration is suspected, patients are often evaluated with video fluoroscopy performed with a speech pathologist. This allows detailed assessment of the phases of swallowing and delineation of barium pooling in the valleculae and piriform sinuses as well as laryngeal and subglottic penetration. Patients with clinically occult aspiration show similar findings on esophagrams performed for other purposes. It is important to note at what point the contrast enters the trachea, since that is essential for determining whether it resulted from laryngeal penetration or from abnormal tracheoesophageal communication.
- **H-type tracheoesophageal fistula (H-TEF).** H-TEF is usually diagnosed on esophagrams performed after the immediate newborn period, whereas TEF with esophageal atresia is diagnosed in utero or in newborns due to the esophageal atresia. H-TEF accounts for only 5% of all TEFs. It has an oblique course, passing upward from the low cervical or upper thoracic esophagus to the trachea. Young infants present with cyanosis, cough, and choking with feeds, whereas older children more likely have recurrent lower respiratory infections. X-rays may show gas in the lower esophagus, scattered parenchymal opacities due to aspiration, and gaseous bowel distension. Diagnosis rests on the esophagram, performed with isotonic water-soluble contrast due to risk of aspiration. However, H-TEF may be difficult to identify and diagnosis delayed, perhaps due to intermittent esophageal occlusion. Repeat esophagrams are often needed. Just before the fistula fills with contrast, a small out-pouching from the anterior esophageal wall may be seen. If contrast is seen in the trachea, it is important to identify the fistulous tract to exclude aspiration. If the tract cannot be identified, a tube esophagram may be performed with gradual pullback of an esophageal catheter.
- **Laryngeal cleft.** This rare congenital anomaly consists of communication between a defect in the posterior wall of the larynx and the anterior hypopharynx or esophagus. Clefts above the level of the vocal cords may present in adults. Lower clefts extending into the cervical or thoracic trachea usually present in infants with severe respiratory symptoms. Over half of patients with laryngeal clefts have other malformations of the gastrointestinal (GI) tract, including esophageal atresia, TEF, and imperforate anus; anomalies elsewhere are also common. Diagnosis is difficult. Clefts may be visualized on esophagrams as a thin tract of contrast extending to the larynx or trachea, or as contrast appearing in the trachea without laryngeal penetration. Final diagnosis relies on direct visualization of a defect in the posterior wall of the airway.

■ Diagnosis

H-type tracheoesophageal fistula.

✓ Pearls

- It is essential to determine whether contrast has entered the trachea due to aspiration or due to an abnormal tracheoesophageal communication.
- H-tracheoesophageal fistula is usually diagnosed in infancy and is often located near the cervicothoracic junction.
- Laryngeal cleft is commonly accompanied with other malformations of the GI tract.

Suggested Readings

Durvasula VS, O'Neill AC, Richter GT. Oropharyngeal dysphagia in children: mechanism, source, and management. Otolaryngol Clin North Am. 2014; 47(5):691–720

Laffan EE, Daneman A, Ein SH, Kerrigan D, Manson DE. Tracheoesophageal fistula without esophageal atresia: are pull-back tube esophagograms needed for diagnosis? Pediatr Radiol. 2006; 36(11):1141–1147

Ng J, Antao B, Bartram J, Raghavan A, Shawis R. Diagnostic difficulties in the management of H-type tracheoesophageal fistula. Acta Radiol. 2006; 47(8):801–805

Windsor A, Clemmens C, Jacobs IN. Rare upper airway anomalies. Paediatr Respir Rev. 2016; 17:24–28

Case 3

Jennifer L. Nicholas

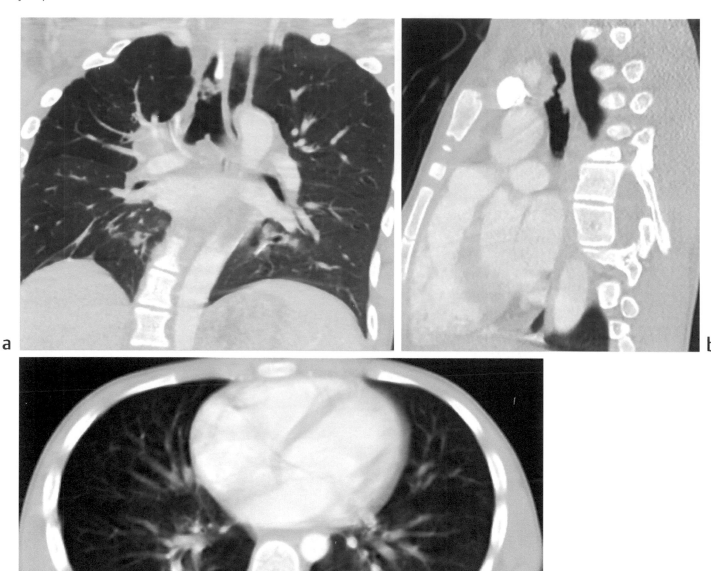

a

b

c

Fig. 3.1 Coronal reformatted contrast-enhanced computed tomography (CT) demonstrates a lobulated soft-tissue mass in the trachea **(a)**. The sagittal reformatted image shows masses arising from both the anterior and the posterior tracheal walls **(b)**. An axial chest CT from several years earlier shows bilateral parenchymal lesions in different stages of cavitation **(c)**. (These images are provided courtesy of Leslie E. Grissom, Nemours/Alfred I. duPont Hospital for Children.)

■ Clinical Presentation

A 15-year-old boy with a chronic illness and recent wheezing (▶Fig. 3.1).

■ Key Imaging Finding

Soft-tissue mass in the airway.

■ Top Three Differential Diagnoses

- **Aspirated foreign body.** The most common intraluminal airway abnormality in a young child is aspirated foreign body. Most aspirated foreign bodies are found on the right, since the course of the right mainstem bronchus is straighter than that of the left. The child may have nonspecific symptoms or present with choking, cough, and unilateral wheezing. The diagnosis is easier when the foreign body is radiodense, but most foreign bodies are radiolucent food material—usually peanuts. Radiographs are often normal. A partially obstructing foreign body may cause lobar or segmental hyperinflation due to air trapping from the ball-valve effect. This suggests the diagnosis even when the foreign body cannot be seen. Larger foreign bodies may completely obstruct the airway, causing atelectasis. The next step is direct visualization of the airway.
- **Subglottic hemangioma.** These are typically seen in the upper trachea of infants younger than 6 months presenting with stridor. Airway narrowing is often asymmetrical, but sometimes the lesions cause circumferential narrowing that mimics croup or subglottic stenosis. CT shows a mass with intense early enhancement. MRI (magnetic resonance imaging) appearance depends on the state of evolution and resembles hemangiomas elsewhere. Most regress spontaneously, but treatment is needed if there is significant airway compromise.
- **Carcinoid.** Primary endobronchial tumors are rare in children. Most, including carcinoid, are malignant. Carcinoid tumors grow slowly and tend to present with wheezing, recurrent pneumonia, and hemoptysis. Findings on chest radiographs mimic those of an aspirated foreign body, but atelectasis is more common than hyperlucency. CT and/or direct visualization with bronchoscopy help differentiate endobronchial carcinoid from aspirated foreign body. The tumors enhance intensely and may be partly calcified. They are ovoid, and their long axis parallels the bronchovascular bundle.

■ Additional Differential Diagnosis

- **Papilloma.** Airway papilloma is typically seen in the setting of juvenile papillomatosis, acquired from perinatal transmission of human papilloma virus or as a result of tracheostomy. One or more lobulated masses may be seen, usually in the larynx but sometimes in the lower trachea and bronchi. Endobronchial lesions may cause atelectasis or air trapping. Patients with papillomas are more likely to have multiple areas of air space abnormalities than are those with aspirated foreign body or carcinoid.

■ Diagnosis

Papillomatosis with endotracheal and parenchymal lesions.

✓ Pearls

- Hyperinflation and/or hyperlucency of one lobe or lung suggest an endobronchial lesion.
- Most aspirated foreign bodies are not visible on radiographs.
- Subglottic hemangiomas are usually eccentric but may be circumferential.
- Primary endobronchial tumors are rare in children and most often carcinoid tumors.

Suggested Readings

Amini B, Huang SY, Tsai J, et al. Primary lung and large airway neoplasms in children: current imaging evaluation with multidetector computed tomography. Radiol Clin North Am. 2013; 51:637-657

Pugmire BS, Lim R, Avery LL. Review of ingested and aspirated foreign bodies in children and their clinical significance for radiologists. Radiographics 2015; 35:1528-1538

Roby BB, Drehner D, Sidman JD. Pediatric tracheal and endobronchial tumors: an institutional review. Arch Otolaryngol Head Neck Surg. 2011; 137:925-929

Yedururi S, Guillerman RP, Chung T, et al. Multimodality imaging of tracheobronchial disorders in children. Radiographics 2008; 28:e29

Case 4

Sandra L. Wootton-Gorges

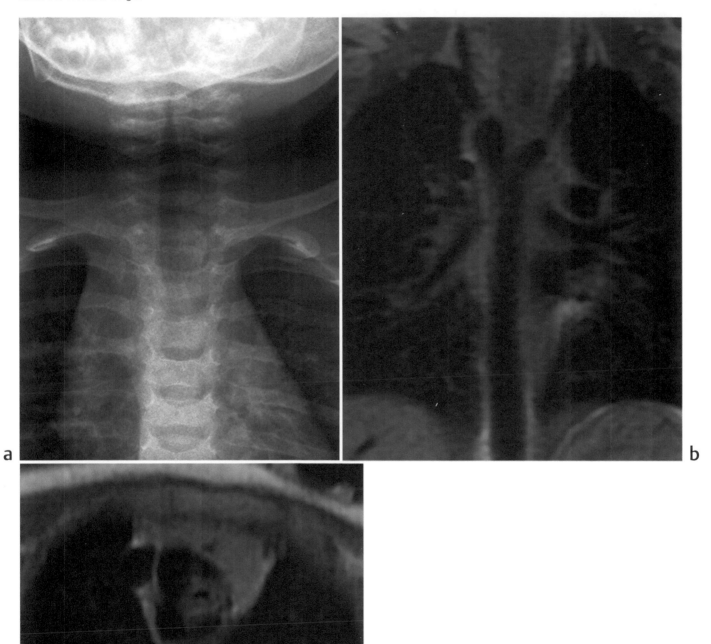

Fig. 4.1 Coned frontal view of the chest shows a large, high, right-sided impression on the trachea **(a)**. Coronal T1-weighted (T1-W) MRI shows a double arch **(b)**. Axial T1-W image shows a dominant right-sided arch and a smaller left-sided arch **(c)**.

◼ Clinical Presentation

A 10-month-old boy with stridor (▶Fig. 4.1).

■ Key Imaging Finding

Vascular anomaly with esophageal and tracheal compression.

■ Top Three Differential Diagnoses

- **Aberrant right subclavian artery (RSCA).** Aberrant RSCA is a common isolated arch anomaly (1% of the population) that is rarely symptomatic. In this anomaly, the RSCA is the last branch of the left aortic arch. It courses behind the esophagus toward the right upper chest, causing posterior indentation on the esophagus during an esophagram. It is not considered a complete vascular ring.
- **Double aortic arch.** This is the most common symptomatic arch anomaly. Two aortic arches are present in this isolated anomaly. The right arch is higher and larger in 75% of cases. The two arches join posteriorly to form the (usually left-sided) descending aorta. The arches thus encircle and may compress the esophagus and trachea, resulting in stridor or problems with feeding. The esophagram will show posterior and bilateral lateral indentation on the esophagus, as well as narrowing of the trachea. MRI and contrast-enhanced CT are excellent modalities to define this vascular anomaly and its effects on surrounding structures.
- **Right aortic arch with aberrant left subclavian artery (LSCA).** In this anomaly, the LSCA arises from the Kommerell diverticulum off a right aortic arch and passes posterior to the esophagus to the left upper extremity. The ductal ligament extends from the LSCA to the left pulmonary artery, completing this often-symptomatic vascular ring.

■ Additional Differential Diagnoses

- **Pulmonary sling.** In this anomaly, the left pulmonary artery arises from the right pulmonary artery and passes between the trachea and esophagus on its way to the left lung. Esophagrams show an anterior indentation on the esophagus and a posterior indentation on the trachea. Associated tracheobronchial anomalies, such as complete tracheal rings, are common and may contribute to respiratory symptoms.
- **Innominate artery compression syndrome.** Compression of the trachea by the crossing innominate artery is a rare cause of respiratory compromise in infants. The innominate artery origin or course may be anomalous in these cases. The patients have a normal left aortic arch. It is uncertain whether this constitutes a real entity, or whether symptoms result from underlying abnormal tracheal development. Surgical reimplantation or suspension may help relieve tracheal narrowing.

■ Diagnosis

Double aortic arch.

✓ Pearls

- Aberrant right subclavian artery is a common anomaly that is rarely symptomatic and is not considered a complete ring.
- Double aortic arch and right arch with aberrant LSCA are the most common symptomatic vascular rings.
- An aberrant left subclavian artery (from a right aortic arch) arises from the diverticulum of Kommerell.
- Pulmonary sling (aberrant origin of the left pulmonary artery) is associated with complete tracheal rings.

Suggested Readings

Castañer E, Gallardo X, Rimola J, et al. Congenital and acquired pulmonary artery anomalies in the adult: radiologic overview. Radiographics. 2006; 26(2):349–371

Hernanz-Schulman M. Vascular rings: a practical approach to imaging diagnosis. Pediatr Radiol. 2005; 35(10):961–979

Kellenberger CJ. Aortic arch malformations. Pediatr Radiol. 2010; 40(6):876–884

Oddone M, Granata C, Vercellino N, Bava E, Tomà P. Multi-modality evaluation of the abnormalities of the aortic arches in children: techniques and imaging spectrum with emphasis on MRI. Pediatr Radiol. 2005; 35(10):947–960

Case 5

Karen M. Ayotte

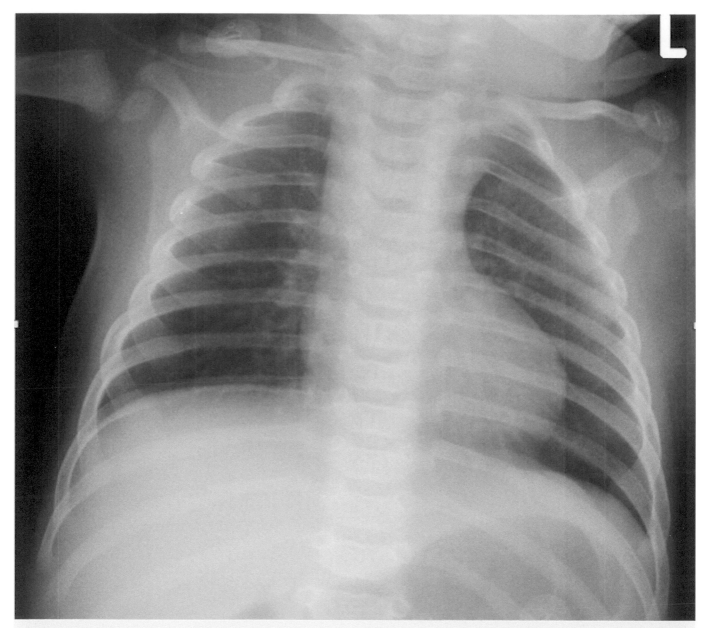

Fig. 5.1 Chest radiograph shows a concave main pulmonary artery contour and elevation of the cardiac apex, resulting in a "boot-shaped" heart. Lungs are relatively oligemic. The aortic arch is on the right.

■ **Clinical Presentation**

A 4-month-old infant with cyanosis (▶Fig. 5.1).

■ Key Imaging Finding

A cyanotic infant with decreased pulmonary flow.

■ Top Three Differential Diagnoses

- **Tetralogy of Fallot.** Tetralogy of Fallot is the most common cyanotic heart condition in children. The four components that define this anomaly are: right ventricular outflow tract obstruction (pulmonic stenosis), ventriculoseptal defect (VSD), overriding aorta, and right ventricular hypertrophy, all resulting from malalignment of the conal septum. Deficiency of the main pulmonary artery segment and elevation of the cardiac apex due to right ventricular hypertrophy lead to the classic radiographic appearance of a boot-shaped heart. Pulmonary vascularity is usually decreased, but severity varies. The aortic arch is on the right in 25% of patients.
- **Pulmonary atresia.** The primary anatomical defect is underdevelopment of the right ventricular outflow tract and pulmonary valve. When present with a VSD, this anomaly is considered a severe variant of tetralogy of Fallot, with similar radiographic findings. When the ventricular septum is intact, there is an obligatory right-to-left shunt at the atrial level. Although the radiographic appearance varies, severe cardiomegaly is common. Pulmonary vascularity is normal to decreased and dependent on a patent ductus arteriosus (PDA).
- **Tricuspid atresia.** In tricuspid atresia, there is no direct path for blood flow between the right atrium and right ventricle. However, there is a right-to-left shunt at the atrial level, usually through a patent foramen ovale. Pulmonic blood flow depends on the presence of a VSD and/or PDA. Associated anomalies occur in up to 30% of affected patients (most commonly transposition of the great arteries). In isolated tricuspid atresia with a small VSD, chest radiographs demonstrate a normal or small heart with decreased pulmonary blood flow. However, when a large VSD is present, there is usually cardiomegaly and increased pulmonary blood flow. A right-sided aortic arch is present in about 10% of patients.

■ Additional Differential Diagnoses

- **Double outlet right ventricle.** Double outlet right ventricle occurs when both the aorta and pulmonary outflow tracts arise from the right ventricle. With 16 described variants, radiographic appearance varies. Some forms mimic tetralogy of Fallot, with pulmonary oligemia and diminished left hilar shadow.
- **Ebstein anomaly.** Ebstein anomaly consists of apical displacement of the tricuspid valve, resulting in atrialization of the right ventricle. Tricuspid regurgitation and stasis of blood flow within the right atrium lead to massive right-sided cardiomegaly with a "box-shaped" heart and pulmonary oligemia. A right-to-left shunt at the atrial level is common.

■ Diagnosis

Tetralogy of Fallot.

✓ Pearls

- Tetralogy of Fallot is the most common cyanotic congenital heart disease.
- Tetralogy is characterized by pulmonic stenosis, ventricular septal defect, right ventricular hypertrophy, and overriding aorta.
- Pulmonary atresia with a ventricular septal defect is considered a severe variant of tetralogy of Fallot.
- Ebstein anomaly leads to massive right-sided cardiomegaly with a "box-shaped" heart.

Suggested Readings

Ferguson EC, Krishnamurthy R, Oldham SA. Classic imaging signs of congenital cardiovascular abnormalities. Radiographics. 2007; 27(5):1323–1334

Kellenberger CJ, Yoo SJ, Büchel ER. Cardiovascular MR imaging in neonates and infants with congenital heart disease. Radiographics. 2007; 27(1):5–18

Lapierre C, Déry J, Guérin R, Viremouneix L, Dubois J, Garel L. Segmental approach to imaging of congenital heart disease. Radiographics. 2010; 30(2):397–411

Schweigmann G, Gassner I, Maurer K. Imaging the neonatal heart: essentials for the radiologist. Eur J Radiol. 2006; 60(2):159–170

Case 6

Karen M. Ayotte

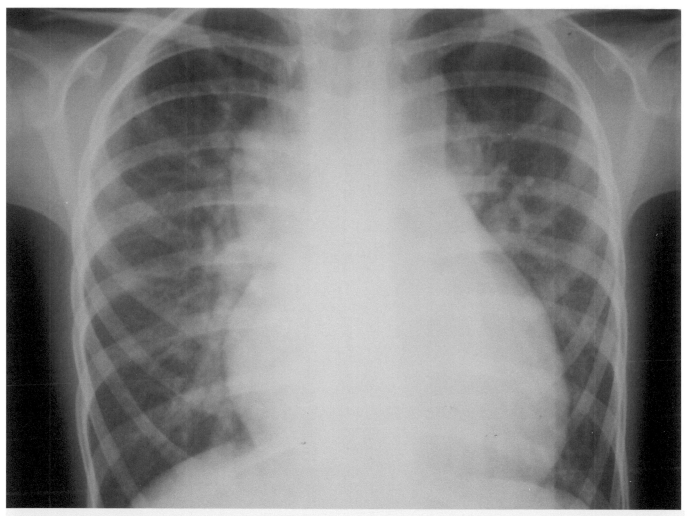

Fig. 6.1 Frontal chest radiograph shows cardiomegaly with a snowman-shaped cardiomediastinal contour. Pulmonary vascularity is markedly increased. There is a left-sided aortic arch. The lungs are hyperinflated.

■ Clinical Presentation

A 2-day-old infant with cyanosis (▶ Fig. 6.1).

■ Key Imaging Finding

A cyanotic infant with increased pulmonary vascularity.

■ Top Three Differential Diagnoses

• **Transposition of the great arteries (TGA).** In d-TGA (dextro-TGA), the aorta arises from the right ventricle and the pulmonary trunk arises from the left ventricle. Without a source for admixture (patent foramen ovale [PFO], ventricular septal defect [VSD], or patent ductus arteriosus [PDA]), this anatomy is incompatible with life. The historical classical radiographic appearance of cardiomegaly, a narrowed mediastinum ("egg on string"), and increased pulmonary vascularity is less common in the current era since patients are now treated in the immediate postnatal period. Instead, in the neonate a normal chest radiograph may be encountered.

• **Truncus arteriosus.** Truncus arteriosus results from failure of division of the primitive single truncal vessel into the aorta and main pulmonary artery. This uncommon lesion accounts for only 1% of cases of congenital heart disease. There is always a large, high VSD. The degree of pulmonary blood flow is initially variable, depending upon pulmonary resistance. When pulmonary resistance drops, usually day 2 to 3 of life, pulmonary blood flow may dramatically increase.

The combination of cardiomegaly, a right-sided arch (30% of cases), and increased pulmonary vascularity suggests the diagnosis.

• **Total anomalous pulmonary venous return (TAPVR).** In TAPVR, the pulmonary veins do not connect normally with the left atrium; instead, they drain into the right heart via various venous pathways. There are three types, classified by the location of pulmonary venous drainage: supracardiac, cardiac, and infracardiac. Supracardiac (usually nonobstructed) type 1 is the most common and may result in the "snowman" configuration of the heart due to an enlarged superior vena cava (SVC) and left vertical vein. In the cardiac type, pulmonary veins drain via the coronary sinus. With infracardiac TAPVR, pulmonary veins drain below the diaphragm into the portal veins or inferior vena cava; typically, this obstructed form of TAPVR demonstrates a normal-sized heart and vascular congestion. Infracardiac TAPVR is associated with heterotaxy. In all three types, intracardiac shunting occurs via a PFO. Imaging and clinical features vary with the type of TAPVR.

■ Additional Differential Diagnoses

• **Tricuspid atresia.** In tricuspid atresia, there is no direct path for blood flow from the right atrium into the right ventricle. There must therefore be a right-to-left shunt at the atrial level, usually through a PFO. Pulmonic blood flow depends on left-to-right shunting through a VSD and/or PDA. When a large VSD is present, there is usually cardiomegaly and increased pulmonary blood flow.

• **Single ventricle.** In this rare malformation, the interventricular septum is absent. The nomenclature describing this diagnosis can be confusing, indicating specific associated anatomy. Patients without pulmonic stenosis demonstrate cardiomegaly, an enlarged main pulmonary artery, and increased pulmonary blood flow.

■ Diagnosis

Supracardiac total anomalous pulmonary venous return.

✓ Pearls

• The superior vena cava and left vertical vein result in the "snowman" configuration in type 1 total anomalous pulmonary venous return.

• Severe pulmonary edema with normal heart size is the classic appearance of infradiaphragmatic total anomalous pulmonary venous return.

• Transposition of the great arteries shows parallel rather than crossing great vessel origins on prenatal ultrasound (US) and—if chronic—"egg on a string" on radiographs.

Suggested Readings

Ferguson EC, Krishnamurthy R, Oldham SA. Classic imaging signs of congenital cardiovascular abnormalities. Radiographics. 2007; 27(5):1323–1334

Lapierre C, Déry J, Guérin R, Viremouneix L, Dubois J, Garel L. Segmental approach to imaging of congenital heart disease. Radiographics. 2010; 30(2):397–411

Schweigmann G, Gassner I, Maurer K. Imaging the neonatal heart: essentials for the radiologist. Eur J Radiol. 2006; 60(2):159–170

Case 7

Karen M. Ayotte

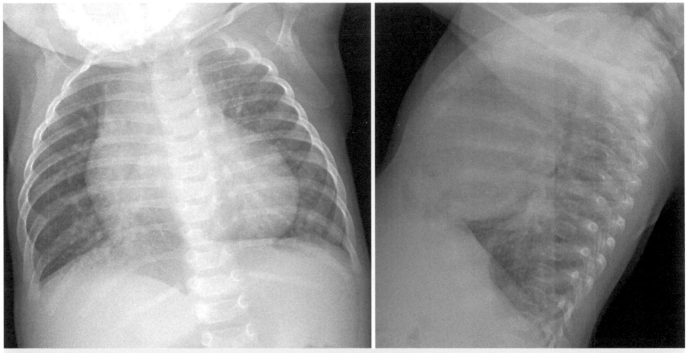

Fig. 7.1 Frontal **(a)** and lateral **(b)** chest radiographs show cardiomegaly with left atrial enlargement, as well as increased and sharply defined pulmonary vasculature. The lungs are hyperinflated, a common finding in patients with congenital heart disease.

■ Clinical Presentation

A 6-month-old acyanotic boy with a systolic heart murmur (▶Fig. 7.1).

■ Key Imaging Finding

Shunt vascularity.

■ Top Three Differential Diagnoses

• **Ventricular septal defect (VSD).** VSD is the most common of the four causes of acyanotic shunt vascularity and is the second most common congenital cardiac malformation after bicuspid aortic valve. Radiographs may be normal when the defect is small. Larger defects are associated with cardiomegaly with left atrial enlargement, increased number and size of visualized, well-defined, "sharp" pulmonary vessels (i.e., shunt vascularity), and an enlarged main pulmonary artery. Hyperinflation is common. Patients typically present after 6 weeks of age with failure to thrive and a holosystolic murmur on physical examination (pulmonary vascular resistance drops at this time, allowing the left-to-right shunt of VSD to manifest). As with any left-to-right shunt, if untreated VSD may lead to severe pulmonary hypertension with eventual reversal of flow across the shunt, referred to as Eisenmenger's physiology.

• **Atrial septal defect (ASD).** As with VSD, radiographic findings may be absent with ASD. Larger ASDs, however, are associated with mild cardiomegaly, enlarged right atrium, normal to enlarged main pulmonary artery, and shunt vascularity. In contrast to an isolated VSD, the left atrium is not enlarged with an ASD. Patients with ASD usually present at an older age than those with VSD, since there is relatively little blood flow across this lower pressure shunt. ASDs are more likely to be clinically occult, and therefore patients are more likely to have severe pulmonary hypertension at presentation.

• **Patent ductus arteriosus (PDA).** The ductus arteriosus normally closes in the perinatal period. Failure to close results in continued left-to-right shunting of blood across the ductus. As an isolated lesion, PDA is commonly seen in premature infants. Radiographic findings include variable degrees of cardiomegaly and shunt vascularity. Over time, left atrial and left ventricular enlargement may develop. When associated with more complex congenital heart disease, PDA may be necessary for survival.

■ Additional Differential Diagnosis

• **Atrioventricular canal defect (aka endocardial cushion defect).** This anomaly is characterized by failure of the atrial and ventricular septa to develop fully; the mitral and/or tricuspid valves are abnormal as well. Nearly 50% of patients have trisomy 21. As with other left-to-right shunts, radiographic findings include cardiomegaly with a squared, enlarged right atrial border, pulmonary artery enlargement, and shunt vascularity.

■ Diagnosis

Ventricular septal defect.

✓ Pearls

• Ventricular septal defect is the most common septal defect; larger lesions result in cardiomegaly and shunt vascularity.
• Patients with atrial septal defect typically present at a later age than ventricular septal defect due to less flow across the shunt.

• Patent ductus arteriosus commonly occurs in premature infants, as well as patients with complex congenital heart disease.
• Nearly half of patients with an atrioventricular canal (endocardial cushion defect) have trisomy 21.

Suggested Readings

Ferguson EC, Krishnamurthy R, Oldham SA. Classic imaging signs of congenital cardiovascular abnormalities. Radiographics. 2007; 27(5):1323–1334
Kellenberger CJ, Yoo SJ, Büchel ER. Cardiovascular MR imaging in neonates and infants with congenital heart disease. Radiographics. 2007; 27(1):5–18
Lapierre C, Déry J, Guérin R, Viremouneix L, Dubois J, Garel L. Segmental approach to imaging of congenital heart disease. Radiographics. 2010; 30(2):397–411
Schweigmann G, Gassner I, Maurer K. Imaging the neonatal heart-essentials for the radiologist. Eur J Radiol. 2006; 60(2):159–170

Case 8

Ernst Joseph and Rebecca Stein-Wexler

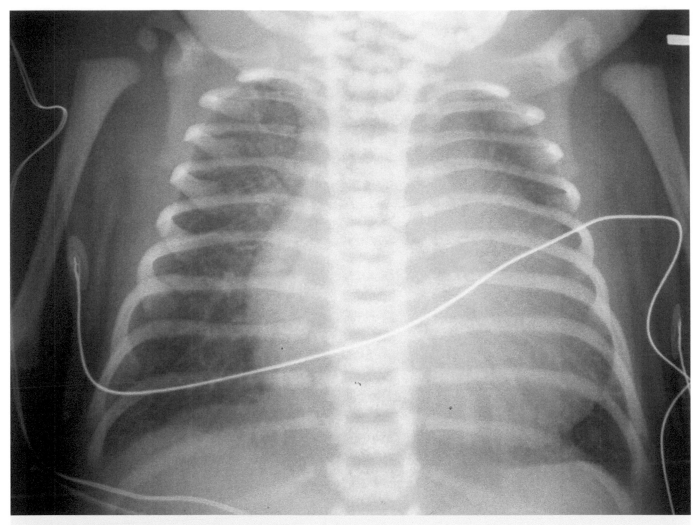

Fig. 8.1 Chest radiograph shows cardiomegaly, vascular congestion, and pulmonary edema.

■ **Clinical Presentation**

A 2-day-old with tachypnea and hypotension (▶Fig. 8.1).

■ Key Imaging Finding

Congestive heart failure (CHF) in an infant.

■ Top Three Differential Diagnoses

• **Hypoplastic left heart syndrome (HLHS).** Underdevelopment of the left heart causes CHF during the first 2 days of life. The principal feature is a very small left ventricle and atresia or stenosis of the aortic valve. In severe cases, the mitral valve may be stenotic, the left atrium small, and the ascending aorta hypoplastic. Most blood leaves the left heart by an obligatory patent foramen ovale (PFO) or atrial septal defect (ASD) to the right heart. It recirculates through pulmonary vasculature, reaching the body via a patent ductus arteriosus (PDA). However, as pulmonary vascular resistance drops and the PDA closes, blood floods the pulmonary vasculature, leading to CHF and systemic hypoperfusion. X-rays are initially normal, but cardiomegaly and vascular congestion develop within a few days.

• **Aortic coarctation (AC).** There are two types of AC. The less common, "tubular," form causes CHF in infants. Also called preductal coarctation, this consists of long segment aortic narrowing beyond the origin of the innominate artery, along with focal constriction before the ductus arteriosus. The aortic valve is often abnormal as well. Neonates present with shock and weak pulses, and chest radiographs show CHF. The more common, localized form of AC presents in older children. This form usually occurs just beyond the origin of the left subclavian artery or ligamentum arteriosum. The brachial pulses are normal, but the femoral pulses are weak. Chest X-ray in localized AC may show the "figure of 3," caused by proximal dilatation of the left subclavian artery and aorta, narrowing at the site of stenosis, and then poststenotic dilatation. AC diagnosed in patients older than 8 years may show notching of ribs 4 through 8 due to collateral blood flow.

• **Critical aortic valvular stenosis.** Most cases of aortic valvular stenosis are diagnosed in later life, but in about 10% the stenosis is so severe that CHF develops in the first 24 hours. In these patients, severely increased left ventricular pressure leads to decreased subendocardial oxygen supply and myocardial ischemia. Radiographs show cardiomegaly and vascular congestion. Echocardiography is diagnostic.

■ Additional Differential Diagnoses

• **Systemic overcirculation.** Infants with hepatic hemangioendothelioma, intracranial arteriovenous (AV) malformation with aneurysmal dilatation of the vein of Galen, or other systemic AV shunts may present with high-output CHF. In this setting, cardiac anatomy is normal but unable to cope with increased blood volume.

• **Endocardial fibroelastosis.** This rare condition usually presents with CHF by age 6 months. It may be primary or it may complicate congenital cardiac diseases, such as HLHS and aortic stenosis, or it may complicate congenital cardiac diseases, such as HLHS and aortic stenosis. Fibrous and elastic tissue in the endocardium and subendocardium is increased, leading to thickening of the heart wall and impaired myocardial contractility. The myocardium appears unusually echogenic at echocardiography. Chest radiography shows CHF. The heart is usually dilated but may be contracted.

■ Diagnosis

Hypoplastic left heart.

✓ Pearls

• Hypoplastic left heart is a spectrum of disorders characterized by underdevelopment of the left side of the heart; it leads to CHF in the first few days of life.

• Tubular, preductal aortic coarctation is much less common than the localized form and leads to CHF in neonates.

• The myocardium affected by endocardial fibroelastosis is extremely echogenic.

Suggested Readings

Ferguson EC, Krishnamurthy R, Oldham SA. Classic imaging signs of congenital cardiovascular abnormalities. Radiographics. 2007; 27(5):1323–1334

Schweigmann G, Gassner I, Maurer K. Imaging the neonatal heart: essentials for the radiologist. Eur J Radiol. 2006; 60(2):159–170

Case 9

Rebecca Stein-Wexler

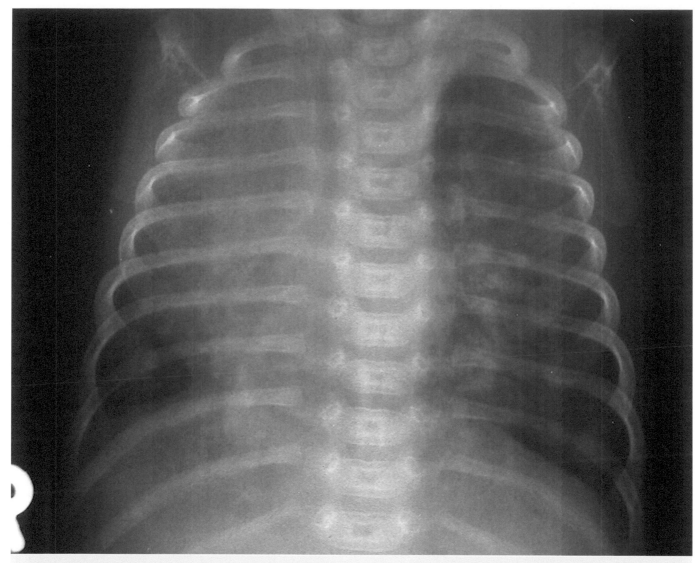

Fig. 9.1 The mediastinum is shifted to the right, and only the right lung base appears aerated. A vertical curvilinear density to the right of the spine at the T8–T9 level overlaps the diaphragm; its size increases as it descends.

■ Clinical Presentation

Infant in respiratory distress (▶Fig. 9.1).

■ Key Imaging Finding

Unilateral small dense lung.

■ Top Three Differential Diagnoses

- **Atelectasis.** It is important to establish whether there is increased or decreased volume of a dense lung and/or pleural space. Shift of the mediastinum toward the denser side indicates ipsilateral decreased volume. This most often results from atelectasis of all or part of the lung. Atelectasis usually affects only one lobe or lobar segment. However, unilateral atelectasis of an entire lung may be seen in patients with asthma, mucus plugging, a foreign body lodged in the mainstem bronchus, a misplaced endotracheal tube, hilar lymphadenopathy, mediastinal mass, and a variety of other pathologies.
- **Unilateral pulmonary hypoplasia/aplasia.** Hypoplastic lung is differentiated from aplastic lung by the presence of underdeveloped parenchyma and hypoplastic vessels; both have rudimentary bronchi. Isolated primary pulmonary hypoplasia, which is most common, usually affects the left lung. Pulmonary hypoplasia/aplasia may be primary or secondary. If primary, there is no identifiable cause, other than hypoplasia of bronchovascular structures. Secondary cases may result from such space-occupying lesions as an ipsilateral mass or congenital diaphragmatic hernia and chest wall deformity. Oligohydramnios or impaired diaphragm motion usually affects both lungs; large masses or hernias and thoracic dystrophy also cause bilateral pathology. CT differentiates between hypoplasia, aplasia, and (much rarer) complete agenesis.
- **Hypogenetic lung (scimitar) syndrome.** The scimitar vein differentiates scimitar syndrome from simple pulmonary hypoplasia/aplasia. This vein drains all or part of the lung, usually into the inferior vena cava but sometimes into a portal or hepatic vein. Its diameter increases as it descends, resembling the Turkish sword. The syndrome consists of the combination of a scimitar vein with lung hypoplasia (virtually always the right), cardiac dextroposition, and right pulmonary artery hypoplasia. The abdominal aorta supplies the affected lung. About one-fourth of patients have other cardiac pathology, but isolated small lesions are usually asymptomatic.

■ Additional Differential Diagnosis

- **Hyperinflation of the contralateral lung.** Mass effect from hyperinflation may lead to volume loss or hypoplasia of the contralateral lung. This may result from air trapping due to an aspirated foreign body. Congenital lobar hyperinflation (CLH) may also cause contralateral mediastinal shift. If the pathology affects only one lobe (usually the case with CLH), there will be adjacent increased density due to compressive atelectasis of the unaffected ipsilateral lobe. However, if the entire lung is hyperinflated, it may be difficult to decide whether the small-volume dense or large-volume lucent side is abnormal. CT may assist with diagnosis.

■ Diagnosis

Scimitar syndrome.

✓ Pearls

- Mediastinal shift toward a dense lung usually indicates atelectasis or hypoplasia, but it may result from hyperinflation of the contralateral lung.
- Asthma, mucus plugging, foreign body, or a misplaced endotracheal tube are common causes of ipsilateral atelectasis.
- Isolated pulmonary hypoplasia affects the left side more often than the right side.
- Scimitar syndrome virtually always affects the right lung and consists of an aberrant draining vein (scimitar), pulmonary hypoplasia, cardiac dextroposition, and hypoplasia of the associated pulmonary artery.

Suggested Readings

Lee EY, Dorkin H, Vargas SO. Congenital pulmonary malformations in pediatric patients: review and update on etiology, classification, and imaging findings. Radiol Clin North Am. 2011; 49(5):921–948

Case 10

Thomas Ray Sanchez

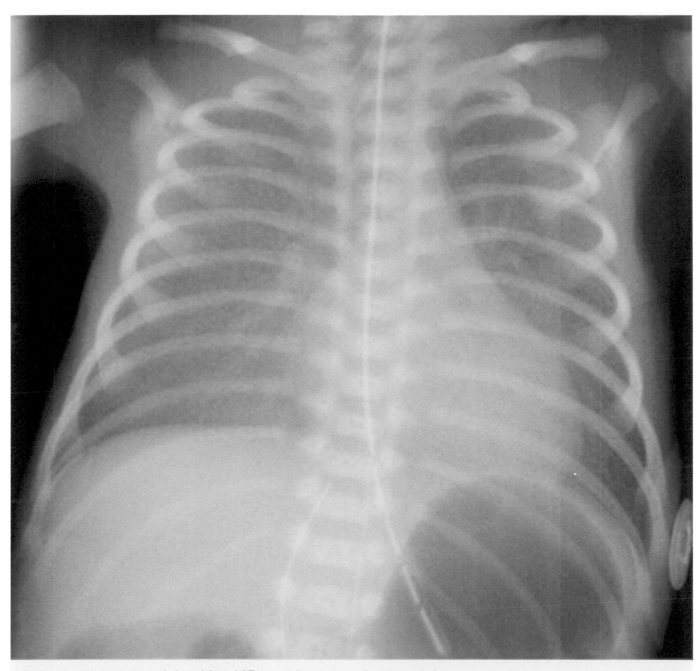

Fig. 10.1 Frontal chest radiograph shows bilateral diffuse granular opacities in this intubated infant.

■ Clinical Presentation

A 4-day-old with tachypnea and grunting (▶ Fig. 10.1).

■ Key Imaging Finding

Neonatal lung disease with diffuse granular opacities.

■ Top Three Differential Diagnoses

• **Surfactant deficiency.** Surfactant deficiency is the most common cause of respiratory distress in preterm infants, especially in those born before 34 weeks of gestation and who weigh less than 1.5 kg. It occurs because immature lungs are unable to produce enough surfactant to keep alveoli open for effective air exchange. Clinical manifestations of grunting, nasal flaring, subcostal retractions, tachypnea, and cyanosis are seen shortly after delivery, and almost always within the first 8 hours of life. Radiographs typically show diffusely hazy, low-volume lungs with air bronchograms. The granularity results from diffuse alveolar collapse, while the air bronchograms represent normal air-filled prealveolar airways. In severe cases (extreme prematurity and very low birth weight), assisted ventilation along with surfactant application may be needed to achieve acceptable gas exchange. Potential complications of positive pressure ventilation include pulmonary interstitial emphysema (PIE), pneumomediastinum, and pneumothorax. Chronic intubation and oxygen administration may eventually result in bronchopulmonary dysplasia (BPD).

• **Neonatal pneumonia.** Bacterial pneumonias, especially those caused by group B *Streptococcus*, predominate in the neonatal period. The more common route of infection is through the birth canal, especially after early rupture of membranes in febrile mothers who are positive for this organism. Since neonatal pneumonia is usually not lobar in distribution, X-ray findings of diffuse haziness and granularity with low lung volumes may mimic surfactant deficiency. However, in patients with neonatal pneumonia caused by organisms other than group B *Streptococcus*, lung volumes are usually normal to slightly expanded (even without mechanical ventilation) due to exudate-filled and distended alveoli. Pleural effusions are rare in surfactant deficiency but are seen in as many as two-thirds of patients with neonatal pneumonia. With adequate antibiotic therapy, complications such as empyema, pulmonary abscess, and pneumatocele are unusual.

• **Transient tachypnea of the newborn (TTNB).** This is the most common cause of respiratory distress in a newborn. Transient and benign, TTNB occurs when immature lymphatic vessels cannot absorb residual lung fluid quickly. Radiographs typically demonstrate central streaky opacities and small pleural effusions, with fluid in the minor fissure. Patients improve clinically within 48 hours of birth, and radiographs normalize within 72 hours. Treatment is limited to supportive care and observation.

■ Diagnosis

Surfactant deficiency.

✓ Pearls

• Surfactant deficiency is the most common cause of respiratory distress in preterm infants.
• Neonatal pneumonia may mimic surfactant deficiency, but neonatal pneumonia often has pleural effusions.

• Transient tachypnea of the newborn is transient and shows rapid clinical improvement; radiographs are normal at 72 hours.

Suggested Readings

Agrons GA, Courtney SE, Stocker JT, Markowitz RI. From the archives of the AFIP: lung disease in premature neonates: radiologic-pathologic correlation. Radiographics. 2005; 25(4):1047–1073

Hermansen CL, Lorah KN. Respiratory distress in the newborn. Am Fam Physician. 2007; 76(7):987–994

Pramanik AK, Rangaswamy N, Gates T. Neonatal respiratory distress: a practical approach to its diagnosis and management. Pediatr Clin North Am. 2015; 62(2):453–469

Case 11

Thomas Ray Sanchez

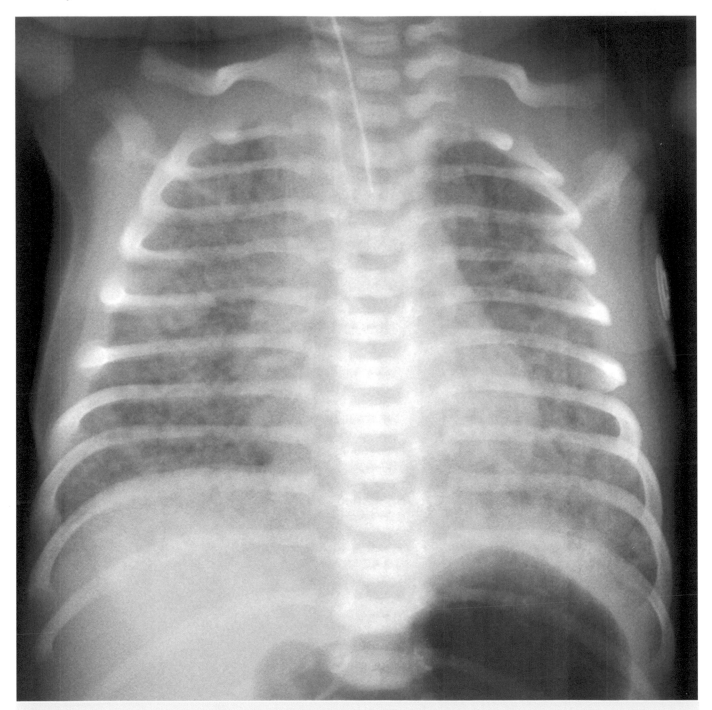

Fig. 11.1 Frontal chest radiograph shows diffuse coarse reticular and nodular opacities in both lungs.

■ Clinical Presentation

A term newborn with respiratory distress (▶ Fig. 11.1).

■ Key Imaging Finding

Neonatal lung disease with diffuse coarse reticulonodular opacities.

■ Top Three Differential Diagnoses

• **Transient tachypnea of the newborn (TTNB).** TTNB is the most common cause of respiratory distress in term newborns. It is caused by delayed absorption of residual fetal lung fluid due to immaturity of lymphatic vessels. The condition is transient and benign. Patients show clinical and X-ray improvement within 72 hours with minimal supportive care. TTNB is more common in term neonates who have undergone cesarean section or precipitous birth. The typical X-ray appearance is hyperinflation, central streaky opacities, and air space disease that resembles edema. Small pleural effusions are common, often limited to the minor fissure. Heart size is normal. Cardiac disease and neonatal pneumonia should be suspected if patients do not improve.

• **Meconium aspiration syndrome (MAS).** MAS usually affects term or post-term infants. Fetal distress causes the anal sphincter to relax, and meconium passed into the amniotic fluid may be aspirated. Airway obstruction results in mixed atelectasis and hyperaeration. Meconium consists of desquamated cells, skin, bile salts, and digestive enzymes. Although aseptic, as an irritant it causes chemical pneumonitis, which predisposes to secondary infection. Infants usually develop respiratory distress a few hours after birth. The chest X-ray shows diffuse, bilateral, but sometimes asymmetric coarse reticulonodular opacities. There is both atelectasis and air trapping. Pneumothorax and pneumomediastinum are common. Persistent pulmonary hypertension may occur in severe cases, sometimes requiring extracorporeal membrane oxygenation (ECMO).

• **Neonatal pneumonia.** Bacterial pneumonia predominates in the neonatal period. Group B *Streptococcal* pneumonia is most common. Other organisms include *Listeria*, *E. coli*, and *Klebsiella*. Infection is usually via the birth canal, especially likely after early rupture of membranes. Radiographic findings of diffuse opacities may resemble meconium aspiration, but opacities may be more patchy, and sometimes radiographs are normal. Lung volumes are usually small with *Streptococcal* pneumonia, whereas with other organisms lungs are usually hyperinflated. Pleural effusions are common. Complications after adequate antibiotic coverage are infrequent but include empyema, pulmonary abscess, and pneumatocele.

■ Additional Differential Diagnosis

• **Congenital heart disease.** Vascular congestion and edema in congenital heart disease may appear as coarse reticulonodular opacities. Lungs are often hyperinflated, and pleural fluid is common. An abnormal cardiomediastinal contour may suggest cardiac pathology, but often the diagnosis rests on echocardiography or MRI.

■ Diagnosis

Meconium aspiration syndrome.

✓ Pearls

• If transient tachypnea of the newborn does not resolve within 3 days, consider neonatal pneumonia or congenital cardiac disease.

• Meconium aspiration syndrome typically shows air space opacities that are more nodular, coarse, and asymmetrical than with transient tachypnea of the newborn.

• Neonatal pneumonia may mimic or complicate meconium aspiration syndrome.

• Air block complications, such as pneumothorax and pneumomediastinum, are common with meconium aspiration.

Suggested Readings

Edwards MO, Kotecha SJ, Kotecha S. Respiratory distress of the term newborn infant. Paediatr Respir Rev. 2013; 14(1):29–36, quiz 36–37

Lobo L. The neonatal chest. Eur J Radiol. 2006; 60(2):152–158

Case 12

Rebecca Stein-Wexler

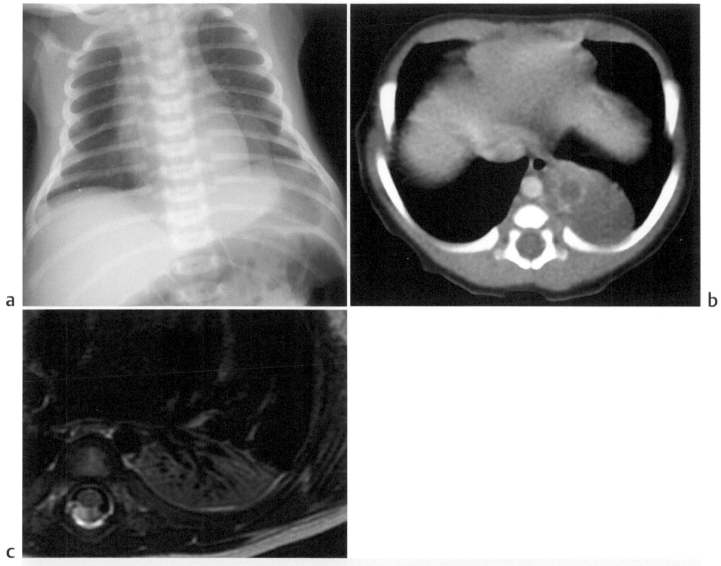

Fig. 12.1 Chest radiograph shows a dense mass at the left lung base **(a)**. Contrast-enhanced axial CT with soft-tissue windows shows the mass appears solid, except for a hypodense cyst **(b)**. Axial T2-W MRI shows small vessels extending from the left side of the aorta into the mass **(c)**.

■ Clinical Presentation

A newborn with chest mass on prenatal US (▶Fig. 12.1).

■ Key Imaging Finding

Dense lung mass in a neonate.

■ Top Three Differential Diagnoses

• **Congenital pulmonary airway malformation (CPAM).** Airway maldevelopment leads to this group of cystic and solid lesions. Type I has microcysts at least 2 cm in diameter. Cysts in type II are between 0.5 and 2 cm. Type III is mostly solid but may have microcysts up to 0.5 cm. Type IV has large air-filled cysts. Type 0 affects all lobes and is lethal. Types IV and 0 are rare. CPAMs are in a spectrum with other lung anomalies, and hybrid lesions may have elements of sequestration. Often detected prenatally, they may present in infants with respiratory distress or in older patients with pneumonia. Type I CPAM appears as cysts filled with fluid or air, whereas type II appears cystic or solid. Type III CPAMs appear solid, with cysts evident only at histology. Types II and III may coexist with other congenital anomalies and hence have a worse prognosis. Large lesions are resected, but management of smaller lesions is controversial.

• **Pulmonary sequestration.** This consists of dysplastic lung whose vascular supply originates from systemic arteries. It is most common in the left lower lobe. Extralobar sequestration presents early in life, drains into the systemic venous system, and has its own pleural covering, whereas intralobar sequestration drains into the pulmonary venous system, lacks a pleural covering, and often presents later in life with recurring infections. Both forms of sequestration appear solid unless they have areas of CPAM or have been superinfected, when tissue breakdown permits communication with the bronchial tree.

• **Diaphragmatic hernia.** Congenital diaphragm defects are most common on the left and lead to herniation of bowel and/or solid organs. Most hernias contain bowel and become lucent as the bowel aerates, but those containing fluid-filled bowel, liver, or other solid organs retain soft-tissue density. They are often diagnosed in utero or in neonates presenting with respiratory distress. Prognosis depends on the degree of pulmonary hypoplasia and the severity of associated anomalies. Surgical consultation is required, regardless of the apparent defect size. Prognosis is worse if lesions contain liver or if there is also a cardiac malformation.

■ Additional Differential Diagnoses

• **Congenital lobar hyperinflation (formerly congenital lobar emphysema).** During the first few days of life—before clearing of trapped fetal lung fluid—this lesion may appear solid. In general, however, it is considered in the differential diagnosis for hyperlucent lesions.

• **Bronchogenic cyst.** Most bronchogenic cysts occur in the middle mediastinum, especially in subcarinal and right paratracheal locations. However, about 10% are parenchymal. Small lesions are asymptomatic, but large cysts may cause chest pain, dysphagia, or respiratory compromise. If superinfected, symptoms may resemble pneumonia. Lesions appear solid and smooth on radiographs. On CT and MRI, they often appear as simple fluid, but if the fluid has high protein content, they may appear bright on T1 and dense on CT.

■ Diagnosis

Extralobar sequestration.

✓ Pearls

• Congenital pulmonary airway malformation is categorized according to cyst size, and if cysts are very small it may appear solid.

• Extralobar sequestration appears solid unless superinfection has resulted in tissue breakdown, allowing communication with bronchi.

• Congenital diaphragmatic hernia that contains fluid-filled bowel or abdominal organs appears solid.

• About 10% of bronchogenic cysts occur in the pulmonary parenchyma.

Suggested Readings

Taylor GA, Atalabi OM, Estroff JA. Imaging of congenital diaphragmatic hernias. Pediatr Radiol. 2009; 39(1):1–16

Thacker PG, Rao AG, Hill JG, Lee EY. Congenital lung anomalies in children and adults: current concepts and imaging findings. Radiol Clin North Am. 2014; 52(1):155–181

Case 13

Karen M. Ayotte

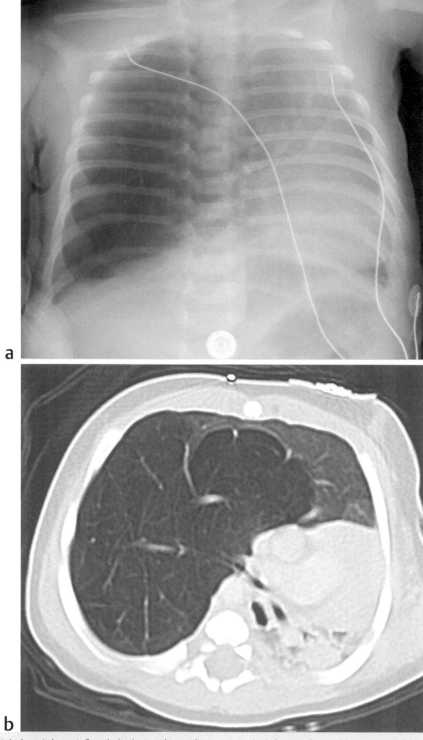

Fig. 13.1 Chest X-ray shows the right lung is hyperinflated, displacing the mediastinum to the left; vascular markings extend almost to the periphery **(a)**. Axial contrast-enhanced CT shows a narrow bronchus leading to a hyperinflated right upper lobe that has attenuated vasculature; the slightly denser normal right middle lobe herniates across the midline anteriorly, and the visualized retrocardiac left lung is severely atelectatic **(b)**.

■ **Clinical Presentation**

A 3-week-old with persistent cough (▶Fig. 13.1).

■ Key Imaging Finding

Lucent lung mass.

■ Top Three Differential Diagnoses

- **Congenital lobar hyperinflation (CLH; formerly congenital lobar emphysema).** CLH constitutes progressive overexpansion of a pulmonary lobe secondary to obstruction of normal airflow, usually due to varying degrees of bronchial underdevelopment or obstruction. Before birth, the lung is filled with fluid. After birth, the radiographic appearance varies as the fluid within the affected lobe is gradually replaced with air. The most common location is the left upper lobe, followed by the right middle lobe and right upper lobe. Parenchyma, vessels, and bronchi are present but attenuated. Patients often present in the neonatal period with respiratory distress. Surgical resection provides definitive treatment.
- **Congenital pulmonary airway malformation (CPAM).** CPAM is a hamartomatous proliferation of terminal bronchioles with abnormal alveolar development. Most of these masses have both cystic and solid components, resulting in varied imaging appearances. The lesions communicate with the tracheobronchial tree and tend to aerate early in life. Internal fluid-fluid levels may be seen in the absence of superimposed infection. Stocker type I CPAM consists of one or more cysts at least 2 cm in size, type II has cysts smaller than 2 cm, and type III is essentially solid. Definitive management is surgical, but treatment of asymptomatic or incidentally discovered lesions is controversial.
- **Congenital diaphragmatic hernia (CDH).** Congenital defects in the diaphragm may lead to intrathoracic herniation of solid and hollow organs of the upper abdomen. Defects are most common on the left. Herniations may appear cystic or solid at birth. If most of the herniated contents are bowel, fluid attenuation will fade as the bowel aerates. Most cases are diagnosed in utero or present in neonates with respiratory distress. Prognosis depends upon the degree of pulmonary hypoplasia, as well as the presence of associated anomalies. Surgical consultation is required, regardless of the apparent defect size.

■ Additional Differential Diagnosis

- **Necrotizing pneumonia.** If parenchymal consolidation becomes necrotic, an abscess may develop, mimicking other cystic lesions. Necrotizing pneumonia is more common in the lower lobes. The cystic areas may be solitary or multiple, as large as 10 cm, and filled with air, fluid, or both. Conservative management is often successful in otherwise healthy children. Bronchopleural fistula may complicate surgical drainage.

■ Diagnosis

Congenital lobar hyperinflation of the right upper lobe.

✓ Pearls

- Prognosis for most chest masses is based primarily on the degree of resultant pulmonary hypoplasia.
- Congenital lobar hyperinflation most commonly occurs within the left upper lobe, followed by the right middle and right upper lobes.
- Congenital pulmonary airway malformations are categorized by the size of cystic components.
- Congenital diaphragmatic hernia may mimic cystic or solid primary thoracic masses and is more common on the left.

Suggested Readings

Biyyam DR, Chapman T, Ferguson MR, Deutsch G, Dighe MK. Congenital lung abnormalities: embryologic features, prenatal diagnosis, and postnatal radiologic-pathologic correlation. Radiographics. 2010; 30(6):1721–1738

Newman B. Congenital bronchopulmonary foregut malformations: concepts and controversies. Pediatr Radiol. 2006; 36(8):773–791

Taylor GA, Atalabi OM, Estroff JA. Imaging of congenital diaphragmatic hernias. Pediatr Radiol. 2009; 39(1):1–16

Case 14

Rebecca Stein-Wexler

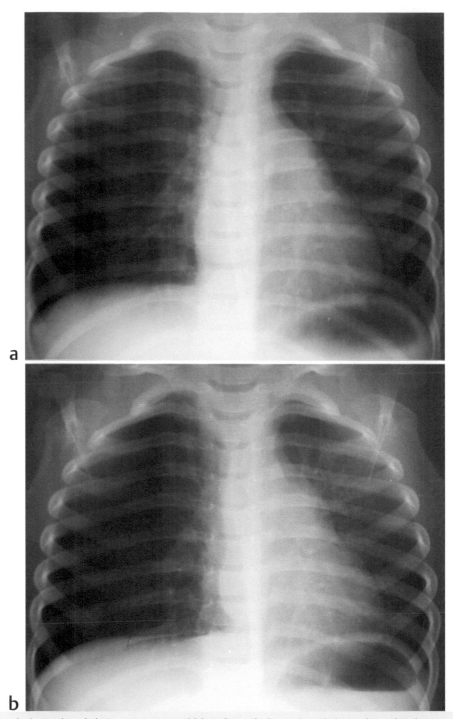

a

b

Fig. 14.1 Chest radiograph obtained in inhalation appears normal **(a)**. Radiograph obtained in exhalation shows that the normal left lung partially collapses and becomes denser, whereas the right lung remains hyperinflated **(b)**.

■ Clinical Presentation

A 2-year-old boy, wheezing (▶ Fig. 14.1).

■ Key Imaging Finding

Asymmetrical lung lucency after infancy.

■ Top Three Differential Diagnoses

- **Aspirated foreign body.** The child with aspirated foreign body often presents with nonspecific symptoms or with choking, cough, and wheezing. Since most foreign bodies are radiolucent food material (usually peanuts), diagnosis rests on secondary findings of lobar or segmental hyperinflation due to air trapping from the ball-valve effect. Larger foreign bodies may completely obstruct the airway, causing atelectasis. Most foreign bodies lodge in the right mainstem bronchus, due to its straight course. If aspiration is suspected—regardless of whether the initial chest radiograph shows unilateral lung/lobar hyperlucency or hyperinflation—expiratory images may show air trapping. Lateral decubitus radiographs, simulating exhalation for the dependent hemithorax, may help in younger patients who cannot inhale and exhale on cue. If hyperlucency and/or hyperinflation persist on the side that is down, air trapping is present.

- **Anterior pneumothorax.** Pleural gas collects anteriorly in supine children, leading to generalized ipsilateral lucency. Clues include an especially sharp cardiomediastinal contour and an accompanying deep sulcus. It is essential to check for mediastinal shift, which indicates tension pneumothorax, an emergency.

- **Unilateral emphysema.** Unilateral emphysematous or bullous disease may develop in patients with a history of prematurity and respiratory distress syndrome (RDS). The acute complication of pulmonary interstitial emphysema (PIE) usually resolves quickly. However, interstitial cysts may persist and enlarge, compressing normal tissue. Alternatively, patients with severe RDS that evolves to bronchopulmonary dysplasia (BPD) may develop large bullae that are sometimes asymmetrical, causing unilateral lucency.

■ Additional Differential Diagnoses

- **Swyer–James syndrome.** Obliterative bronchiolitis due to adenovirus, respiratory syncytial virus (RSV), or *Mycoplasma* causes a (usually unilateral) lucent lung. Radiographs show hyperlucency due to bronchiolar obstruction that causes air trapping. Vessels are relatively few and small, best appreciated at CT. Bronchiectasis is common. Lung volume is usually small, though it may be large if there is collateral ventilation and air

trapping. Mosaic perfusion on CT results from interspersed normal lung tissue.

- **Poland syndrome.** Hypoplasia/aplasia of the pectoralis major muscle and adjacent bony and soft-tissue structures results in hyperlucency of the affected thorax. Fingers may be short (brachydactyly) and fused (syndactyly). The condition is more common in males and is usually seen on the right.

■ Diagnosis

Peanut aspirated into the right mainstem bronchus.

✓ Pearls

- Since most aspirated foreign bodies are radiolucent, inhalation/exhalation or decubitus radiographs are often essential for diagnosis.
- Emphysema and bullae may be unilateral in patients with history of cystic pulmonary interstitial emphysema or with severe bronchopulmonary dysplasia.

- Swyer–James syndrome consists of infectious obliterative bronchiolitis that causes air trapping.
- Brachydactyly and syndactyly hand may accompany Poland syndrome.

Suggested Readings

Dillman JR, Sanchez R, Ladino-Torres MF, Yarram SG, Strouse PJ, Lucaya J. Expanding upon the unilateral hyperlucent hemithorax in children. Radiographics. 2011; 31(3):723–741

Pugmire BS, Lim R, Avery LL. Review of ingested and aspirated foreign bodies in children and their clinical significance for radiologists. Radiographics. 2015; 35(5):1528–1538

Wasilewska E, Lee EY, Eisenberg RL. Unilateral hyperlucent lung in children. AJR Am J Roentgenol. 2012; 198(5):W400–W414

Case 15

Fabienne Joseph and Rebecca Stein-Wexler

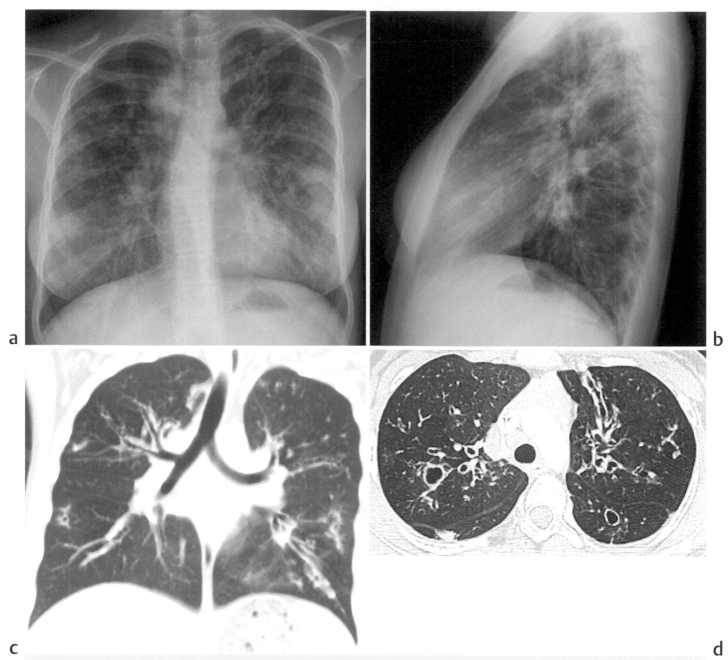

a

b

c

d

Fig. 15.1 Frontal (a) and lateral (b) chest radiographs show dilated, thick-walled bronchi that resemble tram tracks, predominantly in the upper lobes; there are also patchy opacities as well as hilar lymphadenopathy. Coronal reformatted CT shows bronchiectasis in both upper and lower lobes (c). Axial CT shows there is also varicoid bronchiectasis in the left upper lobe and cystic bronchiectasis in the right upper lobe and left lower lobe (d).

■ **Clinical Presentation**

A teenage girl with a chronic cough (▶Fig. 15.1).

■ Key Imaging Finding

Bronchiectasis.

■ Top Three Differential Diagnoses

- **Cystic fibrosis (CF).** CF is a relatively common autosomal-recessive disorder that leads to viscous secretions and affects the lungs, gastrointestinal system, and exocrine glands. The disease is most often encountered in Caucasians. Patients with CF develop airway inflammation that leads to mucus plugging, air trapping, and bronchiectasis that is most severe in the upper lobes. Consolidation is less common. There are three stages of bronchiectasis. Patients may manifest a combination of all three or they may demonstrate only one stage. The mildest form, tubular, is characterized by parallel, thick-walled bronchi that resemble tram tracks. Subtle cases are recognized at CT if the internal diameter of a bronchus exceeds that of the adjacent artery (signet ring sign). The bronchi may fail to taper normally, or they may extend too close to the pleura. Bronchiectasis may progress to the varicoid stage, which appears serpentine and beaded. Finally, in its cystic stage, there is a thick-walled cyst at the end of a dilated, thick-walled bronchus. Superinfection with *Staphylococcus aureus, Haemophilus influenzae, Pseudomonas aeruginosa*, and *Aspergillus fumigatus* is common. There may be mucus plugging within dilated bronchi, along with distal tree-in-bud appearance. Chronic inflammation may lead to bronchial artery neovascularization and subsequent hemoptysis. CT is used to score severity of disease.
- **Postinfectious bronchiectasis.** Pneumonia may impair mucociliary clearance, causing chronic bronchial wall inflammation and injury. This may lead to bronchiectasis, usually tubular, although more advanced stages may also be seen. As with CF, superinfection may lead to a tree-in-bud appearance, as well as consolidation, scattered ground glass opacities, and abscess formation.
- **Primary ciliary dyskinesia (PCD).** This autosomal-recessive disorder is characterized by defective ciliary structure and function, leading to bronchiectasis, abnormal situs, and/or severe sinusitis, as well as dysmotile sperm. Patients usually present with infections of the lungs, sinuses, and middle ear. Bronchiectasis is most common in the right middle lobe, and—unlike with CF—the upper lobes are rarely affected in children. About 50% of patients have normal situs, 40% have situs inversus, and the rest have heterotaxy. Congenital cardiac disease is relatively uncommon. Kartagener syndrome is seen in about 50% of patients with PCD. It is characterized by the triad of bronchiectasis, abnormal situs, and sinusitis.

■ Additional Differential Diagnosis

- **Bronchial dilatation accompanying acute infection or obstruction.** In order for bronchial dilatation to be considered bronchiectasis, it must be irreversible. Thus, the relatively common airway changes that sometimes accompany acute respiratory illness or obstruction are not considered true bronchiectasis, since they are reversible.

■ Diagnosis

Cystic fibrosis.

✓ Pearls

- The stages of bronchiectasis are tubular, varicoid, and cystic.
- In cystic fibrosis, bronchiectasis is most severe in the upper lobes, whereas this area is usually spared with primary ciliary dyskinesia.
- Bronchial artery neovascularization in cystic fibrosis may lead to hemoptysis.
- Patients with Kartagener syndrome have primary ciliary dyskinesia with the triad of bronchiectasis, abnormal situs, and sinusitis.

Suggested Readings

Javidan-Nejad C, Bhalla S. Bronchiectasis. Radiol Clin North Am. 2009; 47(2):289–306

Kennedy MP, Noone PG, Leigh MW, et al. High-resolution CT of patients with primary ciliary dyskinesia. AJR Am J Roentgenol. 2007; 188(5):1232–1238

Murphy KP, Maher MM, O'Connor OJ. Imaging of cystic fibrosis and pediatric bronchiectasis. AJR Am J Roentgenol. 2016; 206(3):448–454

Case 16

Stephen Malutich

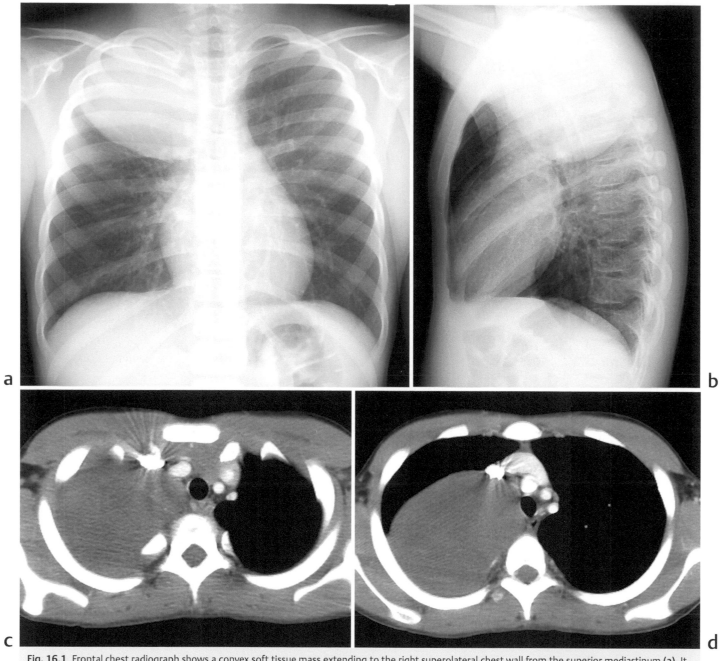

Fig. 16.1 Frontal chest radiograph shows a convex soft tissue mass extending to the right superolateral chest wall from the superior mediastinum **(a)**. It projects over the upper spine on the lateral view **(b)**. Axial contrast-enhanced CT images show a well-demarcated, homogeneous posterior mediastinal soft tissue mass that displaces vascular structures **(c,d)**.

■ **Clinical Presentation**

A 10-year-old boy with chest pain (▶Fig. 16.1).

■ Key Imaging Finding

Posterior mediastinal mass.

■ Top Three Differential Diagnoses

- **Neuroblastic tumor.** Primordial neural crest cells of the sympathetic nervous system give rise to a group of tumors with different degrees of cell maturation. Neuroblastoma, the most undifferentiated and aggressive, occurs in young children (median age 2 years). It is most common in the adrenal; only about one-fifth occur in the posterior mediastinum. Ganglioneuroblastoma is intermediate, containing both mature and immature ganglion cells. Ganglioneuroma is the most mature, usually found in older children and most often in the posterior mediastinum. Mediastinal ganglioneuromas tend to be homogeneous and well circumscribed on CT, whereas the more aggressive tumors tend to appear more invasive. Calcifications occur in most neuroblastomas and in 50% of ganglioneuromas. MRI appearance varies, and the tumors cannot be definitively differentiated with imaging alone. Furthermore, ganglioneuroma may undergo malignant transformation. Norepinephrine receptor imaging with ^{123}I metaiodobenzylguanidine (MIBG) is very useful for confirming the diagnosis of neuroblastoma and for detecting occult metastatic disease.

- **Sequestration.** Bronchopulmonary sequestrations are congenital thoracic malformations that contain abnormal lung tissue with no direct connection to the bronchial tree or pulmonary arterial system. Solid or cystic, they usually occur in the posterior basal segments of the lower lobes (especially the left). They are classified as intra- or extrapulmonary, depending on their vascular drainage and whether they are surrounded by their own pleural layer.

- **Extramedullary hematopoiesis.** Inadequate bone marrow erythrogenesis in the setting of anemia may lead to recruitment of additional sites of erythropoiesis. Involvement of the liver or spleen may cause hepatomegaly or splenomegaly. The posterior mediastinum is less often involved. When affected, there are uni- or bilateral paraspinal masses with lobulated, smooth, sharply delineated borders.

■ Additional Differential Diagnoses

- **Lymphoma.** While uncommonly originating in the posterior mediastinum, lymphoma must be considered due to its prevalence in the pediatric population. On CT, it appears as a homogeneous, well-demarcated soft-tissue mass. The presence of lymphadenopathy elsewhere supports the diagnosis.

- **Foregut duplication cyst.** When epithelium becomes abnormally encased in connective tissue during fetal development, a congenital foregut duplication cyst may result. In the posterior mediastinum, this may be an esophageal duplication or neurenteric cyst. Esophageal cysts may communicate with the esophagus and have air-fluid levels. Neurenteric cysts are associated with vertebral malformations.

■ Diagnosis

Ganglioneuroma.

✓ Pearls

- Ganglioneuroma is a benign, well-differentiated neural crest tumor usually found in the posterior mediastinum.
- Extramedullary hematopoiesis usually causes hepatosplenomegaly but may also cause paraspinal masses.

- Extrapulmonary bronchopulmonary sequestrations usually occur along the left lower mediastinum.

Suggested Readings

Balassy C, Navarro OM, Daneman A. Adrenal masses in children. Radiol Clin North Am. 2011; 49(4):711–727, vi

Lonergan GJ, Schwab CM, Suarez ES, Carlson CL. Neuroblastoma, ganglioneuroblastoma, and ganglioneuroma: radiologic-pathologic correlation. Radiographics. 2002; 22(4):911–934

McCarville MB. Malignant pulmonary and mediastinal tumors in children: differential diagnoses. Cancer Imaging. 2010; (1A):S35–S41

Ranganath SH, Lee EY, Restrepo R, Eisenberg RL. Mediastinal masses in children. AJR Am J Roentgenol. 2012; 198(3):W197–W216

Case 17

Stephen Malutich

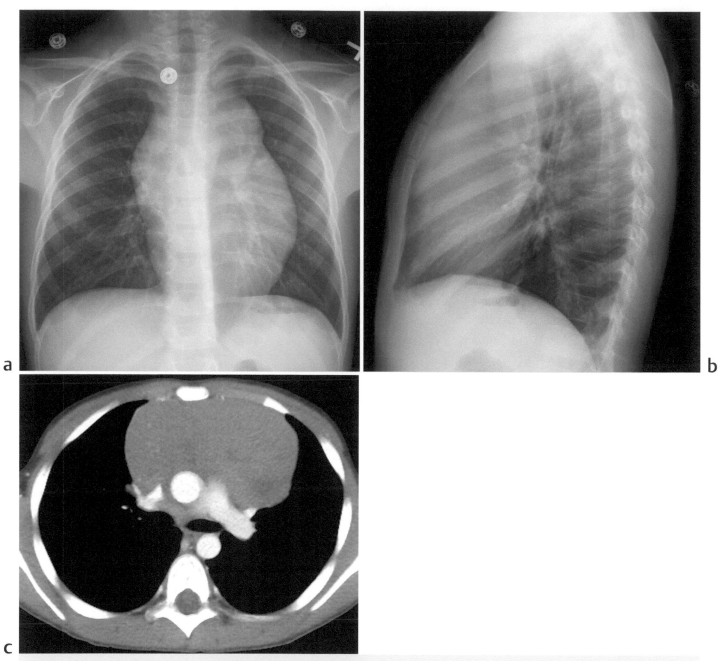

Fig. 17.1 Frontal chest radiograph shows a lobulated anterior mediastinal mass **(a)**. The lateral view shows soft-tissue density filling the retrosternal space **(b)**. Axial contrast-enhanced CT shows a smoothly marginated, predominantly homogeneous soft-tissue mass in the anterior mediastinum, displacing vascular structures and indirectly compressing the trachea **(c)**.

■ **Clinical Presentation**

A 9-year-old boy with cough and shortness of breath (▶ Fig. 17.1).

■ Key Imaging Finding

Anterior mediastinal mass.

■ Top Three Differential Diagnoses

- **Prominent normal thymus.** The normal thymus may cause anterior mediastinal enlargement until about the age of 2 years. It does not cause airway narrowing, and it may show the triangular "sail" sign. The inferior margin is often sharp on lateral views if thymic tissue protrudes into the minor fissure. The ribs may compress the thymus, causing the "wave" sign. Echotexture is similar to liver. The thymus is homogeneous at CT.
- **Lymphoma.** Lymphoma accounts for nearly half of all mediastinal masses in the pediatric population. Since most mediastinal lymphoma is due to Hodgkin disease, with other areas involved as well, the lower neck should be carefully assessed for lymphadenopathy. CT classically shows a smooth, well-demarcated, lobulated, nodular soft-tissue mass. Cystic or ne-

crotic components may be seen with Hodgkin lymphoma. The mass may compress the airway and/or the superior vena cava. Pleural effusions, often unilateral, are seen in up to half the cases. Lung parenchyma is usually spared. Anterior mediastinal involvement is also common in children with non-Hodgkin lymphoma.
- **Leukemia.** Acute lymphocytic leukemia is the most common pediatric malignancy, representing about one-third of oncology cases. The CT appearance of a large, homogeneous, soft-tissue anterior mediastinal mass resembles lymphoma. Large tumors may show central necrosis, and they may compress the airway and adjacent structures. Pleural effusions, mediastinal or lower cervical adenopathy, and bony involvement may also be present.

■ Additional Differential Diagnoses

- **Thymic hyperplasia.** Thymic rebound hyperplasia is usually seen in children recovering from such stresses as chemotherapy and severe illness. The thymus grows back up to 50% larger than its original size. In questionable cases, normal radiotracer uptake helps differentiate thymic rebound from recurrent disease.
- **Teratoma.** Ectopic germ cell tumors represent one-fourth of anterior mediastinal masses and are divided into mature and immature subtypes. Mature teratomas are generally considered benign, with very low risk of malignant transformation. They present as a large, heterogeneous mass of fat and soft tissue that displaces and does not invade adjacent structures.

Most are partly cystic, and one-fourth are partly calcified. Immature teratomas are typically predominantly soft-tissue density with smaller calcific and fatty foci.
- **Thymoma.** Although rare in children, thymoma remains a consideration for an anterior mediastinal mass. CT demonstrates a smoothly marginated soft-tissue mass; larger tumors may have cystic areas or necrosis. The mass is isointense or slightly hyperintense to muscle on T1-W MRI. T2-W MRI shows heterogeneous signal slightly brighter than muscle. Fibrous septa may traverse the mass, hypointense on both T1- and T2-W images; these enhance with contrast administration.

■ Diagnosis

T-cell acute lymphocytic leukemia.

✓ Pearls

- Mediastinal lymphoma and leukemia may enlarge rapidly and cause airway compression.
- Lymphoma and leukemia often cannot be distinguished with imaging alone.

Suggested Readings

Averill LW, Acikgoz G, Miller RE, Kandula VV, Epelman M. Update on pediatric leukemia and lymphoma imaging. Semin Ultrasound CT MR. 2013; 34(6):578–599

Mong A, Epelman M, Darge K. Ultrasound of the pediatric chest. Pediatr Radiol. 2012; 42(11):1287–1297

Nasseri F, Eftekhari F. Clinical and radiologic review of the normal and abnormal thymus: pearls and pitfalls. Radiographics. 2010; 30(2):413–428

Ranganath SH, Lee EY, Restrepo R, Eisenberg RL. Mediastinal masses in children. AJR Am J Roentgenol. 2012; 198(3):W197–W216

Case 18

Aaron Potnick

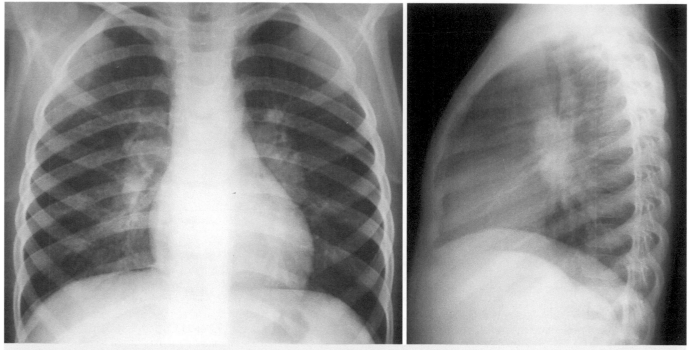

a   b

Fig. 18.1 Frontal **(a)** and lateral **(b)** views of the chest demonstrate enlarged hila with a normal mediastinum and clear lungs.

■ Clinical Presentation

A teenage boy with malaise (▶Fig. 18.1).

■ Key Imaging Finding

Hilar lymphadenopathy.

■ Top Three Differential Diagnoses

- **Mononucleosis.** Most infectious mononucleosis is caused by Epstein–Barr virus (EBV); 10% by cytomegalovirus. It is transmitted via saliva and is most prevalent in adolescents and young adults. Symptoms include general malaise, low-grade fever, lymphadenopathy, and splenomegaly. A characteristic maculopapular rash after administration of *B*-lactam antibiotics (ampicillin, amoxicillin) may be diagnostic of acute infection. Infectious mononucleosis is usually diagnosed clinically. Chest X-ray may show hilar lymphadenopathy. Treatment is supportive. Contact sports should be avoided for at least 3 weeks to avoid splenic injury.
- **Other infections.** Infections most typically associated with hilar lymphadenopathy include tuberculosis (TB), histoplasmosis, and coccidioidomycosis. Primary TB occurs in patients not previously exposed to *Mycobacterium tuberculosis* and is most common in infants and children under the age of 5 years. The distribution of lymphadenopathy is usually unilateral: right-sided hilar and right paratracheal. Although this may be the only manifestation of TB, lower and middle lobe consolidation is also common. Histoplasmosis and coccidioidomycosis both may present with hilar lymphadenopathy. Histoplasmosis is prevalent in the Midwestern and Southeastern United States, and coccidioidomycosis is prevalent in the Southwestern United States.
- **Lymphoma.** Thoracic involvement of both non-Hodgkin and Hodgkin lymphomas typically appears as an anterior mediastinal mass. Hilar involvement is more common with Hodgkin than non-Hodgkin lymphoma and is usually bilateral. Lymphoma may involve almost any organ in the body and should be considered in the differential diagnosis of any puzzling lesion.

■ Additional Differential Diagnosis

- **Sarcoidosis.** This multisystem disorder is characterized by noncaseous epithelioid cell granulomas that may affect almost any organ. The chest is involved in up to 90% of cases. The thoracic lymphadenopathy seen in sarcoidosis is typically symmetrical, bilateral hilar, and right paratracheal in location ("1–2–3 sign," or the "Garland triad"). Pulmonary findings predominate in the upper- and middle-lung zones and include nodules, fibrotic changes (reticular opacities, architectural distortions, traction bronchiectasis), and bilateral perihilar opacities. Sarcoidosis is uncommon in children.

■ Diagnosis

Mononucleosis.

✓ Pearls

- Infectious mononucleosis presents in adolescents and young adults with lymphadenopathy and splenomegaly.
- Tuberculosis should be considered in a patient with hilar lymphadenopathy and lower/middle lobe consolidation.
- Lymphoma most commonly presents in the thorax as an anterior mediastinal mass, and hilar involvement is usually bilateral.
- Thoracic involvement in sarcoidosis is seen in up to 90% of cases.

Suggested Readings

Burrill J, Williams CJ, Bain G, Conder G, Hine AL, Misra RR. Tuberculosis: a radiologic review. Radiographics. 2007; 27(5):1255–1273

Criado E, Sánchez M, Ramírez J, et al. Pulmonary sarcoidosis: typical and atypical manifestations at high-resolution CT with pathologic correlation. Radiographics. 2010; 30(6):1567–1586

Lucas S, Andronikou S, Goussard P, Gie R. CT features of lymphobronchial tuberculosis in children, including complications and associated abnormalities. Pediatr Radiol. 2012; 42(8):923–931

Toma P, Granata C, Rossi A, Garaventa A. Multimodality imaging of Hodgkin disease and non-Hodgkin lymphomas in children. Radiographics. 2007; 27(5):1335–1354

Case 19

Rebecca Stein-Wexler

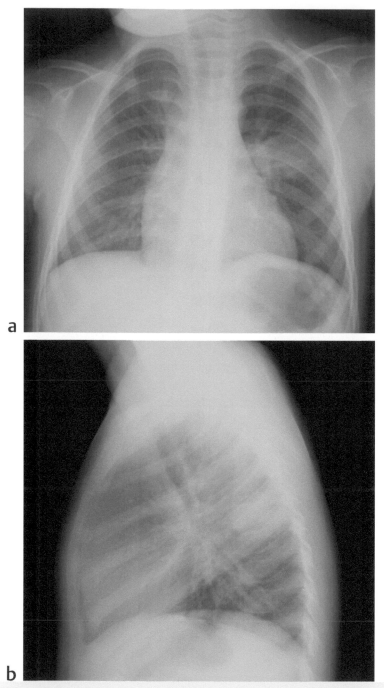

Fig. 19.1 Frontal **(a)** and lateral **(b)** chest radiographs show a rounded density in the superior segment of the left lower lobe.

■ **Clinical Presentation**

A 4-year-old boy with cough and fever (▶ Fig. 19.1).

■ **Key Imaging Finding**

Lung mass.

■ **Top Three Differential Diagnoses**

- **Round pneumonia.** Round pneumonia presents as a well-defined pulmonary opacity in children up to 8 years of age, most often in the superior segment of a lower lobe. Usually caused by *Streptococcus pneumoniae*, the inflammatory process is confined because collateral pathways of airflow (canals of Lambert, pores of Kohn) are less developed in this age group. In the appropriate clinical setting, a follow-up chest radiograph is suggested to ensure resolution with antibiotic therapy.
- **Congenital pulmonary airway malformation (CPAM).** Part of the spectrum of bronchopulmonary foregut malformations, CPAM is often diagnosed in utero. Older patients may present with respiratory distress or recurrent pneumonia. CPAM consists of abnormal proliferation of respiratory elements that communicate with the tracheobronchial tree. Stocker type I contains cysts larger than 2 cm and is most common. Type II contains smaller cysts and is associated with congenital anomalies. Type III appears grossly solid but is truly microcystic. In infants, the mass may appear solid on radiographs, though often it is occult. A solid or cystic mass is seen in older children. CT demonstrates air- or fluid-filled cysts or a solid lesion, depending upon the type. Resection is generally recommended due to increased risk of infection and malignancy.
- **Sequestration.** This congenital lesion consists of dysplastic and nonfunctioning lung tissue with systemic arterial supply. It connects with the tracheobronchial tree only after superinfection. It is often in the left lower lobe. Frequently diagnosed in utero, this too can present with respiratory distress or pneumonia. Extralobar sequestration presents early in life, drains into the systemic venous system, and has its own pleural covering, whereas intralobar sequestration presents later in life with recurring infections, drains into the pulmonary venous system, and lacks a pleural covering. Both appear as a solid mass unless they contain areas of CPAM or have become superinfected, when tissue breakdown permits communication with the bronchial tree.

■ **Additional Differential Diagnoses**

- **Bronchogenic cyst.** This foregut duplication cyst typically presents as a solitary, discrete mediastinal mass, but it occasionally occurs in the pulmonary parenchyma. It contains simple or complex fluid, and its wall is typically thin unless there has been superinfection. Mass effect on mediastinal structures may cause dysphagia or respiratory distress. Older children may complain of chest pain.
- **Pleuropulmonary blastoma.** This rare, aggressive, primitive pleural-based or parenchymal neoplasm presents as a large (> 5 cm) cystic, solid, or mixed soft-tissue mass. Pleural effusion is common, and the disease is often initially diagnosed as pneumonia. Childhood cancers are common in close relatives.

■ **Diagnosis**

Round pneumonia.

✓ **Pearls**

- Round pneumonia presents in children up to 8 years old with less developed collateral airflow pathways.
- Congenital pulmonary airway malformations communicate with the airway and are classified based upon their cystic and/or solid composition.
- Sequestrations have systemic arterial supply and are further classified according to venous drainage and pleural covering.
- Sequestrations are much more common in the lower lobes, especially on the left.

Suggested Readings

Newman B. Congenital bronchopulmonary foregut malformations: concepts and controversies. Pediatr Radiol. 2006; 36(8):773–791

Restrepo R, Palani R, Matapathi UM, Wu YY. Imaging of round pneumonia and mimics in children. Pediatr Radiol. 2010; 40(12):1931–1940

Yikilmaz A, Lee EY. CT imaging of mass-like nonvascular pulmonary lesions in children. Pediatr Radiol. 2007; 37(12):1253–1263

Case 20

Ernst Joseph and Rebecca Stein-Wexler

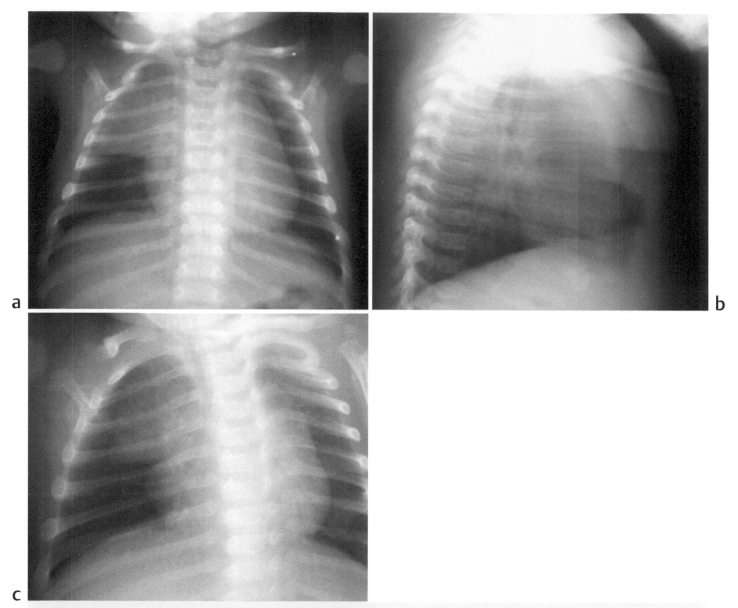

Fig. 20.1 Frontal view shows an opacity at the right upper chest with normal bronchovascular markings projecting through it **(a)**. Lateral view shows increased retrosternal density sharply defined at the minor fissure **(b)**. Oblique view shows the opacity is triangular and has a wavy lateral margin **(c)**.

■ **Clinical Presentation**

A 2-week-old with respiratory distress (►Fig. 20.1).

■ Key Imaging Finding

Right upper lobe (RUL) opacity.

■ Top Three Differential Diagnoses

- **Normal thymus.** The normal thymus reaches maximum weight at puberty, but, compared to chest volume, thymic volume is greatest from infancy through about age 2 years. Its shape is triangular or quadrilateral, and margins should be smooth and not lobular. The thymus may resemble a sail extending from the upper mediastinal border, sometimes mimicking RUL pathology. The normal thymus is soft, so it does not cause airway narrowing. Adjacent ribs distort its contour, resulting in the "thymic wave" sign—most evident on oblique radiographs. The thymus is homogeneous, and the presence of bronchovascular markings behind it helps differentiate thymus from lobar collapse or consolidation as well. On lateral projection, the inferior margin is often sharp due to protrusion of thymic tissue into the minor fissure. Thymic size is exaggerated with hypoventilation, and questionable cases may be clarified by repeat imaging in full inspiration. On CT, the thymus appears homogeneous, and the contour should be smooth and not lobulated. On US, it resembles liver. It is mildly T1 hyperintense and strikingly T2 hyperintense at MRI.
- **RUL collapse.** Lobar collapse is more common in children than in adults. The RUL accounts for more than two-thirds of cases of lobar collapse in neonates and older children hospitalized in intensive care units, whereas in adults the lower lobes are most often affected. These differences are likely due to small-er-sized airways in children, which collapse more easily and are more easily blocked with mucus and debris. Underdeveloped collateral channels contribute as well. Since the RUL bronchus is the most dependent in the supine child, it is the most susceptible to aspiration and resultant collapse. Transient improper endotracheal tube position may contribute as well. Radiographic findings include—in addition to density with possible air bronchograms at the right upper chest—mediastinal shift to the right and elevation of the right hilum. Other signs of volume loss include rib crowding and elevation of the ipsilateral side of the diaphragm. Right middle and lower lobe hyperinflation may be evident as well.
- **RUL pneumonia.** In the setting of pneumonia, lobar consolidation usually indicates bacterial etiology—often *Streptococcus pneumoniae*, sometimes *Haemophilus influenzae*, *Staphylococcus aureus*, or other gram negatives. Lobar pneumonia is most common in children older than 5 years. The presence of air bronchograms helps differentiate pneumonia from normal thymus. Pleural fluid also supports the diagnosis, as does contralateral mediastinal shift. Contrast-enhanced CT may be employed to evaluate for such complications as necrosis, abscess, and empyema. US is very useful for characterizing pleural fluid, and it may help characterize immediately subpleural parenchymal processes.

■ Diagnosis

Normal thymus.

✓ Pearls

- The normal thymus has smooth, nonlobulated margins, and it does not obscure bronchovascular markings.
- RUL collapse is common in acutely ill children; volume loss should suggest the diagnosis.
- Air bronchograms and pleural fluid support the diagnosis of lobar pneumonia.

Suggested Readings

Daltro P, Santos EN, Gasparetto TD, Ucar ME, Marchiori E. Pulmonary infections. Pediatr Radiol. 2011; 41 Suppl 1:S69–S82

Thomas K, Habibi P, Britto J, Owens CM. Distribution and pathophysiology of acute lobar collapse in the pediatric intensive care unit. Crit Care Med. 1999; 27(8):1594–1597

Walker CM, Abbott GF, Greene RE, Shepard JA, Vummidi D, Digumarthy SR. Imaging pulmonary infection: classic signs and patterns. AJR Am J Roentgenol. 2014; 202(3):479–492

Westra SJ, Choy G. What imaging should we perform for the diagnosis and management of pulmonary infections? Pediatr Radiol. 2009; 39 Suppl 2:S178–S183

Case 22

Aaron Potnick

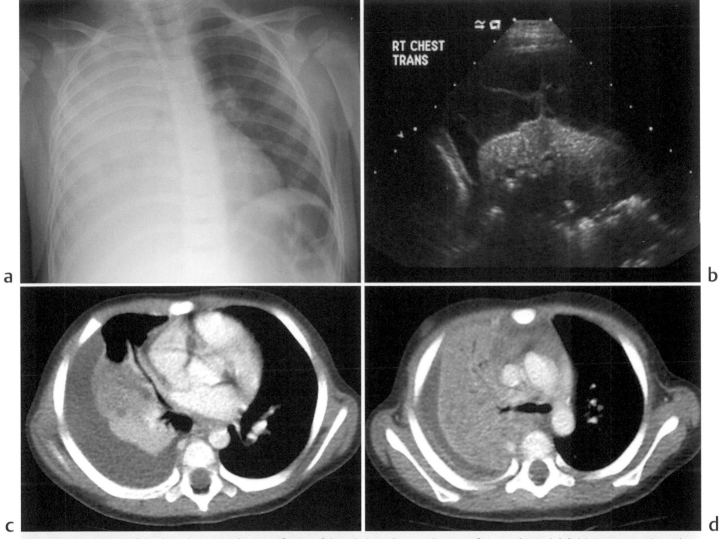

Fig. 22.1 Frontal view of the chest shows complete opacification of the right hemithorax without significant mediastinal shift **(a)**. Transverse US reveals a large right pleural effusion with internal septations, along with consolidated lung **(b)**. Contrast-enhanced CT shows consolidated, necrotic lung parenchyma and a large pleural effusion **(c)**. Another CT image also shows visceral and parietal pleural enhancement **(d)**.

▪ Clinical Presentation

An 18-month-old with 10 days of cough and fever (▶Fig. 22.1).

■ Key Imaging Finding

Unilateral dense chest without volume loss.

■ Top Three Differential Diagnoses

- **Pneumonia.** Lobar pneumonia is most common in children older than 5 years. Most cases are bacterial—often *Streptococcus pneumoniae*, sometimes *Haemophilus influenzae, Staphylococcus aureus*, and other gram negatives. *Mycobacterium tuberculosis* and other organisms may cause lobar consolidation as well. In the setting of a respiratory illness, imaging goals are to distinguish between viral and bacterial pneumonia as well as assess for such complications as abscess and empyema. Contrast-enhanced CT may show necrosis, abscess, and empyema. US can characterize pleural fluid. Viral diseases manifest as increased peribronchial interstitial markings, hyperinflation, and atelectasis. Round pneumonia is seen in children up to 8 years old, usually *S. pneumoniae*. It appears as a well-defined round opacity, usually in the superior segment of a lower lobe. In neonates, pneumonia is most often caused by group B *Streptococcus*. It may resemble surfactant deficiency, with bilateral diffuse granular opacities. However, effusions are common, which helps differentiate. It may alternatively demonstrate perihilar densities, hyperinflation, and/or interstitial opacities.
- **Lymphoma.** Lymphoma affects the chest at presentation in over three-fourths of patients with Hodgkin lymphoma and approximately half of the patients with non-Hodgkin lymphoma. It usually presents as an anterior mediastinal mass. Additional thoracic findings include central airway compression, superior vena cava obstruction, pleural effusion, and pericardial effusion. Lung involvement is relatively rare in children and manifests as nodules, interstitial opacities, or consolidation; this is most often encountered in teens and males.
- **Askin tumor.** Askin tumor, or peripheral primitive neuroectodermal tumor, is part of the Ewing sarcoma family of tumors. These tumors usually develop in the soft tissues of the chest wall and occasionally in the mediastinum or peripheral lung. They should be considered when a child or young adult presents with a heterogeneous soft-tissue chest wall mass accompanied by rib destruction and pleural effusion.

■ Additional Differential Diagnosis

- **Pleuropulmonary blastoma.** This rare, aggressive, malignant primary neoplasm of the pleuropulmonary mesenchyme occurs in early childhood and has a poor prognosis. It usually appears as a large, pleural-based mass but may mimic advanced pneumonia. It is typically on the right and does not invade the
chest wall; pleural effusion is common. Type 1 is purely cystic (usually with a single, large, multiloculated cyst). Type 2 is cystic and solid (multiple small cysts). Type 3 appears solid but is actually composed of multiple microcysts. Type 1 presents earliest in life (less than 1 year) and has the best prognosis.

■ Diagnosis

Pneumonia with empyema.

✓ Pearls

- Viral pneumonia typically causes hyperinflation, peribronchial interstitial opacities, and shifting atelectasis, whereas bacterial pneumonia causes consolidation and pleural effusion.
- Lymphoma usually presents as an anterior mediastinal mass, but pleural, pericardial, and parenchymal involvement may be seen.

- Askin tumor should be considered in a child or young adult with a chest wall mass and rib destruction.
- Pleuropulmonary blastoma presents in a young child with a large, pleural-based mass that does not invade the chest wall; it is often on the right and accompanied with pleural fluid.

Suggested Readings

Eslamy HK, Newman B. Pneumonia in normal and immunocompromised children: an overview and update. Radiol Clin North Am. 2011; 49(5):895–920

Naffaa LN, Donnelly LF. Imaging findings in pleuropulmonary blastoma. Pediatr Radiol. 2005; 35(4):387–391

Toma P, Granata C, Rossi A, Garaventa A. Multimodality imaging of Hodgkin disease and non-Hodgkin lymphomas in children. Radiographics. 2007; 27(5):1335–1354

Case 25

Mike Evens Saint-Louis and Rebecca Stein-Wexler

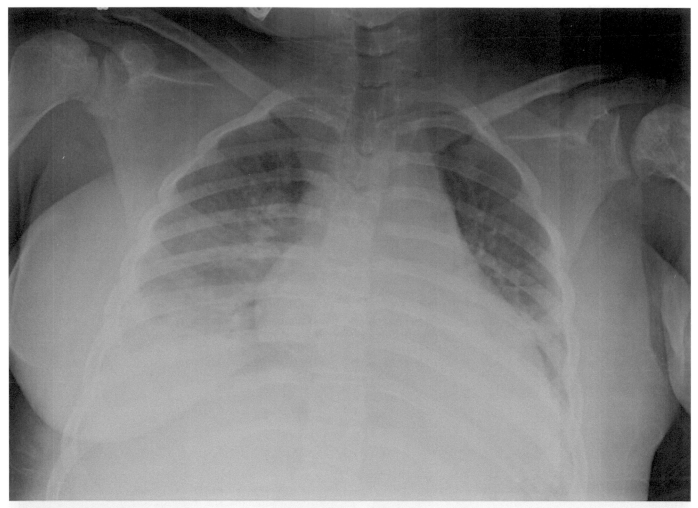

Fig. 25.1 Chest radiograph shows bilateral pleural effusions and basal opacities with associated cardiomegaly and prominent vasculature. Humeral heads are sclerotic and irregular.

■ Clinical Presentation

A 17-year-old girl with sickle cell disease and acute chest pain (▶Fig. 25.1).

■ Key Imaging Finding

Pulmonary opacities in a patient with sickle cell disease.

■ Top Three Differential Diagnoses

• **Pneumonia.** Impaired immune status renders children with sickle cell disease about 100 times more likely to develop pneumonia than unaffected children. These infections are often recurrent. *Streptococcus pneumoniae*, *Haemophilus influenzae*, *Staphylococcus aureus*, *Chlamydia*, and *Salmonella* are the most common pathogens. Children present with cough and fever. Radiographic findings are similar to those in other patients: consolidation and pleural fluid. US may demonstrate a parapneumonic effusion, and if there are septations, pleural thickening, and mass effect on the lung, empyema is likely. Pneumonia may progress to acute chest syndrome. Bones should be evaluated for stigmata of sickle cell disease, such as avascular necrosis of the humeral heads and vertebral body deformities.

• **Acute chest syndrome.** Pneumonia, fat emboli from bone infarct, pulmonary vascular occlusion, and other processes may lead to acute chest syndrome in patients with sickle cell disease. Pneumonia is the most common etiology in children. Acute chest syndrome is the most common reason for hospitalization and death in patients with sickle cell disease. Patients present with fever, chest pain, and usually hypoxemia. Chest radiographs may initially be normal. When opacities develop, they are more common in the middle and lower lobes, and pleural effusions are often present as well. Therapy consists of hydration, blood transfusion, oxygen, and analgesics. If pneumonia precipitated the crisis, antibiotics are also administered.

• **Pulmonary arterial thrombosis.** Risk of pulmonary thrombosis is increased in sickle cell disease due to coagulation and platelet function abnormalities. Pulmonary infarct is caused by small vessel occlusion, and it occurs in the absence of lower extremity venous thrombosis. This phenomenon is more common in older patients with sickle cell disease. Clinical presentation may include fever, tachypnea, and chest pain. As with acute chest syndrome, chest radiographs on admission may be normal, or there may be consolidation. Pleural effusion is relatively uncommon. The radiographic abnormality usually clears within 7 to 10 days.

■ Additional Differential Diagnosis

• **Bone infarct with atelectasis.** Chest pain in patients with sickle cell disease may also result from bone pain due to rib infarct. Chest radiographs may show atelectasis secondary to splinting.

■ Diagnosis

Acute chest syndrome and avascular necrosis of the humeral heads.

✓ Pearls

• Pneumonia is very common in children with sickle cell disease but is otherwise similar to pneumonia encountered in unaffected children.

• Acute chest syndrome most often follows pneumonia in children but may result from fat emboli, vascular occlusion, and other processes.

• Chest radiographs may initially be normal in patients with acute chest syndrome or pulmonary infarct.

Suggested Readings

Dinan D, Epelman M, Guimaraes CV, Donnelly LF, Nagasubramanian R, Chauvin NA. The current state of imaging pediatric hemoglobinopathies. Semin Ultrasound CT MR. 2013; 34(6):493–515

Lonergan GJ, Cline DB, Abbondanzo SL. Sickle cell anemia. Radiographics. 2001; 21(4):971–994

Martin L, Buonomo C. Acute chest syndrome of sickle cell disease: radiographic and clinical analysis of 70 cases. Pediatr Radiol. 1997; 27(8):637–641

Case 27

Rebecca Stein-Wexler

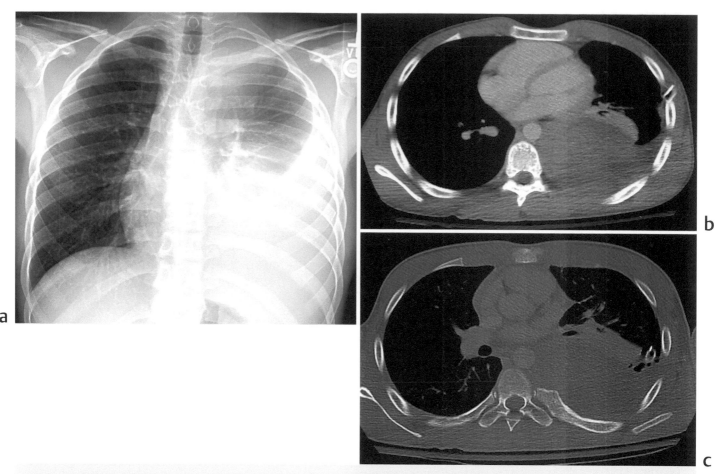

Fig. 27.1 Frontal chest radiograph demonstrates density at the left base, obscuring the heart and diaphragm borders, with a meniscus tracking up the lateral chest wall (**a**). Contrast-enhanced CT shows a minimally enhancing retrocardiac soft-tissue mass that merges with pleural fluid (**b**). Bone windows show mild expansion of the adjacent rib (**c**).

■ Clinical Presentation

A 14-year-old boy with chest pain (▶Fig. 27.1).

■ Key Imaging Finding

Solid soft-tissue chest wall mass in an older child.

■ Top Three Differential Diagnoses

- **Ewing sarcoma (ES).** Primitive neuroectodermal tumor, Askin tumor, and both osseous and extraosseous ES are all in the ES family of tumors (ESFT). These small round cell neoplasms have a translocation between chromosome 11 and 22 and are usually differentiated only by electron microscopy. Common locations of ES in the chest include the clavicle, ribs, and sternum; rib involvement is often posteromedial and may grow along the neural foramen. Most ES occurs in children and adolescents, and the tumor is more common in boys. Patients present with a rapidly growing, painful mass and sometimes also cough, dyspnea, and systemic symptoms such as fever and weight loss. Radiographs show lytic and/or sclerotic bone, often accompanied by a large soft-tissue mass. CT may show dystrophic calcifications. On T1-W MRI, the mass is often hyperintense to muscle; large lesions show hemorrhage and necrosis. The CT and MRI appearance is nonspecific but useful for guiding treatment. Recurrence rate is high, improved by complete resection.

- **Askin tumor.** Also in the ESFT, Askin tumor is defined as extraskeletal ES of the chest wall. Unlike ES, Askin tumor is more common in girls. A large chest wall mass is typical, often merging with extensive pleural fluid that may be loculated and exert considerable mass effect. The adjacent rib may be destroyed or expanded. The mass usually does not calcify. There may be hilar and mediastinal adenopathy.

- **Rhabdomyosarcoma.** This is the most common soft-tissue sarcoma in children, but less than 10% involve the chest wall. Chest wall rhabdomyosarcoma occurs in teens presenting with a rapidly growing mass that may be painful. Most tumors are of the alveolar subtype, which has a worse prognosis than other subtypes. The tumor appears as a soft-tissue mass that enhances heterogeneously, perhaps with areas of necrosis. Adjacent bone may be destroyed. CT/MRI appearance is nonspecific but useful for evaluating disease extent.

■ Additional Differential Diagnoses

- **Desmoid tumor (aggressive fibromatosis).** This infiltrative lesion does not metastasize but is difficult to completely resect, so recurrence is common. It is most common in adolescents and young adults. Usually located in muscle and adjacent fascia, it may encase nerves and vessels. Bones and subcutaneous soft tissues are rarely involved. MRI signal varies with cellularity, vascularity, and the amount of collagen and water.

- **Langerhans cell histiocytosis (LCH).** LCH of the rib may present as a chest wall soft-tissue mass arising from bone. The osseous component initially appears permeative and lytic; there may also be a large soft-tissue mass. However, with healing, margins often appear well circumscribed, and the soft-tissue component resolves. LCH enhances vigorously at MRI.

■ Diagnosis

Askin tumor.

✓ Pearls

- Ewing sarcoma family of tumors usually appear as a large soft-tissue mass associated with lytic or sclerotic clavicle, ribs, or sternum.
- Rhabdomyosarcoma of the chest is usually of the alveolar subtype, with relatively poor prognosis.

- Desmoid tumor does not metastasize but is very infiltrative and hence difficult to resect.
- Bone affected by Langerhans cell histiocytosis may initially appear permeative, but with healing, margins become well circumscribed.

Suggested Readings

Fefferman NR, Pinkney LP. Imaging evaluation of chest wall disorders in children. Radiol Clin North Am. 2005; 43(2):355–370

Restrepo R, Lee EY. Updates on imaging of chest wall lesions in pediatric patients. Semin Roentgenol. 2012; 47(1):79–89

Case 29

Rebecca Stein-Wexler

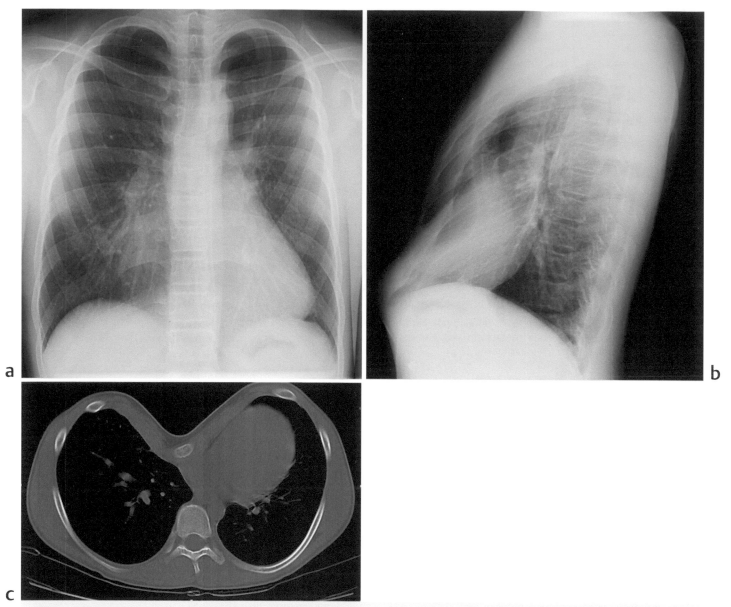

Fig. 29.1 Posteroanterior chest radiograph shows increased soft tissue at the right heart border and a relatively vertical orientation of the ribs (**a**). Lateral view shows the sternum is dorsal to the anterior chest wall, and there is lucency posterior to the chest wall (**b**). Axial CT image shows posterior displacement of the sternum, convexity of the right and left chest wall, and displacement of the heart to the left (**c**).

■ Clinical Presentation

A 14-year-old boy with chest wall deformity (▶ Fig. 29.1).

■ Key Imaging Finding

Chest wall deformity.

■ Top Three Differential Diagnoses

- **Pectus excavatum.** Pectus excavatum is a congenital deformity of the anterior chest wall that may be isolated or familial. The inferior sternum is depressed posteriorly and often tilted to the left, and the ribs protrude anteriorly. The anteroposterior diameter of the chest wall is narrow, displacing the heart to the left. The most common complaint in this condition concerns physical appearance. However, severe cases may be complicated by restrictive lung disease, dyspnea, palpitations, mitral valve prolapse, and pain. Pectus excavatum may be seen in patients with Marfan syndrome. Chest radiographs show increased density along the right heart border due to superimposition of chest wall soft tissue. The heart is displaced to the left, and the lateral view demonstrates displacement of the sternum. The "Haller index," calculated from measurements obtained on axial low-dose CT or MRI, is used to help determine the need for surgery. The Haller index is obtained by dividing the maximum transverse inner diameter of the chest by the distance from the posterior wall of the sternum to the anterior vertebral body. Values greater than 3.25 are associated with an increased need

for surgery. A common surgical approach is to insert a metallic bar across the chest; tension causes gradual remodeling. Possible complications such as migration or angulation of the bar are assessed on chest X-ray.
- **Pectus carinatum.** In this condition, the superior part of the sternum protrudes anteriorly, often as a result of scoliosis. This leads to an unusually convex anterior chest wall. It is associated with congenital heart disease in about 10% of patients. This condition is also more common in patients with Marfan syndrome.
- **Poland syndrome.** Unilateral pectoralis major muscle underdevelopment characterizes this unusual condition. There may also be aplasia of the ipsilateral breast and nipple, and the upper ribs may be dysmorphic. Brachysyndactyly is common as well. The condition usually occurs on the right and is more common in boys. Chest X-ray shows a relatively lucent thorax, along with possible upper rib deformities. Cross-sectional imaging is useful for surgical planning.

■ Diagnosis

Pectus excavatum.

✓ Pearls

- Prominent soft-tissue silhouetting the right side of the heart simulates right middle lobe consolidation in patients with pectus excavatum.
- The Haller index is obtained by dividing the maximum transverse inner diameter of the chest by the distance from the posterior wall of the sternum to the anterior vertebral body; values greater than 3.25 suggest need for surgery.

- Pectus carinatum results from anterior protrusion of the superior portion of the sternum.
- Poland syndrome is characterized by unilateral underdevelopment of the pectoralis major muscle, often accompanied with ipsilateral hand malformation.

Suggested Readings

Donnelly LF, Frush DP, Foss JN, O'Hara SM, Bisset GS III. Anterior chest wall: frequency of anatomic variations in children. Radiology. 1999; 212(3):837–840

Fefferman NR, Pinkney LP. Imaging evaluation of chest wall disorders in children. Radiol Clin North Am. 2005; 43(2):355–370

Restrepo R, Lee EY. Updates on imaging of chest wall lesions in pediatric patients. Semin Roentgenol. 2012; 47(1):79–89

Case 30

Rebecca Stein-Wexler

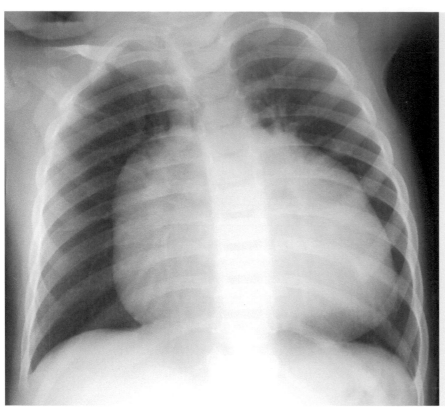

Fig. 30.1 Frontal chest radiograph shows lungs are hyperinflated, vasculature is decreased, and the cardiothymic silhouette is markedly enlarged. The right heart border is strikingly enlarged.

■ Clinical Presentation

An 18-month-old boy with cyanosis (▶Fig. 30.1).

■ Key Imaging Finding

Box-shaped heart.

■ Diagnosis

Ebstein anomaly. In Ebstein anomaly, the septal and posterior leaflets of the tricuspid valve are displaced downward, toward the right ventricle. This results in a large common right ventriculoatrial chamber ("atrialization of the right ventricle") and an initially small right ventricle. The right ventricular outflow is usually reduced, leading to diminished vascularity. The tricuspid valve is incompetent, so there is tricuspid regurgitation, contributing to right atrial enlargement. As the proximal right heart structures dilate, the tricuspid valve becomes even more insufficient, leading to worsening cardiomegaly. The right ventricle also dilates in many patients, as does the right ventricular outflow tract. Meanwhile, right atrial pressure increases, and a right-to-left shunt usually develops across a patent foramen ovale or atrial septal defect, with resulting cyanosis. Left-sided structures remain normal in size.

Pulmonary blood flow is often decreased, though sometimes it is normal. Imaging consistently shows right atrial enlargement, often severe; the right atrium may fill the entire right chest. The left cardiac border may appear shelflike due to a dilated right ventricular outflow tract. The normal convex bulge of the pulmonary outflow tract is not evident, and the aorta is small. These imaging findings combine to create the "box-shaped heart" classically associated with Ebstein anomaly.

Ebstein anomaly accounts for less than 1% of congenital cardiac disease. It is associated with maternal lithium use during the first trimester. Pulmonary blood flow varies with the associated anatomical abnormalities, so patients may be cyanotic or acyanotic. Decreased left ventricular outflow due to right ventricular failure may lead to fatigue and dyspnea. Paroxysmal supraventricular tachycardia is common, and arrhythmias may lead to sudden cardiac death.

Although the box-shaped heart with decreased vascularity is considered essentially diagnostic of Ebstein anomaly, a few other entities could almost mimic this appearance. These include extremely severe lymphadenopathy, a massive pericardial effusion, and an enormous thymus. With these diagnoses, pulmonary vasculature should not be decreased. Isolated pulmonary atresia would not typically cause this configuration of cardiomegaly although it does demonstrate decreased pulmonary vasculature.

✓ Pearls

- In Ebstein anomaly, displacement of the tricuspid valve leads to a common ventriculoatrial chamber (atrialization of the right ventricle).
- Pulmonary vascularity is usually reduced, causing cyanosis.
- An incompetent tricuspid valve causes a vicious cycle of regurgitation, right atrial enlargement, and progressive worsening of the regurgitation and increasing atrial size.
- Ebstein anomaly is associated with maternal lithium use during the first trimester.

Suggested Readings

Ferguson EC, Krishnamurthy R, Oldham SA. Classic imaging signs of congenital cardiovascular abnormalities. Radiographics. 2007; 27(5):1323–1334

Schweigmann G, Gassner I, Maurer K. Imaging the neonatal heart—essentials for the radiologist. Eur J Radiol. 2006; 60(2):159–170

Part 2

Gastrointestinal Imaging

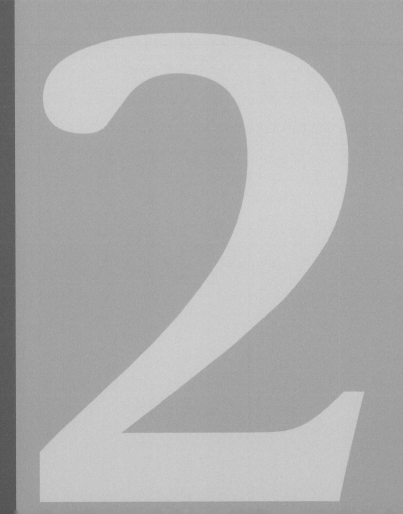

Case 31

Rebecca Stein-Wexler

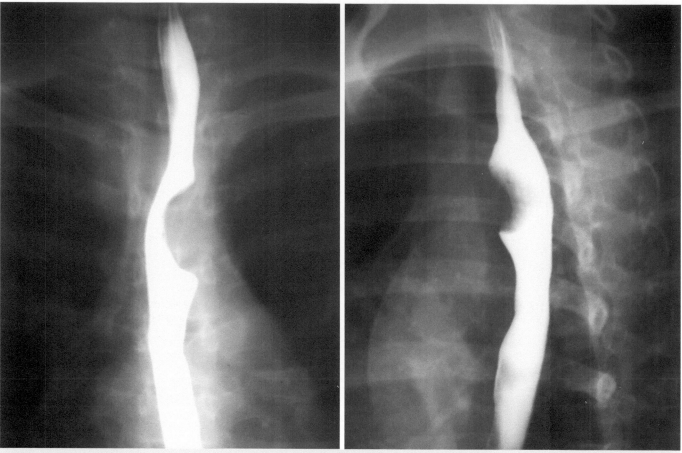

Fig. 31.1 Frontal view from an esophagram demonstrates a well-circumscribed defect that indents the left lateral wall of the esophagus **(a)**. An oblique view shows that the filling defect is anterior **(b)**.

a

b

■ Clinical Presentation

A 10-year-old with difficulty swallowing (▶Fig. 31.1).

■ Key Imaging Finding

Esophageal mass.

■ Top Three Differential Diagnoses

- **Aberrant right subclavian artery.** A left aortic arch with an aberrant right subclavian artery is the most common anomaly of the aortic arch. It is considered an incomplete vascular ring. In 80% of cases, the subclavian artery passes from the left to the right, posterior to the esophagus. It causes symptoms in only 10% of patients (dysphagia lusoria) and is usually identified incidentally on an esophagram.
- **Esophageal duplication cyst.** Esophageal duplications are usually on the right in the distal esophagus, in the posterior mediastinum. Most are asymptomatic, but patients may have respiratory distress or dysphagia, and if there is gastric mucosa in the wall a cyst may bleed. Duplications are rarely complete, and they rarely communicate with the esophagus. Esophageal duplications are the second most common bowel duplication, after the distal ileum. Like bowel duplications elsewhere, they result from abnormal bowel canalization. Cysts in the esophagus

may be isolated or occur along with other bronchopulmonary foregut anomalies. Duplication cysts are near water attenuation on CT and show no central enhancement. On MRI, they are bright on T2 and variable on T1, depending on whether they contain proteinaceous or hemorrhagic fluid.
- **Other foregut cysts.** Neurenteric cysts are formed by CSF-filled leptomeninges protruding through a vertebral defect. These cysts therefore occur in conjunction with vertebral anomalies, such as dysraphism, hemivertebrae, butterfly vertebrae, and split spinal cord malformation. They are most common in the lower cervical and thoracic regions. MRI assesses whether they connect to the thecal sac. Bronchogenic cysts are caused by abnormal budding of the bronchial tree. They are lined with respiratory epithelium and filled with fluid or mucinous material. Seventy percent are located in the middle mediastinum; the rest are located in the hilum or the lung.

■ Additional Differential Diagnosis

- **Vascular ring.** Double-aortic arch and right aortic arch with aberrant left subclavian artery result in a filling defect in the posterior wall of the esophagus at the level of the aortic arch. Esophagrams demonstrate a posterior indentation on the

esophagus on lateral and oblique views and bilateral compression on the frontal view. A double aortic arch is more common than a right arch with an aberrant left subclavian artery.

■ Diagnosis

Esophageal duplication cyst.

✓ Pearls

- Esophageal duplication cysts may be isolated or occur in conjunction with bronchopulmonary foregut malformations.
- The esophagus is the second most common location of bowel duplication cysts, after the distal ileum.

- Neurenteric cysts are accompanied with vertebral anomalies.
- An aberrant right subclavian artery with a left aortic arch is usually asymptomatic.

Suggested Readings

Berrocal T, Torres I, Gutiérrez J, Prieto C, del Hoyo ML, Lamas M. Congenital anomalies of the upper gastrointestinal tract. Radiographics. 1999; 19(4):855–872

Lee NK, Kim S, Jeon TY, et al. Complications of congenital and developmental abnormalities of the gastrointestinal tract in adolescents and adults: evaluation with multimodality imaging. Radiographics. 2010; 30(6):1489–1507

Rao P. Neonatal gastrointestinal imaging. Eur J Radiol. 2006; 60(2):171–186

Case 32

Arvind Sonik

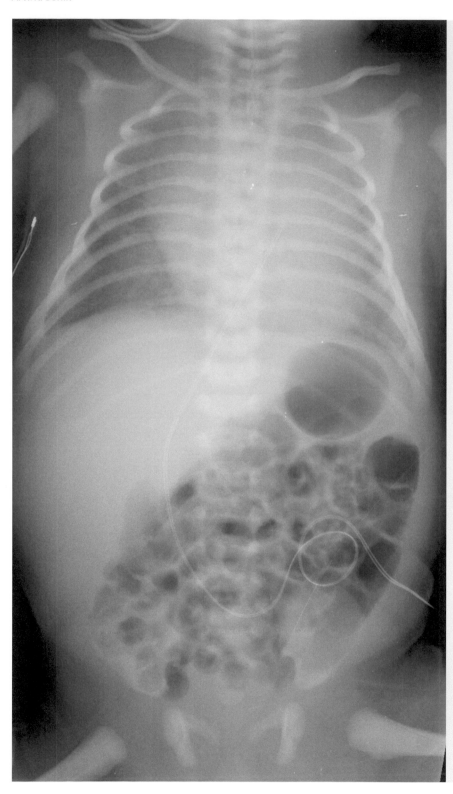

Fig. 32.1 An esophageal catheter ends in a lucent pouch slightly above the carina. Bowel gas is normal. Note the malpositioned umbilical venous catheter.

■ **Clinical Presentation**

A 1-day-old not tolerating oral feedings (▶ Fig. 32.1).

■ Key Clinical Finding

Difficulty feeding.

■ Top Three Differential Diagnoses

- **Tracheoesophageal (TE) fistula/esophageal atresia (EA).** EA is classified based upon the presence and location, or absence, of a TE fistula. Proximal EA with a fistula between the airway and the distal esophageal segment is the most common type. EA is often associated with additional anomalies of the gastrointestinal tract. Cardiac, renal, and vertebral anomalies (including the **V**ertebral anomalies, **A**nal atresia, **C**ardiac defects, Tracheo**E**sophageal fistula, **R**enal anomalies, with or without **L**imb malformations [VACTERL] association) are associated less frequently. Evaluation includes chest radiography after advancement of a feeding catheter to the level of the atresia, along with abdomen radiography to evaluate for intestinal air. If an H-type fistula is suspected (typically in older children who cough while feeding), an esophagram is indicated, preferably with isosmolar water-soluble contrast. Esophageal webs are considered a variant of EA and may be associated with a TE fistula. On esophagrams, webs appear as thin, transverse, or oblique filling defects. In a newborn, EA is the most common cause of difficulty feeding.
- **Foreign body.** Foreign bodies may become lodged in relatively narrow regions of the esophagus: at the level of the thoracic inlet, aortic arch, and less commonly the gastroesophageal (GE) junction. Esophagrams may be useful when a nonopaque foreign body is suspected. Disk batteries should be considered in the differential diagnosis of a disk-shaped metallic foreign body and constitute a medical emergency due to their corrosive properties.
- **Esophageal duplication cyst.** Esophageal duplications generally manifest as cysts, usually on the right and in the posterior mediastinum. They are rarely complete, and they rarely communicate with the esophagus. Duplication cysts are near water attenuation on CT and show no central enhancement. On MRI, they are bright on T2 and variable on T1, depending on their contents.

■ Additional Differential Diagnosis

- **Vascular ring.** The most common vascular anomalies to cause dysphagia are complete vascular rings: (1) double aortic arch and (2) right aortic arch with aberrant left subclavian artery and ligamentum arteriosum arising from the descending aorta. Esophagrams demonstrate a posterior indentation on the esophagus on lateral and oblique views and bilateral compression on frontal views. The double aortic arch is more common than the right arch with aberrant left subclavian artery. A left aortic arch with an aberrant right subclavian artery is the most common anomaly of the aortic arch, but this is an incomplete vascular ring and thus rarely symptomatic.

■ Diagnosis

Esophageal atresia with tracheoesophageal fistula.

✓ Pearls

- Esophageal atresia is classified based upon the presence and location, or absence, of a tracheoesophageal fistula.
- Proximal esophageal atresia with a fistula between the airway and the distal esophagus is most common.
- Foreign bodies typically become lodged at the thoracic inlet, aortic arch, and (less often) gastroesophageal junction.
- Complete vascular rings may cause esophageal compression and dysphagia.

Suggested Readings

Berrocal T, Torres I, Gutiérrez J, Prieto C, del Hoyo ML, Lamas M. Congenital anomalies of the upper gastrointestinal tract. Radiographics. 1999; 19(4):855–872

Lee NK, Kim S, Jeon TY, et al. Complications of congenital and developmental abnormalities of the gastrointestinal tract in adolescents and adults: evaluation with multimodality imaging. Radiographics. 2010; 30(6):1489–1507

Rao P. Neonatal gastrointestinal imaging. Eur J Radiol. 2006; 60(2):171–186

Case 33

Rebecca Stein-Wexler

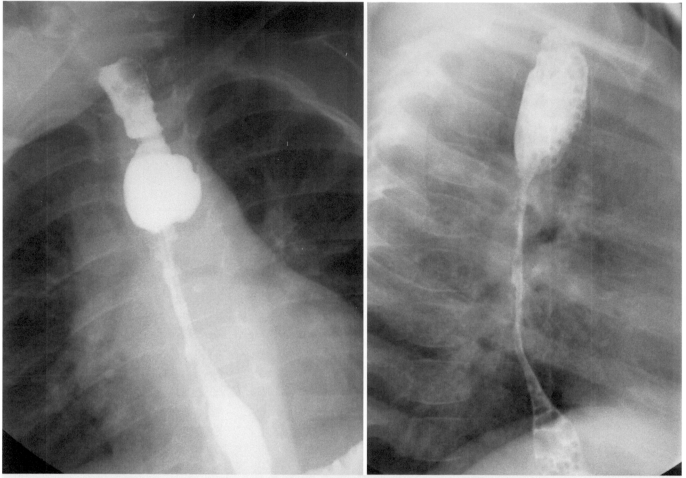

a   b

Fig. 33.1 Frontal view of an esophagram shows severe narrowing of the mid portion of the esophagus, with proximal dilatation and irregularities of the esophageal wall **(a)**. The lateral view shows a smoothly tapered transition between the proximal, dilated esophagus and the area of narrowing **(b)**.

■ **Clinical Presentation**

A 5-year-old boy with difficulty swallowing (▶Fig. 33.1).

■ Key Imaging Finding

Esophageal stricture.

■ Top Three Differential Diagnoses

• **Stricture at site of repaired esophageal atresia.** Approximately one-third of patients with esophageal atresia will develop an anastomotic stricture at the site of repair, regardless of whether a tracheoesophageal fistula was also present. The strictures are caused by tension on the anastomosis, a postoperative leak, and/or gastroesophageal reflux (GER). These strictures are difficult to prevent and are usually treated successfully with progressive esophageal dilatation and possible stenting. Refractory strictures are treated with esophageal anastomosis. In the immediate postoperative period, edema may cause reversible esophageal narrowing that is not considered a stricture.

• **Stricture due to ingestion of caustic material.** Accidental ingestion of caustic materials is most common in children around age 2 years. Household items with pH of 2 or less, or 12 or more, may cause serious esophageal injury. Most ingested caustics are alkaline, with dishwashing soap and disinfectants being the most commonly ingested materials. Patients are treated with antibiotics and steroids. Grade II esophageal burns have a 50% chance of resulting in stricture formation.

• **Stricture secondary to GER.** Chronic GER may lead to similar complications in children as in adults, including stricture formation in those with especially severe disease. It may contribute to reactive airway disease, sinusitis, and sleep apnea. A common finding on upper gastrointestinal (UGI) examinations, clinically significant GER is usually treated with protein pump inhibitors in children. Refractory cases may proceed to fundoplication, with variable success.

■ Additional Differential Diagnoses

• **Eosinophilic esophagitis (EE).** This is a chronic, relapsing, immune-mediated disease characterized by eosinophilic infiltration of the esophageal wall. The incidence is increasing, and EE is now a common cause of GI symptoms in both children and adults. Symptoms are nonspecific in infants and toddlers, including failure to thrive, fussiness, and feeding intolerance, whereas older children and adolescents present with dysphagia that is worse with solid foods. Esophageal rings, strictures, and furrows may develop.

• **Congenital esophageal stenosis.** This rare condition results from congenital malformation of the architecture of the esophageal wall. Up to one-third of patients also have esophageal atresia, other intestinal malformations, or cardiac anomalies. The disorder results from fibromuscular thickening of the wall, tracheobronchial remnants, or a membranous web (in decreasing order of frequency). Dilatation is sometimes successful, especially with fibromuscular thickening.

■ Diagnosis

Esophageal stricture secondary to remote ingestion of lye.

✓ Pearls

• Ingestion of caustic alkaline material such as dishwashing soap may cause esophageal stricture.
• Approximately one-third of patients with esophageal atresia develop stricture at the site of repair.

• Eosinophilic esophagitis in infants and toddlers has nonspecific symptoms, including failure to thrive.
• Congenital esophageal stenosis may coexist with esophageal atresia.

Suggested Readings

Amae S, Nio M, Kamiyama T, et al. Clinical characteristics and management of congenital esophageal stenosis: a report on 14 cases. J Pediatr Surg. 2003; 38(4):565–570

Baird R, Laberge JM, Lévesque D. Anastomotic stricture after esophageal atresia repair: a critical review of recent literature. Eur J Pediatr Surg. 2013; 23(3):204–213

Dellon ES. Eosinophilic esophagitis. Gastroenterol Clin North Am. 2013; 42(1):133–153

Case 35

Karen M. Ayotte

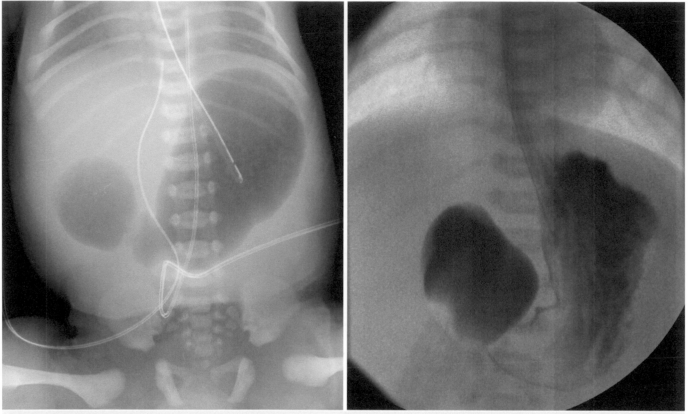

a   b

Fig. 35.1 Supine frontal abdomen radiograph shows a dilated stomach and proximal duodenum with no distal gas, along with an enteric catheter and umbilical vascular catheters **(a)**. Spot image from an upper gastrointestinal (GI) examination shows contrast does not extend beyond the dilated proximal duodenum **(b)**.

■ Clinical Presentation

A newborn boy with no prenatal care presents with emesis (▶Fig. 35.1).

■ Key Imaging Finding

"Double bubble" sign.

■ Top Three Differential Diagnoses

- **Malrotation/midgut volvulus.** Midgut volvulus is a surgical emergency that occurs when bowel twists around a narrow mesenteric pedicle in the setting of malrotation. When the diagnosis is suspected, expedited workup is mandatory to minimize morbidity and mortality. The classic presentation is bilious emesis in an infant in the first month of life, with partial duodenal obstruction. However, both clinical presentation and radiographic findings vary, and the radiographic appearance of volvulus ranges from normal to complete duodenal obstruction, mimicking duodenal atresia. An upper gastrointestinal examination is needed to establish the course of the duodenum and proximal small bowel. With malrotation, the duodenal–jejunal junction (ligament of Treitz) fails to cross to the left of midline and/or is located inferior to the pylorus. With volvulus, the proximal bowel demonstrates a "corkscrew" appearance.
- **Duodenal atresia/stenosis.** Both duodenal atresia and duodenal stenosis result from failure of recanalization of the duodenum, either partial (stenosis) or complete (atresia).

The classic radiographic presentation is the "double bubble" sign. In patients with complete atresia, there is usually no gas distal to the dilated duodenum. Patients present with vomiting in the first few hours of life. In 80% of patients, emesis is bilious, but if the obstruction is proximal to the ampulla of Vater, it is nonbilious. The degree of duodenal dilatation is usually marked, implying long-standing obstruction. Incidence of associated abnormalities is increased, and 30% of patients have trisomy 21. Duodenal stenosis may present in older patients.

- **Annular pancreas.** Annular pancreas often coexists with duodenal atresia or stenosis. Annular pancreas may present in infants with duodenal obstruction or in older children/adults with chronic nausea and vomiting. Cross-sectional imaging shows a soft-tissue mass contiguous with the pancreas, encircling the duodenum. Upper GI examination typically shows circumferential narrowing of the second portion of the duodenum.

■ Additional Differential Diagnoses

- **Duodenal web.** Intraluminal duodenal webs cause a variable degree of obstruction, and thus patients may present as older children and even adults. With severe obstruction in an infant, however, the radiographic appearance resembles other causes of duodenal obstruction. Upper GI examination may show circumferential narrowing of the duodenum or a variable-sized

aperture, allowing a restricted amount of contrast material to pass distally. The web may stretch, leading to a "windsock" appearance.

- **Preduodenal portal vein.** A preduodenal portal vein is a rare anomaly that may obstruct the duodenum. It is usually accompanied by malrotation, duodenal atresia, and other anomalies.

■ Diagnosis

Duodenal atresia.

✓ Pearls

- Malrotation with midgut volvulus is a surgical emergency requiring immediate diagnosis and intervention.
- An upper GI examination establishes the course of the duodenum and position of the ligament of Treitz.

- Duodenal atresia classically presents with the "double bubble" sign; 30% of patients have trisomy 21.
- Annular pancreas results in circumferential narrowing of the second portion of the duodenum.

Suggested Readings

Berrocal T, Lamas M, Gutieérrez J, Torres I, Prieto C, del Hoyo ML. Congenital anomalies of the small intestine, colon, and rectum. Radiographics. 1999; 19(5):1219–1236

Mortelé KJ, Rocha TC, Streeter JL, Taylor AJ. Multimodality imaging of pancreatic and biliary congenital anomalies. Radiographics. 2006; 26(3):715–731

Rao P. Neonatal gastrointestinal imaging. Eur J Radiol. 2006; 60(2):171–186

Strouse PJ. Disorders of intestinal rotation and fixation ("malrotation"). Pediatr Radiol. 2004; 34(11):837–851

Case 37

Rebecca Stein-Wexler

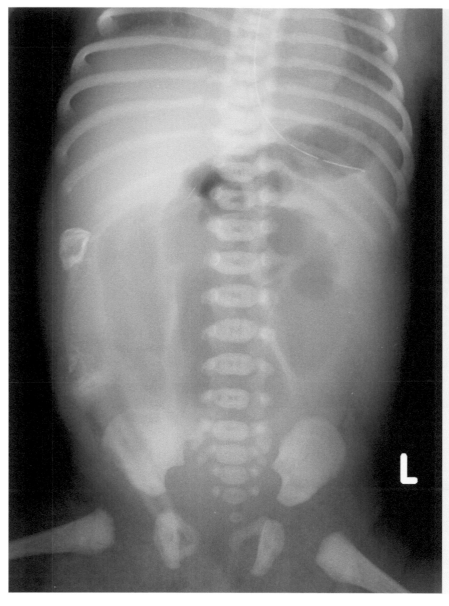

Fig. 37.1 Supine radiograph shows a well-circumscribed calcification in the right lateral abdomen with adjacent more amorphous calcifications as well. Bowel is dilated.

■ Clinical Presentation

A newborn with abdominal distension (▶Fig. 37.1).

■ Key Imaging Finding

Abdominal calcifications in an infant.

■ Top Three Differential Diagnoses

- **Adrenal hemorrhage (AH).** AH initially appears complex and echogenic. As the clot liquefies, the center becomes hypoechoic, and eventually the entire lesion becomes cystic. US shows involution over the course of several months. Curvilinear calcification may develop in the wall as early as 2 weeks post hemorrhage, becoming progressively more prominent. The calcifications eventually contract and appear clumped. AH is the most common adrenal mass in newborns. Seventy percent of cases occur on the right. Neonatal stress, hypoxia, septicemia, and hemorrhagic disorders may precipitate AH. The normal neonatal adrenal gland has a typical "sandwich" appearance at US, with hypoechoic cortex and a thin, echogenic medulla.
- **Meconium peritonitis.** Meconium peritonitis develops after in utero bowel perforation due to atresia, meconium ileus, or other obstruction. Chemical peritonitis leads to ascites and multiple intra-abdominal and intrascrotal calcifications. If a pseudocyst forms, the calcifications appear clustered and, if within the cyst wall, curvilinear. In the absence of pseudocyst formation, they are scattered in the abdomen.
- **Retroperitoneal teratoma (RPT).** RPTs typically occur near the upper pole of the left kidney. They are the third most common retroperitoneal tumor in children, after neuroblastoma and Wilms. Only 5% of pediatric teratomas occur in this location. About half are diagnosed before age 10 years, usually in girls younger than 6 months. Developing from pluripotent cells, they have a low incidence of malignancy. Most RPTs are mature, and of these most are cystic. Almost all contain fat, with foci of (often toothlike) calcification in about half of the cases. Immature RPTs are much less common and tend to be solid. Malignant degeneration is rare and often heralded by elevated serum alpha-fetoprotein.

■ Additional Differential Diagnoses

- **Neuroblastoma (NB).** In the neonatal period, NB and AH may be confused, since both may appear cystic and both may calcify. However, the calcifications of AH are curvilinear, whereas those of NB are typically more stippled in appearance. Since NB in this age group is relatively indolent, it is generally possible to let follow-up US establish the diagnosis. AH shrinks on serial US, whereas NB does not. Urinary vanillylmandelic acid (VMA) is increased with NB.
- **TORSCH infection.** Cytomegalovirus and toxoplasmosis may lead to calcifications in the liver, spleen, and peritoneum.
- **Fetus in fetu.** This benign monozygotic twin fragment is incorporated into the body of its host twin around week 3 of gestation. Usually retroperitoneal in location, it has been reported in the cerebral ventricles, liver, pelvis, and elsewhere. The presence of limbs and vertebral bodies allow differentiation from teratoma.

■ Diagnosis

Meconium peritonitis secondary to jejunal and ileal atresia.

✓ Pearls

- Adrenal hemorrhage is most common on the right and may develop calcifications in the wall by age 2 weeks.
- Neuroblastoma and adrenal hemorrhage may appear similar but are differentiated by follow-up US and urinary vanillylmandelic acid levels.
- Meconium peritonitis follows in utero bowel perforation and may be localized (pseudocyst) or diffuse.
- Retroperitoneal teratomas are most common near the left kidney's upper pole and are usually cystic, with fat and calcification.

Suggested Readings

Lakhoo K. Neonatal teratomas. Early Hum Dev. 2010; 86(10):643–647

Rajiah P, Sinha R, Cuevas C, Dubinsky TJ, Bush WH Jr, Kolokythas O. Imaging of uncommon retroperitoneal masses. Radiographics. 2011; 31(4):949–976

Veyrac C, Baud C, Prodhomme O, Saguintaah M, Couture A. US assessment of neonatal bowel (necrotizing enterocolitis excluded). Pediatr Radiol. 2012; 42 Suppl 1:S107–S114

Case 44

Cathy Zhou

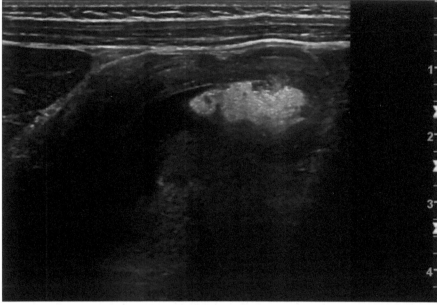

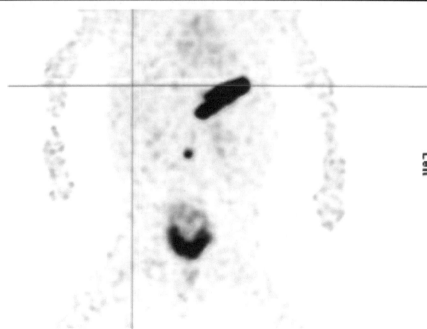

Fig. 44.1 US of the mid abdomen demonstrates a thick-walled bowel loop (a). Image of the abdomen in another patient taken 50 minutes following injection of technetium-99m-labeled sodium pertechnetate shows a discrete focus of radiotracer activity at the midline in the mid abdomen; expected activity in the stomach is due to uptake by gastric cells, and activity in the bladder is due to normal excretion (b).

■ Clinical Presentation

A 2-year-old girl with abdominal pain as well as a history of iron deficiency anemia and two episodes of gastrointestinal bleeding (▶Fig. 44.1).

■ Key Imaging Finding

Focal bowel wall thickening.

■ Top Three Differential Diagnoses

- **Acute appendicitis.** Appendiceal inflammation typically follows obstruction due to lymphoid hyperplasia or an appendicolith. Increased intraluminal pressure leads to ischemia, mucosal compromise, and, if allowed to progress, bacterial invasion and transmural inflammation. US is usually employed for diagnosis in children. Findings that suggest appendicitis include a noncompressible appendix with an outer diameter over 6 mm, a hyperemic wall, and echogenic surrounding fat. If US is inconclusive, CT more clearly shows a dilated appendix with a thick, enhancing wall and periappendiceal inflammation. Adjacent bowel wall may be thickened. Perforation leads to free fluid and possibly abscesses.
- **Meckel diverticulum.** One of the most common congenital abnormalities of the small intestine, this true diverticulum results when the omphalomesenteric duct fails to involute. The diverticulum is found in 2% of the population, in 2-year-olds, 2 feet proximal to the ileocecal valve. It is usually 2 inches long and may contain two types of ectopic tissue: gastric or pancreatic. Most patients are asymptomatic, but a few present with painless intermittent rectal bleeding and/or abdominal pain. It may cause small bowel obstruction, and clinical presentation may resemble appendicitis. Imaging findings vary, depending on whether the diverticulum causes bleeding or inflammation/obstruction. US and CT may show bowel wall thickening and obstruction, and sometimes the diverticulum is demonstrated. If the patient is bleeding, CT angiography may show a persistent omphalomesenteric artery, but the test of choice is the technetium-99m pertechnetate Meckel scan, which demonstrates uptake of pertechnetate by mucin-secreting ectopic gastric mucosa.
- **Crohn disease.** This idiopathic, multifactorial disease results in chronic mucosal and transmural inflammation of the digestive tract with characteristic skip lesions and ulcers that may become fistulas. Both small and large bowel may be involved. In children, sometimes only the terminal ileum is affected, and bowel elsewhere is entirely normal. Extraintestinal manifestations include seronegative spondyloarthropathy, hepatobiliary disease, erythema nodosum, and malnutrition/growth delay. Small bowel follow-through may show mucosal ulcers and with progressive disease bowel wall edema, a cobblestone appearance, strictures, and fistulas. CT readily demonstrates bowel wall thickening, adjacent vascular engorgement, and abscesses. MRI better defines extent of bowel involvement along with transmural inflammation; it also differentiates active inflammation from fibrosis. Direct visualization via capsule or direct endoscopy is diagnostic.

■ Diagnosis

Meckel diverticulum.

✓ Pearls

- US findings of acute appendicitis include a dilated, thick-walled, noncompressible appendix with adjacent echogenic fat.
- Crohn disease often involves only the terminal ileum; it has skip lesions and affects the entire bowel wall.
- Meckel diverticulum may present with rectal bleeding, inflammation, and/or obstruction.

Suggested Readings

McLaughlin PD, Maher MM. Nonneoplastic diseases of the small intestine: differential diagnosis and Crohn disease. AJR Am J Roentgenol. 2013; 201(2):W174–W182

Pepper VK, Stanfill AB, Pearl RH. Diagnosis and management of pediatric appendicitis, intussusception, and Meckel diverticulum. Surg Clin North Am. 2012; 92(3):505–526, vii

Case 47

Rebecca Stein-Wexler

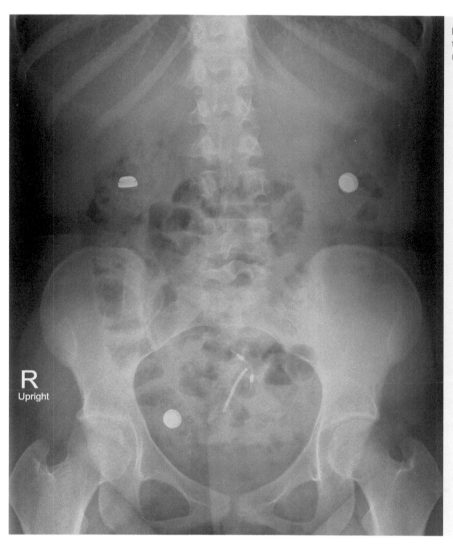

Fig. 47.1 There are three rounded metallic densities that have a bilaminar configuration. There is a fourth metallic density in the pelvis, which has a T shape.

■ Clinical Presentation

A 16-year-old girl with constipation (▶ Fig. 47.1).

■ Key Imaging Finding

Metallic ingested foreign bodies.

■ Top Three Differential Diagnoses

- **Coins.** Coins are by far the most common ingested radiodense foreign body in children, but they are fortunately relatively benign—unless they cause obstruction, remain in the esophagus for more than 24 hours, or persist in the stomach for longer than 28 days. Retention of a large number of pennies in the stomach may mandate removal, since some contain large amounts of zinc. Like other foreign bodies, coins usually lodge in the esophagus—especially at the level of thoracic inlet—or, less commonly, at the pylorus or ileocecal valve.
- **Sharp foreign bodies.** Glass and metallic sharp objects are common ingested foreign bodies. Although radiodense, glass may be too small to recognize on radiographs. Endoscopy is therefore commonly performed if there is a convincing history even if radiographs are normal. Sharp objects retained in the esophagus constitute an emergency due to risk of perforation,

and those that are proximal to the pylorus should be removed as well. Once a sharp object has passed into the small bowel, it should be followed until passage from the gastrointestinal (GI) tract, as perforation may still occur—most often near the ileocecal valve.
- **Disk batteries.** Disk batteries may generate a current, leading to ulceration, fistula formation, and bowel wall perforation. If lodged in the esophagus, damage occurs as quickly as 1 to 2 hours after ingestion, so diagnosis must be made quickly so removal can be prompt. If allowed to remain in the stomach for more than 4 days, they may corrode and release toxic material. Therefore, their position must be followed. The batteries project a double ring when viewed head-on, whereas in profile their beveled edge is readily apparent.

■ Additional Differential Diagnoses

- **Magnets.** Ingestion of multiple magnets is dangerous because they may attract each other across loops of bowel, leading to pressure necrosis and perforation or fistula formation. The risk is greatest with small magnets made of rare earth metals (which may be used in toys). Even without a convincing clinical history, magnet ingestion should be suspected if two or more small metallic objects abut each other.
- **Cylindrical batteries.** Usually AA and AAA, these are less dangerous than disk batteries. However, they can release corrosive

material that may cause perforation, along with poisonous heavy metals such as mercury. If they remain in the stomach for more than 2 days, endoscopic removal is warranted.
- **Lead-containing foreign bodies.** Lead paint dust is the most common cause of lead toxicity in children, but some objects also contain lead. Gastric acid quickly dissolves lead objects, causing lead absorption to start within 90 minutes of ingestion. Distal passage must be confirmed. Symptoms of lead poisoning resemble those of gastroenteritis.

■ Diagnosis

Ingested disk batteries along with an intrauterine contraceptive device.

✓ Pearls

- Sharp foreign objects retained in the esophagus constitute an emergency.
- Magnets may cause pressure necrosis and are suspected if there are two or more adjacent metallic objects.

- Disk batteries lodged in the esophagus for 1 to 2 hours must be endoscopically removed.
- Disk batteries project a double ring en face and a beveled edge in profile.

Suggested Readings

Denney W, Ahmad N, Dillard B, Nowicki MJ. Children will eat the strangest things: a 10-year retrospective analysis of foreign body and caustic ingestions from a single academic center. Pediatr Emerg Care. 2012; 28(8):731–734

Pugmire BS, Lim R, Avery LL. Review of ingested and aspirated foreign bodies in children and their clinical significance for radiologists. Radiographics. 2015; 35(5):1528–1538

Case 50

Cathy Zhou

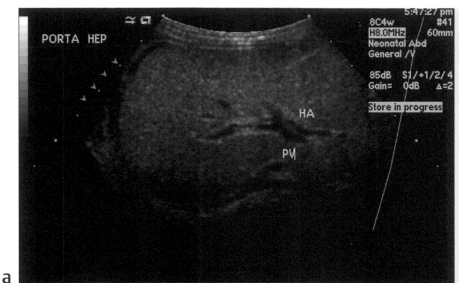

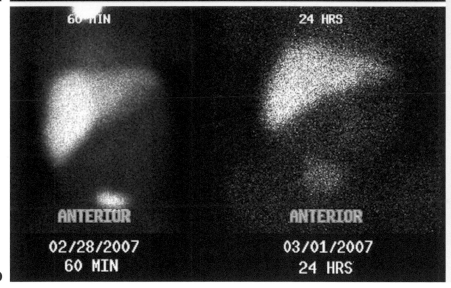

Fig. 50.1 US of the abdomen shows an echogenic liver and thickening of the anterior wall of the right portal vein; neither the common bile duct nor the gallbladder was visualized (a). Hepatobiliary iminodiacetic acid (HIDA) scan images 60 minutes and 24 hours post injection show persistent liver activity and none in the gallbladder or bowel; renal excretion accounts for bladder activity (b).

■ Clinical Presentation

A 19-day-old girl with a history of vomiting, jaundice, and elevated bilirubin (▶Fig. 50.1).

■ Key Clinical Finding

Cholestatic jaundice persisting beyond the first 2 weeks of life.

■ Top Three Differential Diagnoses

- **Biliary atresia.** This is the most common cause of neonatal cholestasis. Inflammation of the biliary tree leads to obliteration of bile ducts, obstruction, and eventual cirrhosis. The right and left hepatic ducts are usually atretic to the level of the porta hepatis, but more proximal or more distal structures may be affected. Syndromic cases, associated with heterotaxy, malrotation, and cardiac or pulmonary malformations, are uncommon and may be diagnosed in utero. Most patients with biliary atresia present at 2 to 4 weeks with cholestatic jaundice, white stools, and dark urine (jaundice in the first week of life is common in normal newborns). US may demonstrate an enlarged, echogenic liver and thickening of the anterior wall of the right portal vein (triangular cord sign). The gallbladder may be absent, malformed, or small and unaffected by oral feeds; more proximal bile ducts are not dilated. There may be cysts in the porta hepatis or—less commonly—the liver. Hepatobiliary iminodiacetic acid (HIDA) scan shows lack of excretion into the bowel at 24 hours. Liver biopsy is required for diagnosis. Definitive treatment is achieved via the Kasai procedure and/or liver transplant.

- **Neonatal hepatitis.** Inflammation of the liver in early infancy is usually idiopathic, with only a small portion of cases attributable to genetic disorders, metabolic causes, or infection. Imaging workup includes US, which may show an enlarged, echogenic liver, and HIDA scan. HIDA scan generally shows delayed uptake of radiotracer from the blood pool, but normal excretion into bowel. However, hepatocellular function may be so greatly impaired that excretion does not occur. Pretreatment with phenobarbital enhances hepatocyte function, facilitating bowel excretion. Treatment is largely supportive, with most cases resolving spontaneously. Neonatal hepatitis is a diagnosis of exclusion.

- **Cystic fibrosis.** This autosomal-recessive disorder results in abnormally folded protein channels and thickened secretions. The disease affects exocrine glands throughout the body, leading predominantly to pulmonary complications and pancreatic insufficiency. Patients may present at birth with meconium ileus or—rarely—with neonatal jaundice due to blockage of the gastrointestinal tract and biliary ducts, respectively. Diagnosis is confirmed with family history, sweat test, and/or genetic testing.

■ Additional Differential Diagnosis

- **Sepsis.** Neonatal sepsis is a leading cause of infant death. Early-onset sepsis results from intrapartum transmission of pathogens, often group B *Streptococcus*. Organ dysfunction may result from hypoxia and hypoperfusion. This may affect the liver, with upregulation of the inflammatory response leading to reduced elimination of toxic compounds and impaired bilirubin metabolism. CT may disclose a source of infection.

■ Diagnosis

Biliary atresia.

✓ Pearls

- Physiological jaundice in the first week of life is common and should improve, but persistent hyperbilirubinemia mandates additional workup.
- Biliary atresia is suggested at US if the gallbladder is absent, small, or abnormal and the common bile duct is not identified; the anterior wall of the right portal vein may be thickened.

- On HIDA scan, biliary atresia usually shows normal uptake of radiotracer and no excretion at 24 hours, whereas with neonatal hepatitis radiotracer uptake is delayed due to impaired hepatocyte function.

Suggested Readings

McKiernan P. Neonatal jaundice. Clin Res Hepatol Gastroenterol. 2012; 36(3):253–256

Nesseler N, Launey Y, Aninat C, Morel F, Mallédant Y, Seguin P. Clinical review: The liver in sepsis. Crit Care. 2012; 16(5):235

Rozel C, Garel L, Rypens F, et al. Imaging of biliary disorders in children. Pediatr Radiol. 2011; 41(2):208–220

Case 51

Rebecca Stein-Wexler

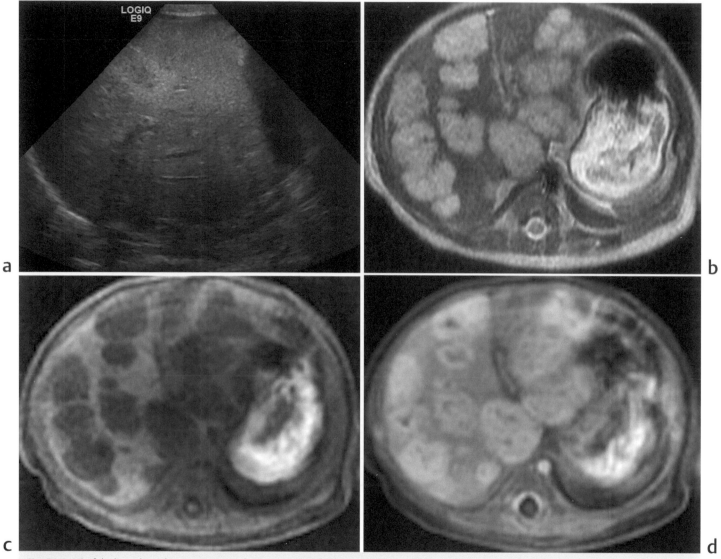

Fig. 51.1 US of the liver shows heterogeneous echotexture and diffuse increased echogenicity with suggestion of small masses (**a**). Axial single-shot fast spin echo (SSFSE) T2-W MRI shows multiple hyperintense, well-defined intrahepatic masses (**b**). These masses are well defined and hypointense on LAVA precontrast T1-W sequence (**c**). Gadolinium-enhanced T1-W arterial phase LAVA image demonstrates intense peripheral enhancement (**d**).

■ Clinical Presentation

A 2-month-old with abdominal distension and shortness of breath (▶ Fig. 51.1).

■ Key Imaging Finding

Multiple hepatic masses.

■ Top Three Differential Diagnoses

- **Infantile hepatic hemangioma (IHH).** This benign tumor consists of fibrous stroma with numerous thin-walled vascular channels. About 90% present by age 6 months, and they gradually involute. When numerous or large, they may cause high-output cardiac failure from vascular shunting. On US, lesions are well circumscribed with lobulated margins, usually hypoechoic and hypervascular. They are often heterogeneous and hypodense to normal liver on CT. Fine or coarse calcifications are common. The lesions are very bright on T2-W MRI. Most enhance, but the pattern varies with lesion size and number—usually initially peripheral and then filling in. Vascular shunting may result in decreased caliber of the infrahepatic aorta.

- **Metastatic disease.** Hepatic metastases—typically neuroblastoma and Wilms tumor in young children—usually result from hematogenous spread. Nodules are usually hypoechoic or (with neuroblastoma) heterogeneous due to hemorrhage and calcification. They often enhance less than hepatic parenchyma at CT/MRI and are typically mildly T2-hyperintense. Urine catecholamines are elevated with metastatic neuroblastoma.
- **Lymphoma.** Secondary hepatic lymphoma typically occurs in the setting of Hodgkin disease with accompanying splenic involvement and para-aortic lymphadenopathy (which is an important diagnostic clue). Lesions are hypoechoic at US and show variable, sometimes peripheral, enhancement at CT and MRI. Primary hepatic lymphoma may also be multifocal.

■ Additional Differential Diagnoses

- **Multifocal hepatoblastoma.** This is the most common pediatric primary liver tumor, usually seen before age 6 years. About 20% of cases have satellite lesions. Vascular invasion is more common with multifocal tumors. Lesions are heterogeneous and enhance less than liver; they may have calcifications. Serum alpha-fetoprotein is elevated. Hepatocellular carcinoma may also be multifocal but is usually seen after age 5 years.
- **Infection.** Pyogenic abscesses—especially *Staphylococcus aureus* and *Entamoeba histolytica*—are the most common infection to cause multiple liver lesions in children, though

candidiasis is common in premature infants and the immunosuppressed. Early on, most lesions are hypoechoic on US and hypodense on CT. On MRI, abscesses are hypointense on T1 and hyperintense on T2, with surrounding edema. In immunocompetent patients, there is peripheral enhancement.
- **Focal nodular hyperplasia.** These hamartomatous lesions are seen with increased frequency in children treated with chemotherapy or abdominal radiation, and in this setting are often multiple. The US appearance is nonspecific. CT/MRI shows a T2-hyperintense central scar with delayed enhancement.

■ Diagnosis

Multifocal infantile hepatic hemangioma.

✓ Pearls

- Infantile hepatic hemangioma usually enhances centripetally and may present with high-output cardiac failure.
- Neuroblastoma and Wilms tumor are the most common pediatric neoplasms to metastasize to the liver.

- Calcifications are seen with infantile hepatic hemangioma, neuroblastoma metastases, and hepatoblastoma.
- Multifocal focal nodular hyperplasia is usually encountered in children who have survived cancer.

Suggested Readings

Duigenan S, Anupindi SA, Nimkin K. Imaging of multifocal hepatic lesions in pediatric patients. Pediatr Radiol. 2012; 42(10):1155–1168, quiz 1285

Hegde SV, Dillman JR, Lopez MJ, Strouse PJ. Imaging of multifocal liver lesions in children and adolescents. Cancer Imaging. 2013; 12:516–529

Case 52

William T. O'Brien, Sr

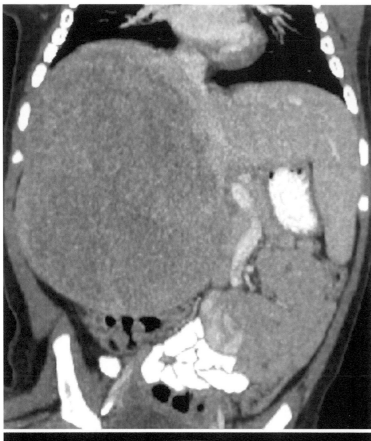

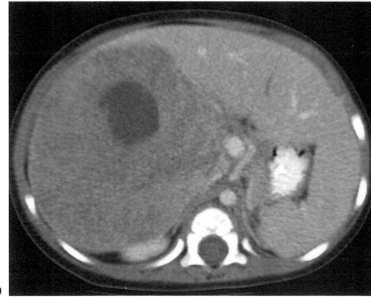

Fig. 52.1 Coronal reformatted contrast-enhanced abdomen CT shows a heterogeneous moderately enhancing mass essentially replacing the right lobe of the liver (**a**). The axial CT demonstrates central hypodensity, either necrosis or a central cyst; note the mass effect on the kidney (**b**).

■ Clinical Presentation

A 3-month-old with hepatomegaly on physical exam (▶ Fig. 52.1).

■ Key Imaging Finding

Liver mass in an infant.

■ Top Three Differential Diagnoses

• **Hepatoblastoma.** Hepatoblastoma is the most common primary hepatic neoplasm in infancy, with the vast majority of cases occurring within the first 3 years of life. Patients usually present with a painless abdominal mass. More than 90% of patients have elevated levels of serum AFP, a useful discriminator. The lesion is typically large, solitary, heterogeneous, and well circumscribed, although it may appear ill defined. The tumor is hypodense on CT, with calcifications in about 50% of cases. The calcifications are "chunky," compared to fine or coarse calcifications of hemangio-endothelioma. Solid elements enhance slightly. On US, hepato-blastoma is heterogeneous and may have calcifications.

• **Hemangioendothelioma.** Hemangioendothelioma is a vascular liver lesion that occurs in neonates, with approximately 90% of cases presenting in the first 6 months of life. The tumor is often large, in which case vascular shunting may cause high-output cardiac failure as well as enlargement of the suprahepatic aorta and decreased caliber of the infrahepatic aorta. The lesion appears heterogeneous and hypodense to surrounding normal liver parenchyma on CT. Fine or coarse calcifications are common. Enhancement is the rule, although the pattern varies depending on lesion size and number.

• **Mesenchymal hamartoma.** Mesenchymal hamartoma is an uncommon, benign hepatic mass that typically presents in infancy. It is usually large, well circumscribed, cystic, and multiloculated. If there are solid components, the tumor resembles hepatoblastoma or hemangioendothelioma.

■ Additional Differential Diagnoses

• **Metastases.** Neuroblastoma metastases typically arise from primary adrenal lesions, although the primary may occur anywhere along the sympathetic chain. Metastatic foci are commonly heterogeneous secondary to hemorrhage and calcification. Metastatic foci from Wilms tumor (less common than from neuroblastoma) are hypodense on CT.

• **Abscess.** A large abscess infrequently mimics a hepatic mass. Liver abscess is hypodense on CT with peripheral enhancement. Abscess results from direct or hematogenous spread.

• **Hematoma.** Hepatic hematomas vary in size and appearance. They are usually hypodense to normal liver parenchyma on CT. Care should be taken to look for areas of active extravasation of contrast. Follow-up imaging will show regression. In addition to abdominal trauma and bleeding disorders, etiology includes malpositioned umbilical venous catheters.

■ Diagnosis

Mesenchymal hamartoma.

✓ Pearls

• Hepatoblastoma is the most common primary hepatic malignancy of infancy and has elevated AFP levels.

• Hemangioendothelioma may be associated with vascular shunting and high-output cardiac failure.

• Mesenchymal hamartoma is usually large, multiloculated, and cystic.

• Neuroblastoma and Wilms tumor are the most common malignancies to metastasize to the liver.

Suggested Readings

Helmberger TK, Ros PR, Mergo PJ, Tomczak R, Reiser MF. Pediatric liver neoplasms: a radiologic-pathologic correlation. Eur Radiol. 1999; 9(7):1339–1347

Keup CP, Ratnaraj F, Chopra PR, Lawrence CA, Lowe LH. Magnetic resonance imaging of the pediatric liver: benign and malignant masses. Magn Reson Imaging Clin N Am. 2013; 21(4):645–667

Woodward PJ, Sohaey R, Kennedy A, Koeller KK. From the archives of the AFIP: a comprehensive review of fetal tumors with pathologic correlation. Radiographics. 2005; 25(1):215–242

Case 53

Rebecca Stein-Wexler

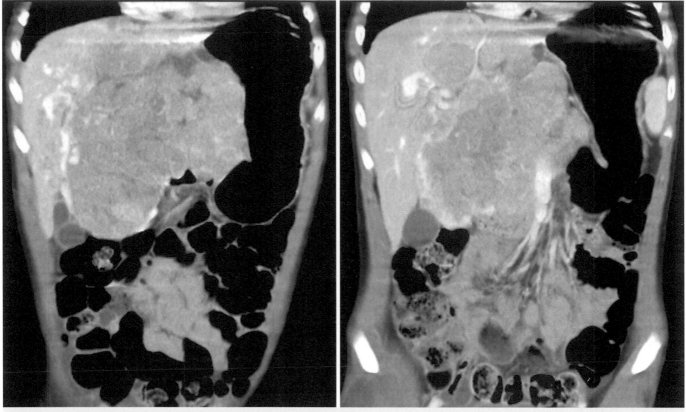

a   b

Fig. 53.1 Coronal reformatted contrast-enhanced CT images show a lobulated, heterogeneous hepatic mass with areas of necrosis and prominent peripheral vascularity **(a,b)**.

■ Clinical Presentation

A 13-year-old boy with anorexia and abdominal pain (▶Fig. 53.1).

■ Key Imaging Finding

Liver mass in an older child.

■ Top Three Differential Diagnoses

- **Metastatic disease.** Liver metastases in children are usually due to Wilms tumor, neuroblastoma, or lymphoma, and infrequently intrahepatic spread of biliary and hepatic primaries. As a rule, metastases are more common than primary liver tumors. Metastases are usually multiple.
- **Hepatocellular carcinoma (HCC).** This is the most common hepatic primary malignancy in teenagers and is more common than hepatoblastoma even in children as young as 6 years old. The serum AFP is usually elevated. Predisposing factors include biliary atresia, familial cholestatic jaundice, glycogen storage disease, and cirrhosis. Imaging resembles HCC in adults. The tumor is heterogeneous and predominantly solid at US. CT and MRI may show necrotic areas. There is intense arterial enhancement and delayed washout. Pediatric HCC is insensitive to chemotherapy, and prognosis is poor.
- **Hepatoblastoma.** Patients with hepatoblastoma are usually younger than 6 years of age and present with a painless mass and weight loss. Serum AFP is elevated in 90% of patients. Hepatoblastoma is typically large, solitary, heterogeneous, and well circumscribed, though it may be ill-defined. Often hemorrhagic and necrotic, it is heterogeneous on US and hypodense on CT, with chunky calcifications in about 50%. Solid elements enhance slightly. On T1- and T2-W sequences, and also after gadolinium, the tumor appears heterogeneous. Invasion of hepatic vessels and inferior vena cava is common, limiting surgical options.

■ Additional Differential Diagnoses

- **Focal nodular hyperplasia (FNH).** This benign hamartomatous tumor contains functioning hepatocytes, does not hemorrhage, has no malignant potential, and is usually discovered incidentally. It may form in utero as an arteriovenous malformation, or in children who have survived childhood cancer. The tumor is isoechoic to liver on US. CT shows intense, early homogeneous enhancement, with rapid washout so most of the tumor resembles liver on delayed imaging. A central scar is seen in 30% of patients, initially hypodense and then filling in. On MRI, FNH looks like liver, though it may be slightly hypointense on T1 and slightly hyperintense on T2. The central scar is bright on T2-W imaging and shows delayed enhancement.
- **Hepatocellular adenoma.** This uncommon tumor composed of hepatocytes and sinusoids occurs in adults and sometimes in teens. Imaging appearance is usually nonspecific, but dual gradient echo imaging may show signal drop-off due to intracellular lipid. It is often resected due to risk of hemorrhage.
- **Fibrolamellar carcinoma.** This rare, painful tumor occurs in adolescents without prior liver disease. Collagen and fibrosis form a central scar that may calcify and is dark on both T1 and T2. The scar does not enhance (unlike with FNH). Calcifications are present in 40% of patients. Prognosis is better than with HCC.

■ Diagnosis

Hepatocellular carcinoma.

✓ Pearls

- Hepatocellular carcinoma is the most common hepatic primary malignancy in teenagers and resembles hepatocellular carcinoma in adults.
- Wilms tumor, neuroblastoma, and lymphoma most often metastasize to the liver.
- Fibrolamellar carcinoma has a central scar that may calcify; its prognosis is better than hepatocellular carcinoma.

Suggested Readings

Keup CP, Ratnaraj F, Chopra PR, Lawrence CA, Lowe LH. Magnetic resonance imaging of the pediatric liver: benign and malignant masses. Magn Reson Imaging Clin N Am. 2013; 21(4):645–667

Rasalkar DD, Chu WC, Cheng FW, Hui SK, Ling SC, Li CK. A pictorial review of imaging of abdominal tumours in adolescence. Pediatr Radiol. 2010; 40(9):1552–1561, quiz 1589–1590

Tran VT, Vasanawala S. Pediatric hepatobiliary magnetic resonance imaging. Radiol Clin North Am. 2013; 51(4):599–614

Case 54

Rebecca Stein-Wexler

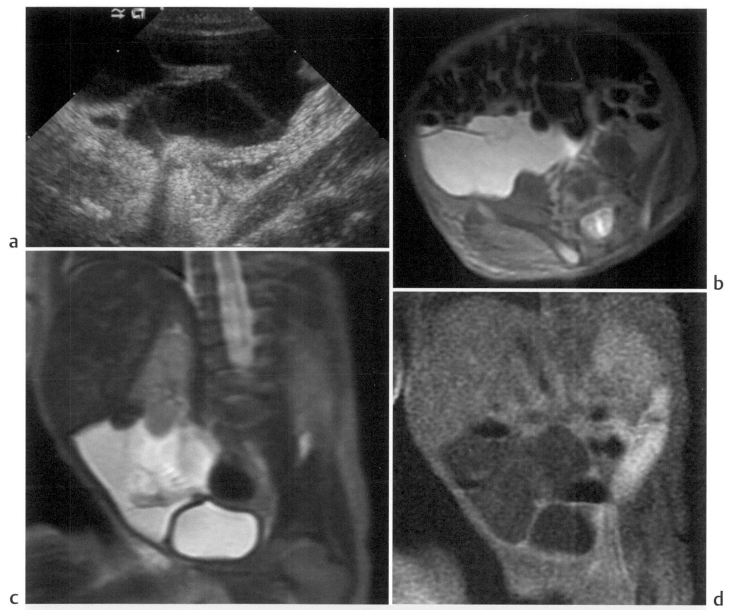

a

b

c

d

Fig. 54.1 US of the right lower quadrant shows a multiseptated cystic lesion with low-level echogenic debris (**a**). Axial fast imaging employing steady-state acquisition (FIESTA) MRI confirms the cystic nature of the lesion (**b**). Coronal single-shot fast spin echo (SSFSE) image shows the mass fills the right lower quadrant (**c**). Coronal gadolinium-enhanced T1-W fat-suppressed image shows that the septa enhance, but the fluid areas do not (**d**).

■ **Clinical Presentation**

An 8-year-old girl with abdominal pain and jaundice (▶Fig. 54.1).

■ Key Imaging Finding

Right abdominal cystic mass.

■ Top Three Differential Diagnoses

- **Ovarian cyst.** Functional cysts and cystic neoplasms (especially benign cystic teratomas) account for about three-fourths of ovarian masses. When large, these lesions may extend from the pelvis to the liver. Girls typically complain of insidious abdominal pain and distension, though if the cyst has undergone torsion, pain may be acute.
- **Choledochal cyst.** This congenital cystic malformation of the intra- and/or extrahepatic biliary tree usually presents by age 10 years. Only one-fourth of patients have the classic triad of intermittent abdominal pain, right upper quadrant (RUQ) mass, and jaundice. Diagnosis rests on identifying a cystic RUQ mass that is distinct from the gallbladder and that has bile duct(s) leading to or from it. US and MR cholangiopancreatography (MRCP) are optimal for diagnosing the specific type of lesion (the Todani classification has more than five). Radionuclide imaging is also useful to confirm biliary origin. Risks of ascending cholangitis, calculi, and malignancy mandate resection.
- **Pancreatic pseudocyst.** Pseudocyst accounts for 75% of cystic lesions of the pancreas in children. It usually results from traumatic pancreatic injury and subsequent leakage of fluid that is then contained by a fibrous capsule. This well-circumscribed, unilocular, thin-walled cystic mass is usually located near the body or tail of the pancreas, but it can be found anywhere. Septations and debris suggest hemorrhage or infection. Pancreatic pseudocyst is usually anechoic on US and near water attenuation on CT. Congenital pancreatic cysts are rare.

■ Additional Differential Diagnoses

- **Gallbladder hydrops.** This probably results from transient cystic duct obstruction or inefficient emptying. It is associated with respiratory infections, gastroenteritis, and Kawasaki syndrome. The gallbladder appears massively distended without wall thickening, pericholecystic fluid, calculi, or dilated bile ducts.
- **Mesenteric cyst.** Mesenteric cysts are part of a spectrum with lymphatic malformations and omental cysts. One-third are diagnosed in children younger than 15 years, who may present with pain, mass, vomiting, or fever. The lesions occur in small or large bowel mesentery and may be massive (up to 40 cm).

If complicated by hemorrhage or infection, the normally anechoic fluid becomes complex, and there may be calcifications and septations. MRI allows optimal delineation of lesion extent.
- **Duplication cyst.** Bowel duplication cysts most often involve the distal ileum, but other areas may be affected. Patients present with a mass, obstruction, or—in the 20% in whom gastric mucosa is present—hemorrhage. Cysts are usually spherical or tubular and adjacent to bowel, sometimes communicating with it. There may be intraluminal debris. CT/MRI show mild mural enhancement.

■ Diagnosis

Mesenteric cyst.

✓ Pearls

- Large ovarian cysts may extend into the upper abdomen.
- Diagnosis of choledochal cyst depends on identifying bile ducts leading to or from a cyst that is separate from the gallbladder.
- Most pancreatic pseudocysts in children result from trauma.

Suggested Readings

Ranganath SH, Lee EY, Eisenberg RL. Focal cystic abdominal masses in pediatric patients. AJR Am J Roentgenol. 2012; 199(1):W1–W16

Rao P. Neonatal gastrointestinal imaging. Eur J Radiol. 2006; 60(2):171–186

Wootton-Gorges SL, Thomas KB, Harned RK, Wu SR, Stein-Wexler R, Strain JD. Giant cystic abdominal masses in children. Pediatr Radiol. 2005; 35(12):1277–1288

Case 55

Rebecca Stein-Wexler

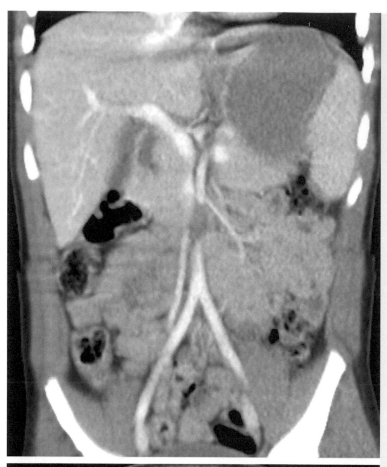

a

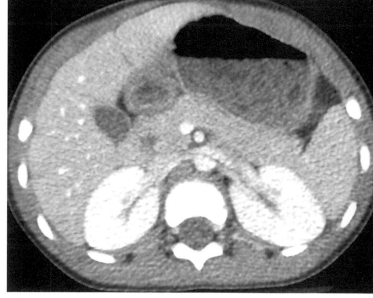

b

Fig. 55.1 Coronal reformatted contrast-enhanced CT shows soft-tissue density lateral to the hypodense lumen of the second portion of the duodenum; part of the normal gallbladder drapes over the lateral margin on the soft-tissue mass **(a)**. Axial image shows a soft-tissue mass in continuity with the pancreas, surrounding the duodenal lumen **(b)**.

■ Clinical Presentation

A 3-year-old boy with abdominal pain (►Fig. 55.1).

■ Key Imaging Finding

Pancreatic head mass.

■ Top Three Differential Diagnoses

- **Pancreatitis.** The most common cause of pancreatitis in children is trauma due to nonaccidental injury, bicycle handlebar accidents, and automobile accidents. Infection and systemic disease are less common. The gland may show focal or diffuse enlargement. US appearance varies considerably. CT shows ill-defined margins, adjacent fluid, and—if there is necrosis—focal hypodensity and lack of enhancement.
- **Annular pancreas.** Fifty percent of patients with annular pancreas present as newborns with duodenal obstruction, the others presenting later with pain/obstruction. Most newborns with annular pancreas have other congenital anomalies as well, such as duodenal stenosis/atresia, trisomy 21, tracheoesophageal fistula, and heart disease. Imaging shows soft tissue partly or completely surrounding the duodenum, in continuity with the

pancreatic head. Circumferential narrowing of the second portion of the duodenum is seen on upper gastrointestinal tract.
- **Solid pseudopapillary tumor.** This nonendocrine pancreatic tumor is most common in the pancreatic head. It usually presents as a palpable, sometimes painful mass in teenage girls and young women. Usually larger than 5 cm, it appears solid and well defined, but may be partly cystic if necrotic. Unlike other pancreatic masses, this tumor is often hemorrhagic. A hypointense capsule or rim of residual pancreatic tissue may be seen on T1-W MRI, and the central signal intensity varies considerably depending on the presence of hemorrhage and necrosis. Metastases in children are uncommon, and prognosis is relatively good.

■ Additional Differential Diagnoses

- **Lymphoma.** Non-Hodgkin lymphoma—especially Burkitt—is the most common tumor to metastasize to the pancreas, but even that is rare. The most likely location for a single metastatic focus is the pancreatic head.
- **Pancreatoblastoma.** This is the most common exocrine pancreatic tumor in children. Mean age at presentation is 4 years, and the tumor is more common in boys. Children usually present with a large abdominal mass. Serum AFP is often increased, and the tumor may also secrete adrenocorticotropic hormone. The mass appears large, solid, and well defined, with variable calcification. Although the tumor may occur in

the pancreatic head, it more often protrudes into the lesser sac. It tends to encase arteries and invade veins. Metastases often involve the liver and are noted at presentation in one-third of patients.
- **Islet cell neoplasms.** Functioning endocrine tumors, such as insulinoma and gastrinoma, are often quite small, coming to medical attention because of symptoms due to hormonal hypersecretion. Gastrinomas are more likely to be in the pancreatic head, whereas insulinomas favor the body and tail. Pancreatic endocrine tumors are associated with multiple endocrine neoplasia and with von Hippel–Lindau syndrome.

■ Diagnosis

Annular pancreas.

✓ Pearls

- Pancreatitis in children usually results from direct trauma and may be seen with child abuse.
- Annular pancreas appears as soft tissue surrounding the duodenum, continuous with the pancreas.
- Solid pseudopapillary tumor occurs in teenage girls and is most common in the pancreatic head.
- Pancreatoblastoma is most common in young boys; it may cause elevated AFP.

Suggested Readings

Alexander LF. Congenital pancreatic anomalies, variants, and conditions. Radiol Clin North Am. 2012; 50(3):487–498

Nijs E, Callahan MJ, Taylor GA. Disorders of the pediatric pancreas: imaging features. Pediatr Radiol. 2005; 35(4):358–373, quiz 457

Shet NS, Cole BL, Iyer RS. Imaging of pediatric pancreatic neoplasms with radiologic-histopathologic correlation. AJR Am J Roentgenol. 2014; 202(6):1337–1348

Case 56

Rebecca Stein-Wexler

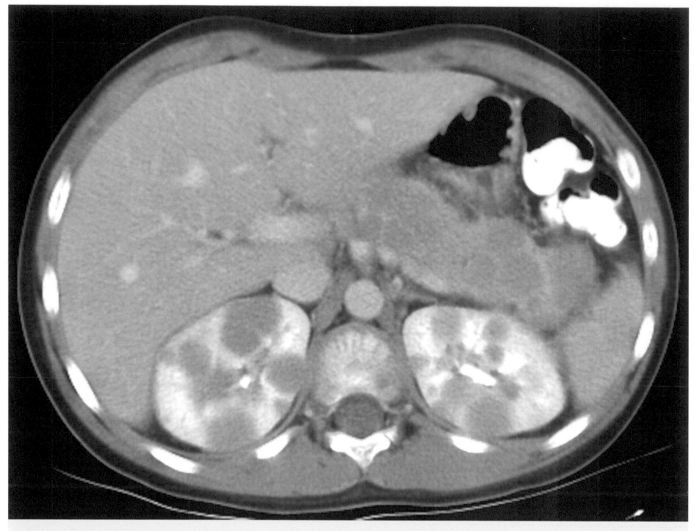

Fig. 56.1 Axial contrast-enhanced CT shows multiple hypodense masses in the pancreas, as well as in the kidneys.

■ Clinical Presentation

A 16-year-old boy with abdominal pain (▶ Fig. 56.1).

■ Key Imaging Finding

Multiple pancreatic hypodensities.

■ Top Three Differential Diagnoses

- **Lymphoma.** The most common nonepithelial pancreatic tumor in children is lymphoma, but even this is relatively rare. Cell type is usually non-Hodgkin lymphoma, either large cell or Burkitt lymphoma. Primary pancreatic lymphoma is even less common. Imaging may show a single hypodense mass, multiple masses, or diffuse enlargement of the gland.
- **Autosomal-dominant polycystic kidney disease (ADPKD).** This common inherited disease usually presents in adults, with diagnosis in childhood usually serendipitous. If even one renal cyst is seen in a genetically predisposed child, ADPKD is likely; the presence of three cysts establishes the diagnosis. ADPKD is characterized by normal to slightly enlarged kidneys with multiple round cysts that are found throughout the nephron. Cysts may also develop in the pancreas, as well as in the liver, spleen, and seminal vesicles. Brain aneurysms occur in about 10%.
- **von Hippel–Lindau disease.** Non-neoplastic, epithelial-lined pancreatic cysts may develop in up to about 50% of patients with this autosomal-dominant disorder. Pancreatic cysts may be the only abdominal manifestation of the disease, and the cysts may be single or multiple. Von Hippel–Lindau disease is also characterized by CNS hemangioblastomas, retinal angiomas, pheochromocytomas, renal cysts and tumors, and pancreatic endocrine and other neoplasms.

■ Additional Differential Diagnoses

- **Metastases.** Neuroblastoma may metastasize to the pancreas, and contiguous spread may also occur. Autopsy findings report alveolar rhabdomyosarcoma metastasizes to the pancreas in about two-thirds of cases. Synovial sarcoma may also be considered.
- **Pancreatitis.** The most common cause of pancreatitis in children is trauma due to nonaccidental injury, bicycle handlebar accidents, and automobile accidents. Anomalies, systemic disease, and toxins are less common causes. Focal pancreatitis may result in multiple lesions. US appearance varies considerably. The lesions are ill-defined on CT, and there may be adjacent fluid. If there is necrosis, lesions will be hypodense and not enhance.

■ Diagnosis

Burkitt lymphoma.

✓ Pearls

- Pancreatic lymphoma is usually secondary and due to either large cell or Burkitt lymphoma.
- Multiple pancreatic cysts may be the only abdominal manifestation of von Hippel–Lindau syndrome.
- Neuroblastoma and various sarcomas may metastasize to the pancreas.

Suggested Readings

Alexander LF. Congenital pancreatic anomalies, variants, and conditions. Radiol Clin North Am. 2012; 50(3):487–498

Nijs E, Callahan MJ, Taylor GA. Disorders of the pediatric pancreas: imaging features. Pediatr Radiol. 2005; 35(4):358–373, quiz 457

Shet NS, Cole BL, Iyer RS. Imaging of pediatric pancreatic neoplasms with radiologic-histopathologic correlation. AJR Am J Roentgenol. 2014; 202(6):1337–1348

Case 59

Cathy Zhou

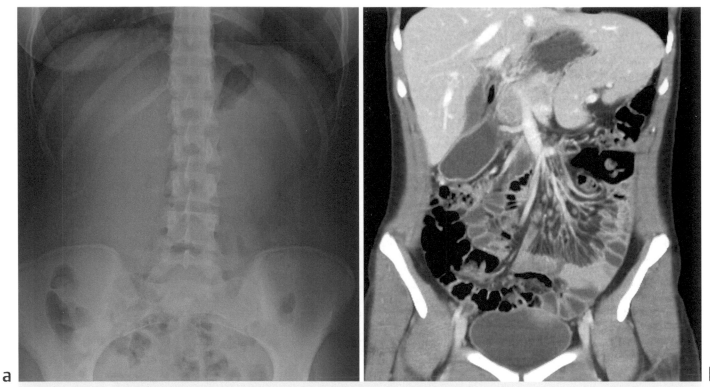

a b

Fig. 59.1 The gastric bubble is displaced medially by a soft-tissue mass **(a)**. Coronal reformatted contrast-enhanced CT shows the spleen positioned relatively medially in the left upper quadrant; the orientation of the splenic hilum is abnormal, facing inferolaterally **(b)**.

■ Clinical Presentation

A 15-year-old girl status post motor vehicle crash (▶Fig. 59.1).

■ Key Imaging Finding

Splenic ectopy.

■ Top Three Differential Diagnoses

• **Wandering spleen.** In children, wandering spleen usually results from absence or elongation of one or more splenic suspensory ligaments. It is more common in patients with prune-belly syndrome, renal agenesis, gastric volvulus, diaphragmatic eventration, and other congenital abnormalities. The spleen migrates from its normal position to anywhere in the pelvis or abdomen. Patients younger than 1 year of age usually present with an abdominal mass, whereas older children more often have abdominal pain due to torsion (discussed later). Fifteen percent of cases are diagnosed incidentally. Physical examination usually reveals a palpable mass. Chronic hypersplenism occasionally leads to pancytopenia. Abdomen radiographs may show absence of the normal splenic shadow and mass effect elsewhere, but cross-sectional imaging is usually needed for diagnosis. US shows no spleen in the splenic fossa. Instead, elsewhere in the abdomen there is a spleenlike mass with a central vascular hilum. Blood flow is intact. CT and MRI show similar findings. Treatment is splenopexy.

• **Splenic torsion.** Splenic torsion develops in over half of children with wandering spleen. Torsion may be intermittent, and abdominal pain may therefore be acute, chronic, or episodic. Prolonged torsion leads to splenomegaly, pancytopenia, and ultimately infarction. Splenic torsion may be diagnosed with US. The ectopic spleen tends to be relatively large, perhaps due to chronic, recurrent torsion and venous congestion. In

the absence of infarction, parenchyma should appear homogeneous. There may be adjacent fluid. Doppler shows absent blood flow, and the vascular pedicle may appear torsed. CT may show the highly specific "whorl" sign, representing the twisted vascular pedicle alternating with fat and ectopic pancreatic tissue. MRI is also diagnostic. Treatment is detorsion with splenopexy or splenectomy if the spleen cannot be saved.

• **Splenic infarction.** If torsion persists, splenic infarction may develop, with global interruption of blood supply. Patients present with an acute abdomen. Prolonged venous occlusion leads to localized peritonitis, venous thrombosis, and hypersplenism. If there is arterial occlusion, hemorrhagic infarction, subcapsular and intrasplenic hemorrhage, gangrene, fibrosis, and functional asplenia may follow. Doppler US demonstrates absent blood flow in the parenchyma, with elevated resistive index in the proximal splenic artery. Parenchymal echogenicity is inhomogeneous. Similar findings are seen at CT, with the addition of the whorl sign. Of course, splenic infarction also occurs in the absence of splenic ectopy. In that case, infarction may be segmental or global, predominantly due to hematologic abnormalities, thromboembolic events, trauma, infection, and pancreatitis. Both US and CT are diagnostic, revealing classic wedge-shaped peripheral or global hypoechoic/hypoenhancing defects.

■ Diagnosis

Wandering spleen.

✓ Pearls

• Infants with wandering spleen usually present with an abdominal mass, whereas older children present with abdominal pain.
• The wandering spleen may be found anywhere in the abdomen.

• The CT "whorl sign" is specific for splenic torsion.
• Splenic parenchyma appears heterogeneous if torsion has progressed to infarction.

Suggested Readings

Ayaz UY, Dilli A, Ayaz S, Api A. Wandering spleen in a child with symptoms of acute abdomen: ultrasonographic diagnosis. Case report. Med Ultrason. 2012; 14(1):64–66

Brown CV, Virgilio GR, Vazquez WD. Wandering spleen and its complications in children: a case series and review of the literature. J Pediatr Surg. 2003; 38(11):1676–1679

Lombardi R, Menchini L, Corneli T, et al. Wandering spleen in children: a report of 3 cases and a brief literature review underlining the importance of diagnostic imaging. Pediatr Radiol. 2014; 44(3):279–288

Case 62

Rebecca Stein-Wexler

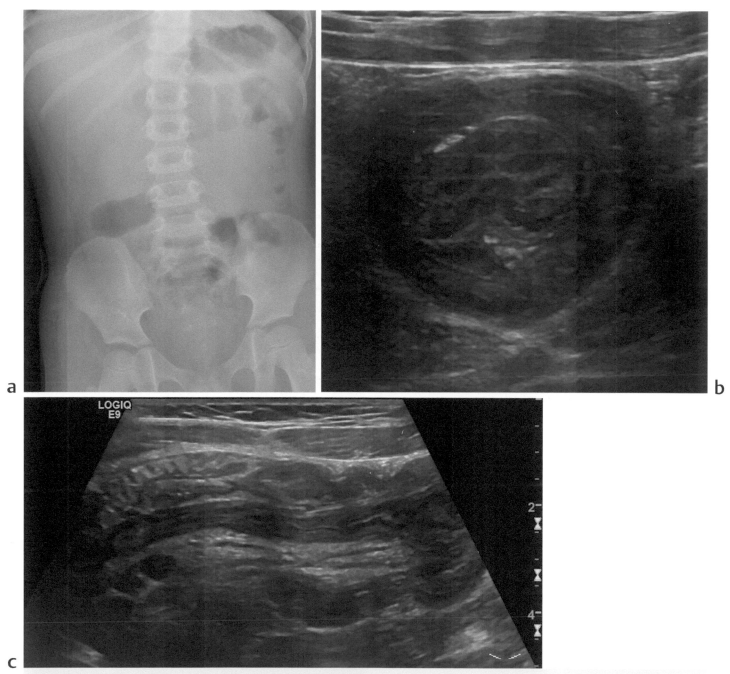

Fig. 62.1 Supine radiograph shows a few dilated bowel loops with suggestion of a rounded soft-tissue density in the right mid abdomen and with no rectal gas (a). Abdominal US shows a donut-type appearance of bowel, with multiple echogenic and hypoechoic layers (b). Longitudinal image of this area shows a layered, pseudokidney appearance of telescoping thick-walled bowel loops, along with a small amount of interloop and free fluid (c).

■ Clinical Presentation

A 3-year-old child with colicky abdominal pain (▶Fig. 62.1).

■ Key Imaging Finding

Telescoping bowel.

■ Diagnosis

Ileocolic intussusception. Ileocolic intussusception is a radiographic and surgical emergency that occurs when small bowel telescopes into large bowel, causing obstruction and, if allowed to progress, bowel ischemia. It is usually "idiopathic" (caused by hyperplastic distal ileal lymphoid tissue) and most common between the ages of 3 and 24 months. The presence of a pathologic lead point, such as bowel duplication, Meckel diverticulum, polyp, cystic fibrosis, Henoch–Schönlein purpura, or lymphoma, is more likely in children outside this age range.

The classic triad of episodic colicky abdominal pain, currant jelly stool, and a palpable abdominal mass is rarely present. Symptoms vary from vomiting, diarrhea, rectal bleeding, listlessness, and irritability to cardiovascular collapse. US allows highly accurate diagnosis of this common disorder. When intussusception is viewed transversely, there is a target appearance of layered bowel loops (the intussusceptum telescopes into the receiving intussuscipiens). Viewed longitudinally, a more reniform appearance is evident. Although ileocolic intussusception begins in the ileocecal region, the bowel may telescope as far as the rectum, and therefore evaluation of the entire abdomen is essential. Free fluid, interloop fluid, bowel wall thickening and vascularity, and obstruction should be assessed. Radiographs may demonstrate bowel obstruction or a soft-tissue mass at the site of intussusception but are sometimes normal and do not exclude the diagnosis.

There are four different kinds of intussusception. Small bowel–small bowel intussusception is very common and resolves if there is no lead point—and sometimes even if there is. It is recognized on US or CT as a short segment and narrow diameter intussusception; follow-up US confirms resolution. Ileocolic intussusception accounts for most clinically significant intussusceptions. Ileoileocolic intussusception occurs when small bowel telescopes into small bowel and the entire mass also prolapses inside large bowel. This form of intussusception is relatively difficult to reduce with enema, often needing surgical reduction. Finally, colocolic intussusception is an unusual intussusception, usually associated with a pathologic lead point.

Ileocolic and ileoileocolic intussusception are first treated with enema reduction, usually with fluoroscopic guidance in the United States, but US monitoring may be used. Liquid or air reduction may be performed. Air has the advantages that perforations are smaller, radiation exposure is less, the process is less messy, and reduction may be more successful. With air reduction, the maximum pressure is 120 mm Hg, and a needle must be available to release the rare complication of tension pneumoperitoneum. The "rule of three" applies to liquid reduction: no more than three attempts of 3 minutes each with the contrast material 3 feet above the patient. However, this rule was developed for barium, and if iodinated contrast is employed the height of 5 feet yields similar pressure. Many modify this rule of three to apply to air reduction, limiting the number of attempts to three to and the duration of each (with the intussuscipiens not moving) to 3 minutes. Failed reduction results in surgery.

✓ Pearls

- Presentation of intussusception is highly variable and radiographs may be normal, but US provides a sensitive and specific means of diagnosis.
- On transverse US, intussusception shows a target or donut sign of multiple telescoped bowel loops; longitudinal views show a reniform (pseudokidney) appearance.
- Air reduction employs less radiation, results in smaller perforations, and may be more successful than liquid.

Suggested Readings

Daneman A, Navarro O. Intussusception. Part 1: a review of diagnostic approaches. Pediatr Radiol. 2003; 33(2):79–85

Daneman A, Navarro O. Intussusception. Part 2: an update on the evolution of management. Pediatr Radiol. 2004; 34(2):97–108, quiz 187

Lioubashevsky N, Hiller N, Rozovsky K, Segev L, Simanovsky N. Ileocolic versus small-bowel intussusception in children: can US enable reliable differentiation? Radiology. 2013; 269(1):266–271

Case 63

Rebecca Stein-Wexler

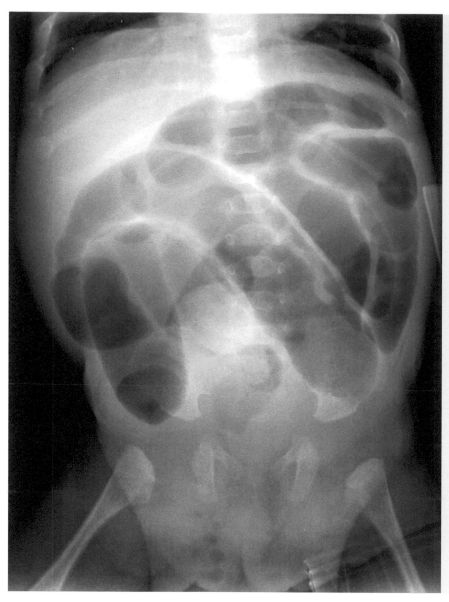

Fig. 63.1 Supine radiograph shows dilated bowel loops filling the abdomen. There are also several small foci of gas in the right scrotum. Both inguinal folds are bulging.

■ Clinical Presentation

Premature boy with distended abdomen (▶Fig. 63.1).

■ Key Imaging Finding

Dilated bowel loops along with scrotal gas.

■ Diagnosis

Incarcerated inguinal hernia causing bowel obstruction.
Inguinal hernias are very common in newborns and especially common in premature infants. They are much more common in boys than in girls. Most hernias are diagnosed clinically as an asymptomatic bulge in the groin, scrotum, or labia. The hernia is more obvious with Valsalva maneuvers, such as crying.

Inguinal hernias are almost always indirect, and they form if the normal processus vaginalis fails to close. In normal boys, between gestational weeks 25 and 35, the testes descend from the retroperitoneum through the inguinal canal. They bring peritoneum with them, forming the processus vaginalis, which is an outpouching of the peritoneum that extends to the scrotum or labium majora. In most newborn boys, the processus vaginalis is patent, but it is normally obliterated by age 2 years, becoming the tunica vaginalis. If the processus vaginalis is patent, fluid, omentum, and bowel may enter the scrotum. Hernias are more common on the right, because the right testicle descends later than the left.

Inguinal hernias develop differently in girls. In girls, the patent processus vaginalis usually obliterates at 8 months of gestation. It may fail to do so and then persist as a peritoneal outpouching adjacent to the round ligament, termed the "diverticulum of Nuck." Inguinal hernias in girls are usually bilateral, and in the preschool age group about 20% contain an ovary.

If the processus vaginalis is narrow, only fluid will traverse the hernia, resulting in a communicating hydrocele. If it is widely patent, bowel and omentum may extend into the scrotum or labia. Inguinal hernias are often diagnosed by physical examination, but US is useful in difficult or equivocal cases. It is also helpful for identifying bowel within the hernia and assessing its vascularity and reducibility. These factors help determine whether bowel is incarcerated or strangulated. Gas in the scrotum, peristalsis, and/or "gut signature" in the scrotum or inguinal canal indicate the presence of bowel within the hernia. Hydroceles that communicate with the abdominal cavity are considered to be hernias.

It is difficult to predict which hernias will lead to bowel incarceration/strangulation and gonadal infarction, and therefore essentially all pediatric inguinal hernias are surgically repaired. Delayed repair is associated with increased risk of these complications. However, surgical risks are also high in preterm infants, many of whom have—and may outgrow—inguinal hernias. The approach to timing of surgical repair therefore varies. A small percentage of patients will eventually develop a contralateral hernia, and opinions differ about the need for routine exploration.

✓ Pearls

- Inguinal hernias are common in boys younger than 2 years and extremely common in premature infants.
- Inguinal hernias usually occur on the right in boys and are usually bilateral in girls.
- US helps assess whether the hernia contains bowel and whether strangulation is present.

Suggested Readings

Basta AM, Courtier J, Phelps A, Copp HL, MacKenzie JD. Scrotal swelling in the neonate. J Ultrasound Med. 2015; 34(3):495–505

Cascini V, Lisi G, Di Renzo D, Pappalepore N, Lelli Chiesa P. Irreducible indirect inguinal hernia containing uterus and bilateral adnexa in a premature female infant: report of an exceptional case and review of the literature. J Pediatr Surg. 2013; 48(1):e17–e19

Graf JL, Caty MG, Martin DJ, Glick PL. Pediatric hernias. Semin Ultrasound CT MR. 2002; 23(2):197–200

Wang KS; Committee on Fetus and Newborn, American Academy of Pediatrics. Section on Surgery, American Academy of Pediatrics. Assessment and management of inguinal hernia in infants. Pediatrics. 2012; 130(4):768–773

Case 64

Rebecca Stein-Wexler

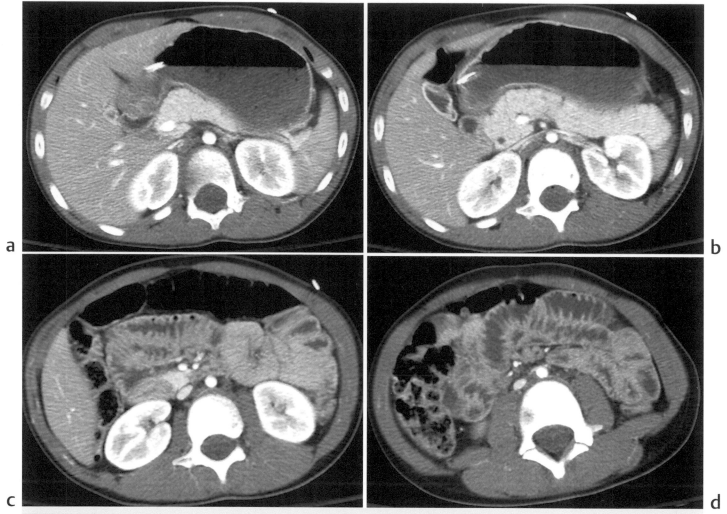

Fig. 64.1 Axial contrast-enhanced CT shows hyperintense adrenal glands, pancreas, and kidneys. The aorta and inferior vena cava are relatively small. Bowel is mildly dilated, and its wall enhances intensely **(a–d)**.

■ Clinical Presentation

A 12-year-old after a motor vehicle accident (▶ Fig. 64.1).

■ Key Imaging Finding

Intense enhancement of adrenals, pancreas, kidneys, and bowel wall with small caliber great vessels.

■ Diagnosis

Hypoperfusion complex. Hypoperfusion complex usually occurs with severe blunt trauma, often in patients with significant neurologic impairment from intracranial injury. It develops in badly injured children who are in a state of hypovolemic shock. The condition may be diagnosed on abdomen CT of patients who appeared stable after receiving fluid resuscitation for arterial hypotension, but in whom the administered fluid temporarily masks underlying hypotension. These children are at extremely high risk for rapid and unpredictable hemodynamic decompensation. Twenty percent may develop hypotension while still in the CT suite.

This condition develops when vessels supplying skin, viscera, and muscles progressively constrict in order to preserve blood flow to the brain, heart, and kidneys. In addition, administered intravenous contrast is more concentrated than usual since the intravascular volume is relatively small. These patients are usually on the brink of collapse, and the mortality rate may approach 50%. It is very important to correctly diagnose this constellation of findings so that clinical care is directed toward rapid resuscitation.

Typical CT findings include fluid-filled bowel and intense enhancement of the bowel wall, aorta, and inferior vena cava.

Both the aorta and the inferior vena cava are small. The aorta is considered narrow when its anteroposterior diameter is less than 6 mm 1 cm below the origin of the superior mesenteric artery. The inferior vena cava is considered narrow if it is flattened over the course of at least 3 cm. The kidneys are typically hyperdense, but infrequently in severe cases there may be no renal enhancement at all (the "black kidney"). Periportal edema may be seen, along with intense enhancement of the pancreas, adrenals, and mesentery. However, sometimes the pancreas and spleen show decreased enhancement. Fluid may be present in the abdomen and retroperitoneum and bowel wall thickened.

Bowel wall thickening that occurs in hypoperfusion complex may be mistaken for traumatic bowel wall injury. However, with hypoperfusion complex the thickening is diffuse and the intestines are dilated. Furthermore, only the small bowel is usually involved. In addition, the aforementioned ancillary findings will be present. Missed bowel wall injury and a variety of other processes may lead to diffuse bowel wall thickening and enhancement, but again the presence or absence of ancillary findings of hypoperfusion complex should allow differentiation.

✓ Pearls

- Patients with hypoperfusion complex may decompensate suddenly if fluid resuscitation has temporarily masked severe underlying hemodynamic decompensation.
- Classic findings are dilated bowel with intense enhancement of bowel wall, aorta, and inferior vena cava as well as narrow caliber aorta and inferior vena cava.

- Pancreas, adrenals, and mesentery may enhance intensely, and kidneys are often hyperdense as well.
- Hypoperfusion complex involves bowel diffusely, whereas with bowel wall injury usually only a limited area is affected.

Suggested Readings

Sheybani EF, Gonzalez-Araiza G, Kousari YM, Hulett RL, Menias CO. Pediatric non-accidental abdominal trauma: what the radiologist should know. Radiographics. 2014; 34(1):139–153

Sivit CJ. Imaging children with abdominal trauma. AJR Am J Roentgenol. 2009; 192(5):1179–1189

Strouse PJ, Close BJ, Marshall KW, Cywes R. CT of bowel and mesenteric trauma in children. Radiographics. 1999; 19(5):1237–1250

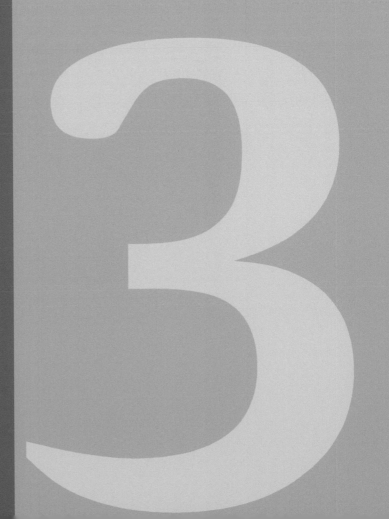

Part 3

Genitourinary Imaging

Case 65

Shruthi Ram

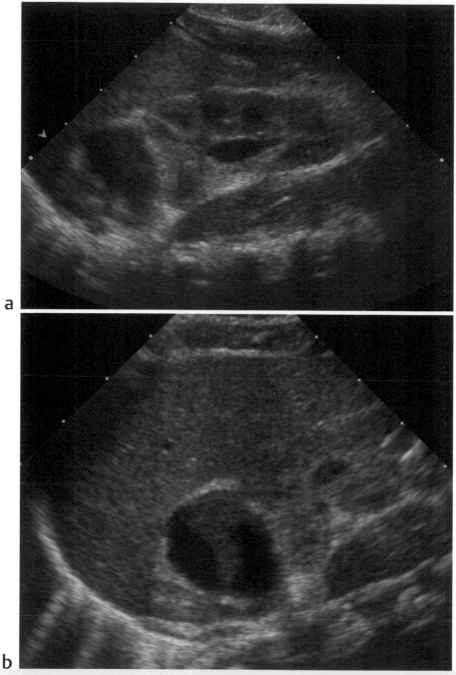

Fig. 65.1 Longitudinal US of the right upper quadrant shows a complex hypoechoic suprarenal mass **(a)**. Transverse image shows the lesion is predominantly anechoic **(b)**. Color flow images (not shown) demonstrated no internal vascularity.

■ Clinical Presentation

Newborn baby with anemia (▶Fig. 65.1).

■ Key Imaging Finding

Suprarenal mass in a newborn.

■ Top Three Differential Diagnoses

- **Adrenal hemorrhage.** Difficult labor, hypoxia, septicemia, and hemorrhagic disorders may cause a normal adrenal to hemorrhage in the perinatal period. Clinical manifestations include a palpable mass, anemia, jaundice, hypovolemic shock, and eventual adrenal insufficiency, but adrenal hemorrhage is occasionally diagnosed incidentally on renal US. It is more common on the right. The normal neonatal adrenal gland is relatively large and readily imaged by US, where it appears Y- or V-shaped with layers of hypoechoic cortex and thin echogenic medulla. With acute adrenal hemorrhage, the normal adrenal is replaced by a complex echogenic mass. As the hematoma evolves, the central portion becomes more hypoechoic and then completely cystic before eventual involution and subsequent calcification. This dynamic pattern of progressively decreasing echogenicity helps differentiate hemorrhage from other adrenal lesions.
- **Neuroblastoma (NB).** NB derives from sympathetic ganglion cells of the neural crest and is the most common malignancy of infancy. In newborns, the origin is usually adrenal. On US, NB typically appears solid, heterogenous, and predominantly hyperechoic. Calcifications are common, contributing to diffuse increased echogenicity. Infrequently, the tumor appears cystic. NB shares imaging features with adrenal hemorrhage. On serial imaging, both lesions may decrease in size, since neonatal NB may involute. However, NB becomes more complex in appearance, whereas adrenal hemorrhage becomes more cystic. Neonatal NB may be widely metastatic but has an excellent prognosis that is not affected by the delay entailed by limited follow-up imaging. CT and MRI are useful for staging purposes. Urine catecholamines are often normal in neonatal NB, though elevated in older children with NB.
- **Intra-abdominal extralobar sequestration.** Extralobar sequestration may occasionally be found in the abdomen, usually above the left kidney. Like extralobar sequestration elsewhere, it consists of nonfunctional bronchopulmonary tissue that is separate from the tracheobronchial tree and that has its own systemic arterial blood supply arising from the aorta, as well as venous drainage into the systemic system. The diagnosis of intra-abdominal extralobar sequestration is typically made on prenatal US as early as 16 weeks' gestation. Characteristic imaging features include a solid, well-defined, triangular echogenic mass, usually just below the left diaphragm. It may have small cysts. The normal adrenal gland is visualized separate from the sequestration. Vascular supply may be shown by US, CT, or MRI.

■ Diagnosis

Adrenal hemorrhage.

✓ Pearls

- Gradual decrease in echogenicity helps differentiate hemorrhage from neuroblastoma.
- Neonatal adrenal neuroblastoma has an excellent prognosis that is not affected by limited serial imaging.
- Intra-abdominal extralobar pulmonary sequestration consists of nonfunctional bronchopulmonary tissue with systemic arterial blood supply, systemic venous drainage, and its own pleural covering.
- Adrenal hemorrhage and neonatal neuroblastoma are often on the right, whereas sequestration is typically on the left.

Suggested Readings

Dhingsa R, Coakley FV, Albanese CT, Filly RA, Goldstein R. Prenatal sonography and MR imaging of pulmonary sequestration. AJR Am J Roentgenol. 2003; 180(2):433–437

Jordan E, Poder L, Courtier J, Sai V, Jung A, Coakley FV. Imaging of nontraumatic adrenal hemorrhage. AJR Am J Roentgenol. 2012; 199(1):W91–W98

Papaioannou G, McHugh K. Neuroblastoma in childhood: review and radiological findings. Cancer Imaging. 2005; 5:116–127

Yao W, Li K, Xiao X, Zheng S, Chen L. Neonatal suprarenal mass: differential diagnosis and treatment. J Cancer Res Clin Oncol. 2013; 139(2):281–286

Case 66

Karen M. Ayotte

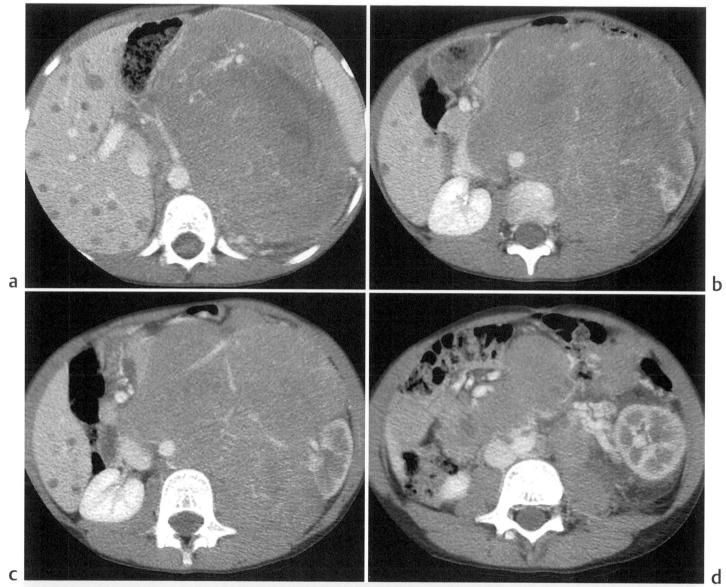

Fig. 66.1 Axial contrast-enhanced CT images show a large left upper quadrant mass that displaces the liver, bowel, spleen, and left kidney **(a–d)**. Vessels are encased and displaced, but not invaded. Multiple engorged collateral vessels are evident medial to the left kidney, and perfusion of the left kidney is delayed. There are numerous hypodense, round lesions in the liver.

■ Clinical Presentation

A 7-year-old girl with abdominal mass and malaise (▶Fig. 66.1).

■ Key Imaging Finding

Suprarenal mass in a child.

■ Top Three Differential Diagnoses

- **Neuroblastoma.** Neuroblastoma is a malignant tumor of primitive neural crest cells. It accounts for approximately 10% of all pediatric neoplasms. Average age at diagnosis is approximately 2 years, and nearly all cases are diagnosed by age 10 years. Affected children are typically quite ill. They may present with paraneoplastic syndromes, such as profuse, watery diarrhea due to vasoactive intestinal peptide (VIP) secretion. The tumor may arise anywhere along the sympathetic chain, but it usually arises from the adrenal gland. Imaging features include an infiltrative soft-tissue mass that commonly calcifies, encases rather than invades vessels, and metastasizes to liver and bone.

- **Pheochromocytoma.** Approximately 70% of pheochromocytomas arise from the adrenal gland. These tumors are rare in children, usually presenting with hypertension. Most occur spontaneously, but incidence is increased in patients with multiple endocrine neoplasia (MEN) syndrome and von Hippel–Lindau syndrome. These tumors are usually metaiodobenzylguanidine avid and are classically very bright on T2-W MRI.
- **Extralobar sequestration.** Although far more common in the lower lobes, sequestrations may occur below the diaphragm, usually above the left kidney. Always extralobar in this location, they drain into the systemic venous system. As with all sequestrations, arterial supply is directly from the aorta.

■ Additional Differential Diagnoses

- **Adrenal hemorrhage.** In the perinatal period, adrenal hemorrhage is a significantly more common cause of a suprarenal mass than is neuroblastoma, but in the absence of trauma it is uncommon in older children. Classic US findings are a hypo- or anechoic, avascular suprarenal mass, although in the acute phase hemorrhage may appear complex. Serial imaging shows progressive decrease in size, often eventually leading to radiographically evident coarse calcification.
- **Adrenocortical carcinoma.** Although a rare tumor of childhood, adrenocortical carcinomas are more common than simple adenomas. They are usually hormonally active. The tumors are typically greater than 5 cm in diameter at presentation.

Internal necrosis and calcification are common, yielding an irregular, heterogeneous mass.
- **Renal or hepatic mass.** Determining whether a suprarenal mass is adrenal, exophytic renal, or hepatic may be difficult, especially on axial imaging. Coronal and sagittal CT/MRI is helpful. Wilms tumor is the most common renal tumor, except in the neonatal period, when mesoblastic nephroma is encountered most often. Younger patients are more likely to have infantile hepatic hemangioma or hepatoblastoma, whereas hepatocellular carcinoma is more common in older children.

■ Diagnosis

Adrenal neuroblastoma with hepatic metastases.

✓ Pearls

- Neuroblastoma often calcifies, encases vessels, and metastasizes to liver and bone.
- Adrenal hemorrhage is common in the perinatal period and decreases in size over time.

- Pediatric pheochromocytomas are most common in children with underlying syndromes.

Suggested Readings

Balassy C, Navarro OM, Daneman A. Adrenal masses in children. Radiol Clin North Am. 2011; 49(4):711–727, vi

Nour-Eldin NE, Abdelmonem O, Tawfik AM, et al. Pediatric primary and metastatic neuroblastoma: MRI findings: pictorial review. Magn Reson Imaging. 2012; 30(7):893–906

Paterson A. Adrenal pathology in childhood: a spectrum of disease. Eur Radiol. 2002; 12(10):2491–2508

Case 67

Rebecca Stein-Wexler

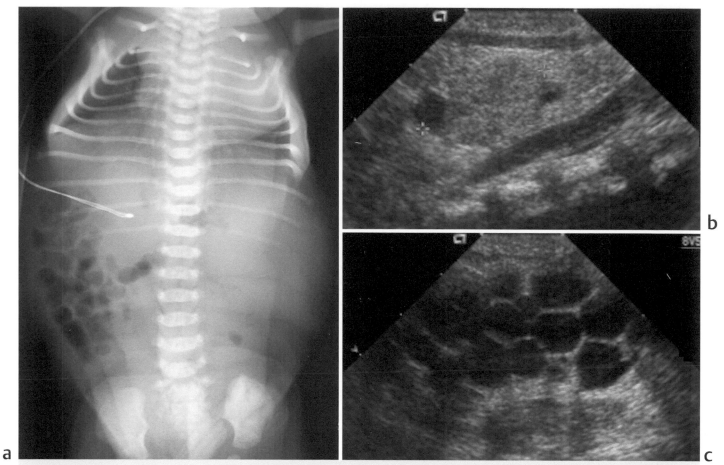

Fig. 67.1 Supine radiograph shows an extremely small thorax and disproportionally large abdomen (**a**). Longitudinal right renal US shows the kidney is small and hyperechoic (length 2 cm) and has several small cysts (**b**). Longitudinal US of the left kidney shows it consists of multiple cysts that do not communicate with each other (**c**).

■ Clinical Presentation

Newborn with abnormal prenatal US (▶Fig. 67.1).

■ Key Imaging Finding

Pulmonary hypoplasia secondary to oligohydramnios.

■ Top Three Differential Diagnoses

- **Bilateral multicystic dysplastic kidneys (MCDK).** MCDK is thought to result from intrauterine obstruction of the fetal renal collecting system or altered induction of renal tissue due to an abnormal ureteropelvic junction. US findings include multiple cysts of varying sizes that do not communicate with one another, along with echogenic, dysplastic-appearing intervening parenchyma. Renal size varies. Bilateral MCDK causes anuria and extreme oligohydramnios, leading to bilateral pulmonary hypoplasia, facial compression, and limb malformations (Potter sequence). The condition is fatal.
- **Bilateral renal agenesis.** Bilateral renal agenesis is most common if at least one parent has unilateral renal agenesis or a renal anomaly. It too causes Potter sequence.

- **Severe bladder outlet obstruction.** Posterior urethral valves (PUV) are the most common cause of congenital urethral obstruction. They occur only in boys. Wolffian duct tissue forms a thick, valvelike membrane that courses from the verumontanum to the distal prostatic urethra. Voiding cystourethrography (VCUG) demonstrates a dilated and elongated prostatic urethra that balloons above abrupt narrowing at the external sphincter. The bladder is often thick walled and trabeculated. Severe unilateral or bilateral hydroureteronephrosis is often seen. There may be renal cysts, and parenchyma may appear heterogeneous and echogenic due to cystic dysplasia. In utero oligohydramnios, hydronephrosis, bladder distension, and sometimes urinary ascites lead to prenatal diagnosis. Severe cases may demonstrate typical findings of Potter sequence.

■ Additional Differential Diagnosis

- **Autosomal-recessive polycystic kidney disease (ARPKD).** About half of the cases of ARPKD are diagnosed prenatally with severe renal disease and oligohydramnios that may lead to pulmonary hypoplasia. Perinatal US shows massively enlarged, echogenic kidneys that lack normal corticomedullary differentiation; there may also be rosettes of tiny, dilated tubular ducts. Renal involvement is generally less severe in cases presenting later in childhood, when hepatic pathology dominates.

■ Diagnosis

Potter sequence with multicystic dysplastic kidneys.

✓ Pearls

- Intrauterine renal obstruction or altered induction of renal tissue leads to multicystic dysplastic kidney.
- Posterior urethral valves usually lead to a dilated prostatic urethra, bladder wall thickening, and severe hydroureteronephrosis.

- Renal cystic dysplasia may accompany posterior urethral valves.
- Extreme oligohydramnios due to a variety of causes results in Potter sequence: bilateral pulmonary hypoplasia, facial compression, and limb malformations.

Suggested Readings

Avni FE, Hall M. Renal cystic diseases in children: new concepts. Pediatr Radiol. 2010; 40(6):939–946

Berrocal T, López-Pereira P, Arjonilla A, Gutiérrez J. Anomalies of the distal ureter, bladder, and urethra in children: embryologic, radiologic, and pathologic features. Radiographics. 2002; 22(5):1139–1164

Case 68

Rebecca Stein-Wexler

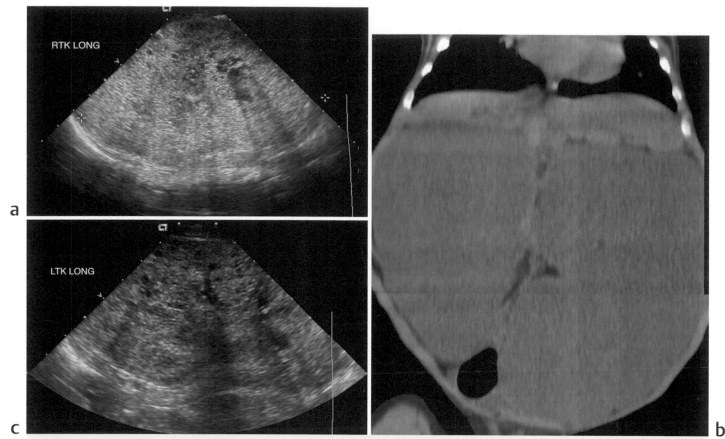

Fig. 68.1 US of the right kidney shows an enlarged (11 cm) echogenic kidney with multiple tiny cysts (**a**). The left kidney appears similar (**b**). Coronal CT without contrast shows massively enlarged kidneys that fill the abdomen (**c**).

■ **Clinical Presentation**

A 1-month-old with decreased urine output and bulging abdomen (▶ Fig. 68.1).

■ Key Imaging Finding

Bilateral nephromegaly.

■ Top Three Differential Diagnoses

- **Autosomal-recessive polycystic kidney disease (ARPKD).** This ciliopathy leads to nonobstructive dilatation of the renal collecting ducts and portobiliary fibrosis. The extent of renal and hepatic involvement varies greatly. Mean age at presentation is 2.5 years, but about half of the cases are diagnosed prenatally with severe renal disease and oligohydramnios that may lead to pulmonary hypoplasia. Perinatal US shows massively enlarged, echogenic kidneys that lack normal corticomedullary differentiation; it may show rosettes of tiny, dilated tubular ducts. There may be a hypoechoic halo of normal, compressed cortex. At MRI, the kidneys are relatively T1-hypointense and T2-hyperintense; they demonstrate innumerable tiny tubular cystic foci and sometimes a few macrocysts. Renal involvement is generally less severe in cases presenting later in childhood, when hepatic findings dominate, including intrahepatic biliary ductal dilatation or cysts, relatively large left hepatic lobe, and eventual portal venous hypertension.

- **Lymphoma/leukemia.** Lymphocytic leukemia may infiltrate the kidneys diffusely, causing renal enlargement. Corticomedullary differentiation is decreased, and cortical enhancement reduced. Non-Hodgkin Burkitt lymphoma is the most common lymphoma to affect the kidneys. Renal involvement usually results from either hematogenous spread or direct extension. There may be multiple bilateral soft-tissue nodules, a solitary mass, or diffuse nephromegaly.

- **Meckel–Gruber syndrome.** This perinatally lethal disorder typically presents with cystic renal dysplasia, postaxial polydactyly, and occipital encephalocele. It may be diagnosed in utero, during the late first or early second trimester (earlier than ARPKD). The medullary pyramids appear enlarged and hypoechoic.

■ Additional Differential Diagnoses

- **Bilateral multicystic dysplastic kidneys (MCDK).** MCDK is thought to result from intrauterine obstruction of the fetal renal collecting system or altered induction of renal tissue due to an abnormal ureteropelvic junction. US findings include multiple cysts of varying sizes that do not communicate with one another, along with echogenic, dysplastic-appearing intervening parenchyma. Renal size varies. Bilateral MCDK leads to intrauterine Potter sequence due to anuria and severe oligohydramnios.

- **Autosomal-dominant polycystic kidney disease (ADPKD).** This usually presents in older children but is occasionally encountered in infants and young children with enlarged, echogenic kidneys that mimic ARPKD. However, high-resolution US shows round cysts, rather than the tiny tubular cysts of ARPKD, and the cortex is not spared. Cysts are also common in the liver, spleen, pancreas, and seminal vesicles. ADPKD is the most common inherited cause of end-stage renal disease.

■ Diagnosis

Autosomal-recessive polycystic kidney disease.

✓ Pearls

- Kidneys affected by autosomal-recessive polycystic kidney disease are enlarged and diffusely echogenic, with mostly medullary tubular cysts.
- Hepatic disease predominates in autosomal-recessive polycystic kidney disease presenting in older children.

- Renal lymphoma appears as multiple nodules, a solitary mass, or diffuse nephromegaly.
- Autosomal-dominant polycystic kidney disease may mimic autosomal-recessive polycystic kidney disease but cysts are usually larger, round, and both cortical and medullary.

Suggested Readings

Avni FE, Hall M. Renal cystic diseases in children: new concepts. Pediatr Radiol. 2010; 40(6):939–946

Chung EM, Conran RM, Schroeder JW, Rohena-Quinquilla IR, Rooks VJ. From the radiologic pathology archives: pediatric polycystic kidney disease and other ciliopathies: radiologic-pathologic correlation. Radiographics. 2014; 34(1):155–178

Lee EY. CT imaging of mass-like renal lesions in children. Pediatr Radiol. 2007; 37(9):896–907

Case 71

Rebecca Stein-Wexler

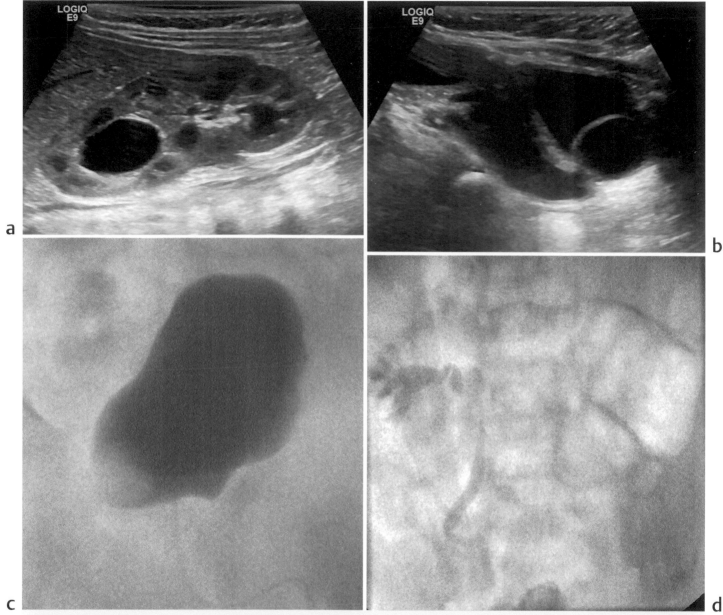

Fig. 71.1 Longitudinal right renal US shows a single cyst in the upper pole (a). Longitudinal US of the urinary bladder shows a thin-walled intraluminal cystic structure, which is closely related to a dilated, cystic tubular structure (b). Oblique view of the bladder from a VCUG shows a rounded filling defect at the right bladder base (c). After voiding, contrast is seen in the collecting system, which has a drooping lily configuration (d).

■ Clinical Presentation

A 2-month-old girl with a urinary tract infection (UTI) (▶Fig. 71.1).

■ Key Imaging Finding

Cystic upper pole of the kidney.

■ Top Three Differential Diagnoses

- **Duplex kidney with upper pole hydronephrosis.** Duplex collecting systems are relatively common, encountered in about 10% of children with UTI. According to the Weigert–Meyer rule, the upper pole ureter inserts ectopically, inferomedial to the normal position; the collecting system is more likely to obstruct and to terminate in a ureterocele. The lower pole collecting system is more likely to reflux. Therefore, either or both collecting systems may be dilated. The lower pole of a duplex system has relatively few calyces. Hence, the configuration of the contrast-filled lower pole calyces suggests a "drooping lily."
- **Segmental multicystic dysplastic kidney (MCDK).** Sometimes part of the kidney is normal, and only a portion is affected by multicystic dysplasia. Furthermore, multicystic

dysplasia may affect a portion of a duplex kidney, suggested by the presence of a ureterocele. The presence of dysplastic, echogenic parenchyma helps with the diagnosis, but sometimes functional renal nuclear imaging is required to differentiate between a large cyst due to upper pole hydronephrosis (which will show activity) and segmental MCDK (which will not).
- **Cystic renal mass.** Multilocular cystic nephroma is a rare entity that affects young males and older adult females. Patients present with a multiloculated cystic renal mass that characteristically herniates into the renal pelvis/collecting system. Wilms tumor is more common, but, although there is often central necrosis and hemorrhage, Wilms tumor is rarely purely cystic. Similarly, mesoblastic nephroma and clear cell renal carcinoma are rarely completely cystic.

■ Additional Differential Diagnoses

- **Renal cyst.** Simple cysts are uncommon in children. Three or more may indicate the presence of cystic renal disease.
- **Cystic adrenal mass.** Occasionally, it is difficult to differentiate a suprarenal adrenal mass from an upper pole renal mass, although clarification is almost always possible with coronal

or sagittal CT or MRI. Depending on its phase of evolution, adrenal hemorrhage may appear cystic. Although neuroblastoma is usually solid and often partly calcified, it may be cystic when presenting in the perinatal period.

■ Diagnosis

Vesicoureteral reflux into the lower pole of the kidney with associated ureterocele and hydroureter.

✓ Pearls

- According to the Weigert–Meyer rule, the upper pole ureter inserts ectopically inferomedial to its normal position, may be obstructed, and may terminate in a ureterocele.
- Reflux is more common in the lower pole of a duplex system.

- Segmental multicystic dysplasia may develop in a normal kidney or in part of a duplex kidney.
- Wilms tumor may be hemorrhagic and necrotic, but it is rarely purely cystic.

Suggested Readings

Avni FE, Hall M. Renal cystic diseases in children: new concepts. Pediatr Radiol. 2010; 40(6):939–946

Muller LS. Ultrasound of the paediatric urogenital tract. Eur J Radiol. 2014; 83(9):1538–1548

Case 72

William T. O'Brien Sr.

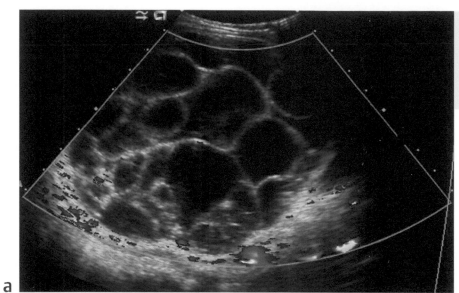

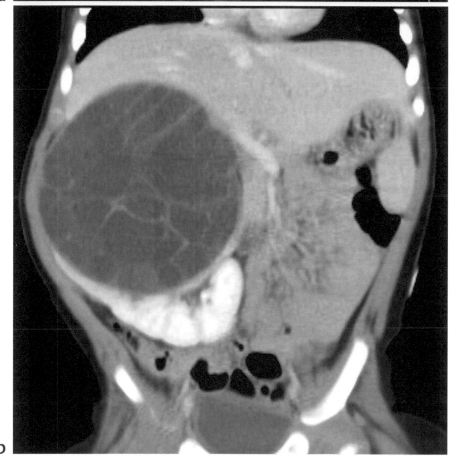

Fig. 72.1 Transverse US of the upper right kidney shows a mass consisting of multiple noncommunicating cysts (**a**). Coronal reformatted contrast-enhanced CT shows a multiloculated cystic mass extending to the renal hilum, replacing the upper pole of the right kidney, with normal lower pole parenchyma stretched about the lesion in the "claw" sign (**b**).

■ Clinical Presentation

A 10-month-old with a right-sided palpable abdominal mass on routine physical examination (▶Fig. 72.1).

■ Key Imaging Finding

Unilateral cystic renal mass.

■ Top Three Differential Diagnoses

- **Hydronephrosis.** Hydronephrosis is the most common cause of a renal mass in a child. Unilateral disease is most often due to ureteropelvic junction (UPJ) obstruction or extrinsic compression on the ureter. Bilateral hydronephrosis is usually due to bladder outlet obstruction (posterior urethral valves in boys). On US, the cystic lesions, which are the dilated collecting system, communicate centrally at the renal pelvis, a key distinguishing feature.
- **Multicystic dysplastic kidney (MCDK).** MCDK is thought to result from intrauterine obstruction of the fetal renal collecting system or altered induction of renal tissue due to an abnormal UPJ. US findings include multiple cysts of varying sizes that do not communicate with one another. The affected renal segment is nonfunctioning. The other kidney should be closely evaluated, since contralateral anomalies, such as UPJ obstruction, are common.
- **Multilocular cystic nephroma.** This rare entity has a bimodal age distribution and affects young males and older adult females. Patients present with a multiloculated cystic renal mass that characteristically herniates into the renal pelvis/collecting system. Septations within the lesion may enhance on CT. The tumor is surgically resected.

■ Additional Differential Diagnoses

- **Cystic Wilms tumor.** Wilms tumor is the most common renal malignancy of childhood, with a peak incidence of age 3 years. Patients typically have a large abdominal mass that is solid and heterogeneous, but especially in infants Wilms tumor may be cystic. Rarely, both kidneys are involved. Local spread includes the renal vein, inferior vena cava, and lymph nodes. Unlike neuroblastoma, Wilms tumor invades vessels rather than encasing them. It usually metastasizes to the lungs and liver. The tumor is typically sporadic but may be associated with cryptorchidism, hemihypertrophy, aniridia, Denys–Drash, and other syndromes.
- **Renal abscess.** Renal abscesses are rare but serious complications of UTIs. They usually occur in children with chronic infections from persistent vesicoureteral reflux. US shows an ill-defined hypoechoic region, usually at the corticomedullary junction. Abscesses are hypoechoic on US and hypodense on CT.

■ Diagnosis

Multilocular cystic nephroma.

✓ Pearls

- Hydronephrosis is the most common cause of a renal mass in childhood.
- Multicystic dysplastic kidney consists of multiple noncommunicating cysts; incidence of contralateral anomalies is increased.
- Multilocular cystic nephroma has a bimodal age distribution and typically herniates into the renal pelvis.
- Wilms tumor, the commonest renal malignancy of childhood, may occasionally be cystic, especially in infants.

Suggested Readings

Avni FE, Hall M. Renal cystic diseases in children: new concepts. Pediatr Radiol. 2010; 40(6):939–946

Chung EM, Conran RM, Schroeder JW, Rohena-Quinquilla IR, Rooks VJ. From the radiologic pathology archives: pediatric polycystic kidney disease and other ciliopathies: radiologic-pathologic correlation. Radiographics. 2014; 34(1):155–178

Lowe LH, Isuani BH, Heller RM, et al. Pediatric renal masses: Wilms tumor and beyond. Radiographics. 2000; 20(6):1585–1603

Case 73

Rebecca Stein-Wexler

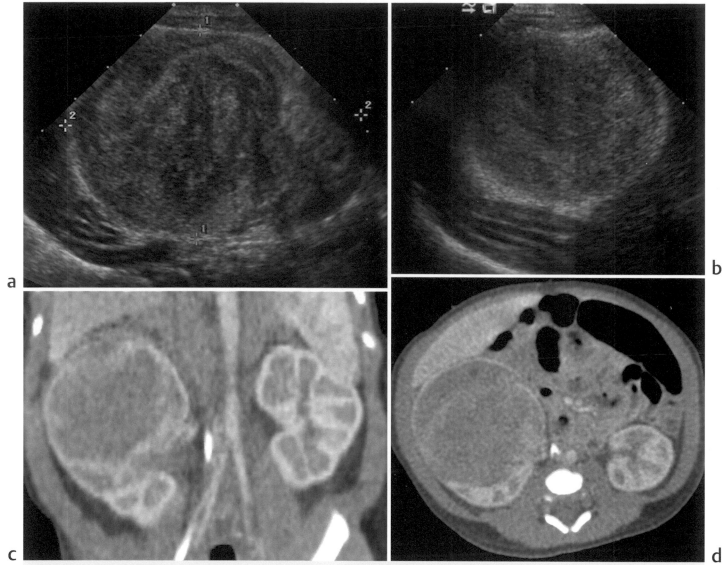

Fig. 73.1 Longitudinal **(a)** and transverse **(b)** US of the right upper quadrant shows a solid mass with the suggestion of concentric rings of alternating increased and decreased echogenicity, adjacent to a normal adrenal. Coronal reformatted contrast-enhanced CT shows the mass is partly surrounded by claws of renal tissue, indicating it arose from the kidney **(c)**. Axial contrast-enhanced CT shows the mass is well circumscribed, compressing a thin rim of renal tissue **(d)**.

■ Clinical Presentation

A 2-month-old with a palpable abdominal mass (▶Fig. 73.1).

■ Key Imaging Finding

Solid renal mass in a young infant.

■ Top Three Differential Diagnoses

• **Mesoblastic nephroma.** Mesoblastic nephroma is a hamartomatous tumor of the kidney and is the most common solid renal mass in neonates. Mean age at presentation is 2 months. Patients are typically asymptomatic except for a palpable mass, although they may have hypercalcemia. Since imaging findings of mesoblastic nephroma are indistinguishable from Wilms tumor, it must be resected.

• **Wilms tumor.** Wilms tumor is the most common renal malignancy of childhood, with peak incidence at age 3 years. After age 2 months, it is the most common renal mass in infants. Tumors usually present as an asymptomatic abdominal mass. They are typically well defined and round, arising from the renal cortex. When large, they may appear heterogeneous and partly cystic, with internal necrosis and hemorrhage. Calcification is relatively uncommon, and intratumoral fat is extremely rare. Wilms tumor spreads locally through the ipsilateral renal vein, via lymphatics to local lymph nodes, and hematogenously to the lungs and liver. Bilateral disease is seen in about 5% of patients, more common in those with nephroblastomatosis or associated congenital anomalies such as cryptorchidism, hypospadias, horseshoe kidney, hemihypertrophy, and aniridia. Incidence is increased with numerous syndromes.

• **Rhabdoid tumor.** This very aggressive renal malignancy usually occurs before age 2 years and presents with hematuria or fever. Increased parathormone levels may cause hypercalcemia, leading to medullary nephrocalcinosis in the contralateral kidney. The tumor is usually at least 9 cm at presentation. In general, it resembles Wilms tumor. However, rhabdoid tumor is more central than Wilms tumor, arising from the medulla and often involving the hilum. Subcapsular fluid collections are more common than with Wilms tumor. Lung and liver metastases are common, but the tumor also spreads to bone and brain. There is an increased incidence of posterior fossa medulloblastoma and primitive neuroectodermal tumor, as well as other CNS tumors. Mortality is about 75%.

■ Additional Differential Diagnosis

• **Neuroblastoma.** Under some circumstances, an adrenal neuroblastoma may mimic a renal mass at US, though CT and MRI should allow differentiation. Neuroblastoma derives from sympathetic ganglion cells of the neural crest. In newborns, neuroblastoma is more common than Wilms tumor. At US, it typically appears solid, heterogenous, and predominantly hyperechoic. Calcifications are common, contributing to diffuse echogenicity and helping differentiate this tumor from Wilms tumor. Infrequently, the tumor appears cystic. Neonatal neuroblastoma may be widely metastatic but has an excellent prognosis. Urine catecholamines are often normal in neonatal neuroblastoma, though elevated in older children with the disease.

■ Diagnosis

Mesoblastic nephroma.

✓ Pearls

• Mesoblastic nephroma is the most common solid renal mass in neonates.
• Rhabdoid tumor is extremely aggressive and is often accompanied with posterior fossa tumors.

• Bilateral Wilms tumor is more common in patients with nephroblastomatosis, congenital anomalies, and numerous syndromes.
• Neuroblastoma is more common than Wilms tumor in neonates.

Suggested Readings

Gee MS, Bittman M, Epelman M, Vargas SO, Lee EY. Magnetic resonance imaging of the pediatric kidney: benign and malignant masses. Magn Reson Imaging Clin N Am. 2013; 21(4):697–715

Geller E, Kochan PS. Renal neoplasms of childhood. Radiol Clin North Am. 2011; 49(4):689–709, vi

Paterson A. Adrenal pathology in childhood: a spectrum of disease. Eur Radiol. 2002; 12(10):2491–2508

Case 74

John P. Lichtenberger III

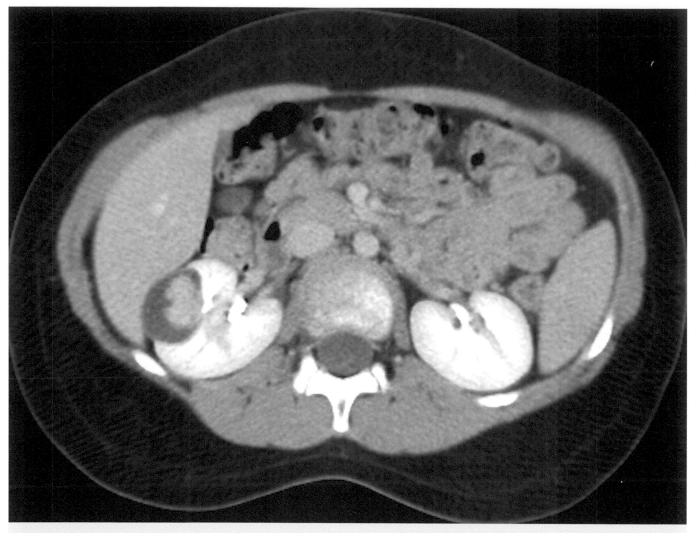

Fig. 74.1 Axial image from a contrast-enhanced CT shows a small right renal mass that has a solid, nodular enhancing component within a well-circumscribed cyst.

■ Clinical Presentation

A 5-year-old girl status post motor vehicle accident (▶ Fig. 74.1).

■ Key Imaging Finding

Solid renal mass in an older child.

■ Top Three Differential Diagnoses

- **Wilms tumor.** Wilms tumor is the most common renal malignancy of childhood, with peak incidence at age 3 years. Patients often present with an abdominal mass. The tumor characteristically appears as a well-defined, round mass that arises from renal cortex and causes mass effect. It generally enhances less than surrounding renal parenchyma. Renal origin is confirmed by noting compressed renal parenchyma along the margin of the tumor, referred to as the "claw sign." When large, Wilms tumor may appear heterogeneous and partly cystic, with internal necrosis and hemorrhage. Calcification is relatively uncommon. Intratumoral fat is extremely rare. Wilms tumor spreads locally through the ipsilateral renal vein, via lymphatics to local lymph nodes, and hematogenously to the lungs and liver. Associated syndromes include WAGR (Wilms tumor, aniridia, genital anomalies, and mental retardation) and Beckwith–Wiedemann syndrome. Staging is surgical.

- **Nephroblastomatosis.** Persistence of nephrogenic rests is termed nephroblastomatosis. The lesions typically present as bilateral, confluent, plaquelike or rounded, peripheral solid renal masses in infants. Surveillance is required to evaluate for malignant degeneration to Wilms tumor.

- **Lymphoma.** Although primary renal lymphoma is rare, secondary involvement is common. Patients may present with multiple bilateral homogeneous hypodense parenchymal masses (most common), a solitary renal mass, or diffuse infiltration of the renal parenchyma. Bulky adjacent extrarenal lymphadenopathy is a diagnostic clue.

■ Additional Differential Diagnoses

- **Renal cell carcinoma (RCC).** RCC is relatively rare in childhood, except in the setting of von Hippel–Lindau disease. Patients are typically older and present with flank pain or hematuria. The tumor is usually hypervascular and may be solid or cystic. Calcifications are seen in 25% of cases. RCC spreads locally through the ipsilateral renal vein, via lymphatics to local lymph nodes, and hematogenously to the liver, lungs, and bones.

- **Mesoblastic nephroma.** This hamartomatous solid tumor of the kidney is the most common solid renal mass in neonates but is rare in older children. Patients are typically asymptomatic except for a palpable mass, although hypercalcemia may occasionally be detected clinically. Since mesoblastic nephroma is indistinguishable from Wilms tumor based upon imaging findings, treatment is surgical.

■ Diagnosis

Renal cell carcinoma.

✓ Pearls

- Wilms tumor may spread by direct extension (renal vein), lymphatic spread, and hematogenous spread.
- Mesoblastic nephroma is a benign, hamartomatous lesion with a peak incidence of 2 to 3 months of age.

- Nephroblastomatosis is usually bilateral and may degenerate into Wilms tumor.
- Renal cell carcinoma is rare in childhood, except in patients with von Hippel–Lindau disease.

Suggested Readings

Geller E, Kochan PS. Renal neoplasms of childhood. Radiol Clin North Am. 2011; 49(4):689–709, vi

Lowe LH, Isuani BH, Heller RM, et al. Pediatric renal masses: Wilms tumor and beyond. Radiographics. 2000; 20(6):1585–1603

McHugh K. Renal and adrenal tumours in children. Cancer Imaging. 2007; 7:41–51

Siegel MJ, Chung EM. Wilms' tumor and other pediatric renal masses. Magn Reson Imaging Clin N Am. 2008; 16(3):479–497, vi

Case 75

Ellen Cheang

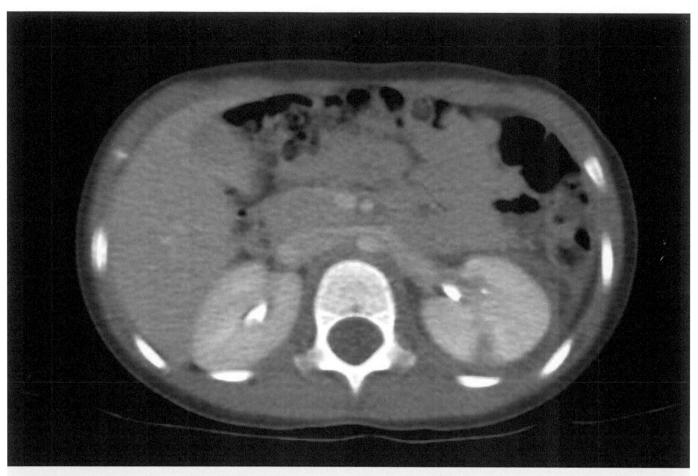

Fig. 75.1 Contrast-enhanced CT demonstrates a wedge-shaped area of hypoattenuation in the left kidney, without extension to the collecting system. There is also subcapsular fluid.

■ Clinical Presentation

A 4-year-old girl with left flank pain after a motor vehicle crash (▶Fig. 75.1).

■ Key Imaging Finding

Renal hypodensity.

■ Top Three Differential Diagnoses

- **Pyelonephritis.** Pyelonephritis results from ascending or hematogenous infection. Most cases are diagnosed by clinical and laboratory findings. Imaging is warranted for atypical presentations, persistent symptoms, poor response to medical treatment, and suspected abscess formation. CT reveals focal or multiple wedge-shaped area(s) of hypoattenuation resulting from edema and microvascular occlusion. Similar findings are seen on MRI, but US is relatively insensitive. Imaging may remain abnormal for up to 5 months.
- **Contusion/laceration.** Renal trauma in children usually results from blunt injury, is low grade, and responds well to conservative treatment. The American Association for the Surgery of Trauma grades injury according to depth of damage and involvement of the collecting system/vessels. CT criteria for grade 1 injury include normal imaging with hematuria, intrarenal contusion, and/or nonexpanding subcapsular hematoma. Grade 2 injuries have a superficial cortical laceration less than 1 cm deep without collecting system injury and/or a nonexpanding perinephric hematoma confined to the retroperitoneum. Grade 3 injuries are defined as lacerations greater than 1 cm in depth that spare the collecting system; perinephric hematoma is nonexpanding. Grade 4 injuries include lacerations extending into the collecting system, injuries involving the renal vasculature, and segmental infarctions without associated lacerations. Grade 5 injuries include shattered/devascularized kidney, ureteropelvic junction avulsion, and/or complete main renal artery or vein laceration/thrombosis.
- **Wilms tumor.** Wilms tumor is the most common pediatric renal mass, typically occurring in early childhood with peak incidence at age 3 years. Most cases are sporadic, but the tumor may be associated with cryptorchidism, hypospadias, hemihypertrophy, Beckwith–Wiedemann syndrome, and WAGR (Wilms tumor, aniridia, genital anomalies, and mental retardation) syndrome. Patients often present in good health with a painless abdominal mass. US typically shows a mostly homogeneous, well-circumscribed mass that may invade the renal vein. CT and MRI better define tumor extent and show limited enhancement. About 20% of patients have lung metastases at diagnosis.

■ Additional Differential Diagnosis

- **Angiomyolipoma (AML).** AMLs are benign neoplasms composed of vessels, smooth muscle, and fat. Most are sporadic, with a strong female predilection. About 20% are associated with phakomatoses, including tuberous sclerosis, neurofibromatosis type 1, and von Hippel–Lindau syndrome. Usually an incidental finding, occasionally AMLs cause spontaneous retroperitoneal hemorrhage. The risk of bleeding is greater in lesions more than 4 cm. The presence of macroscopic fat on CT or MRI is essentially diagnostic of AML. The lesions may enhance, depending on the degree of vascularity. US shows a well-defined, round, hyperechoic mass.

■ Diagnosis

Grade 3 renal laceration.

✓ Pearls

- If grade 4 or higher injury is suspected on routine portal phase CT, a delayed series at 5 to 15 minutes should be considered to exclude collecting system injury.
- If patients with pyelonephritis respond to antibiotic therapy, imaging is not required.
- Wilms tumor, the commonest renal mass in children, may invade the renal vein.
- The risk of hemorrhage is significantly higher in angiomyolipomas that are larger than 4 cm.

Suggested Readings

Kawashima A, Sandler CM, Corl FM, et al. Imaging of renal trauma: a comprehensive review. Radiographics. 2001; 21(3):557–574

Lowe LH, Isuani BH, Heller RM, et al. Pediatric renal masses: Wilms tumor and beyond. Radiographics. 2000; 20(6):1585–1603

Park SJ, Kim JK, Kim KW, Cho KS. MDCT findings of renal trauma. AJR Am J Roentgenol. 2006; 187(2):541–547

Case 77

Ernst Joseph and Rebecca Stein-Wexler

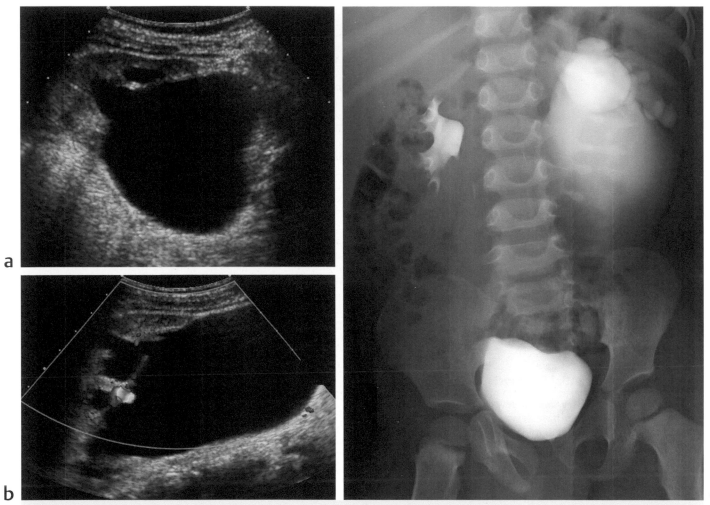

Fig. 77.1 Transverse US of the left kidney shows the renal pelvis is very dilated **(a)**. Longitudinal US of the same kidney shows massive enlargement of the renal pelvis, with moderate dilatation of the calyces and infundibula **(b)**. A 2-hour delayed image from an intravenous pyelogram shows that contrast is diluted in a massively dilated renal pelvis, there are moderately dilated calyces, and no contrast is seen in the left ureter; the right collecting system appears normal **(c)**.

■ Clinical Presentation

A 2-year-old boy with hematuria (▶ Fig. 77.1).

■ Key Imaging Finding

Hydronephrosis.

■ Top Three Differential Diagnoses

- **Ureteropelvic junction obstruction (UPJO).** With UPJO, hydronephrosis develops due to obstruction at the junction between the renal pelvis and the ureter. In neonates, this usually results from abnormal collagen and muscle at the UPJ, whereas in older children a crossing vessel is often responsible. The condition is bilateral in about one-third of patients, and in those with unilateral disease the left side is affected in about two-thirds of patients. Incidence of vesicoureteral reflux (VUR) is increased, as is contralateral multicystic dysplastic kidney. US shows variable amounts of calyceal dilatation, with an enlarged renal pelvis but no hydroureter. Extent of hydronephrosis does not necessarily correlate with the severity of obstruction. Intravenous pyelogram, nuclear medicine imaging, and MR urography evaluate function and offer quantitative estimates of the obstruction. CT or MR imaging delineates crossing vessels. Hydronephrosis improves somewhat after surgical correction but does not resolve.
- **Obstructed duplex collecting system.** If the upper and lower pole renal segments fail to fuse, renal duplication results. In symptomatic patients, two complete ureters are usually present as well, whereas if ureteral duplication is partial the condition is clinically silent. A bridge of normal parenchyma separates the upper and lower collecting systems at cross-sectional imaging. According to the Weigert–Meyer rule, the upper collecting system is more likely to obstruct and have an ectopic ureter and a ureterocele. The lower collecting system is more likely to reflux. Hydronephrosis may be seen in either pole but is more common in the upper pole, due to obstruction or VUR. Coexistent UPJO may also cause hydronephrosis. US delineates hydronephrosis, and VCUG or sometimes US is used to evaluate for VUR.
- **Congenital megacalycosis.** Underdevelopment of medullary renal pyramids results in ballooning of calyces. Lack of enlargement of the renal pelvis differentiates this condition from hydronephrosis. Congenital megacalycosis often coexists with polycalycosis, wherein the calyces are more numerous than usual and have a mosaic appearance due to crowding.

■ Additional Differential Diagnosis

- **Urolithiasis.** Urinary stasis, UTI, metabolic abnormalities, and enteric disease predispose children to stone formation. Calculi usually lodge at the UPJ or distal ureter and sometimes at the calyces or mid ureter. They are usually identified by US, and CT is rarely needed. Those larger than 5 mm usually show posterior acoustic shadowing. Color Doppler US may show "twinkle" artifact, rapidly changing color Doppler signal. The degree of dilatation does not necessarily correlate with the severity of obstruction.

■ Diagnosis

Ureteropelvic junction obstruction on the left.

✓ Pearls

- Ureteropelvic junction obstruction is bilateral in one-third of patients and is more common on the left.
- The degree of hydronephrosis does not necessarily correlate with severity (or even presence) of obstruction.
- In duplex systems, the upper pole is more likely to obstruct, and the lower pole more likely to reflux.
- In congenital megacalycosis, unlike hydronephrosis, the renal pelvis appears normal.

Suggested Readings

Epelman M, Victoria T, Meyers KE, Chauvin N, Servaes S, Darge K. Postnatal imaging of neonates with prenatally diagnosed genitourinary abnormalities: a practical approach. Pediatr Radiol. 2012; 42 Suppl 1:S124–S141

Kraus SJ, Lebowitz RL, Royal SA. Renal calculi in children: imaging features that lead to diagnoses: a pictorial essay. Pediatr Radiol. 1999; 29(8):624–630

Case 78

Mike Evens Saint-Louis and Rebecca Stein-Wexler

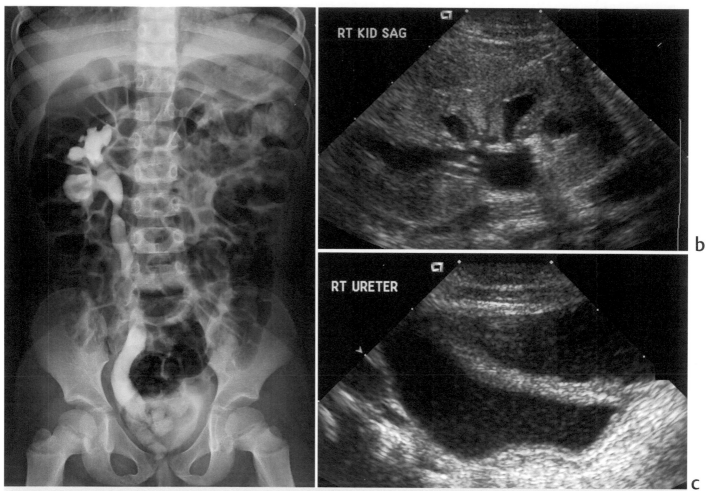

Fig. 78.1 A 45-minute image from an intravenous pyelogram shows dilated calyces and ureter, with ureteral narrowing at the vesicoureteral junction; contrast has cleared from the left kidney (a). US shows hydronephrosis (b). Sagittal US of the bladder shows marked right hydroureter with distal tapering; there is debris within the ureter and within the urinary bladder (c).

■ **Clinical Presentation**

A 5-year-old girl with recurrent UTIs (▶Fig. 78.1).

■ Key Imaging Finding

Hydroureter.

■ Top Three Differential Diagnoses

• **Primary vesicoureteral reflux (VUR).** Primary VUR results from a short submucosal distal ureteral segment, leading to abnormal formation of the one-way distal ureteral valve that should prevent passive reflux. VUR is common in patients with UTI, and it leads to such complications as pyelonephritis and renal scarring. The VCUG allows grading of VUR: grade 1—reflux is confined to the ureter; grade 2—reflux extends into a nondilated renal collecting system; grade 3—the calyces are blunted; grade 4—pelvis and calyces are moderately dilated, and the ureter moderately tortuous and dilated; grade 5—calyces are massively dilated, and the ureter is grossly dilated and tortuous. Routine US may be normal in the setting of significant VUR. However, dilatation of the ureter may indicate the presence of high-grade VUR. Low-grade VUR often resolves spontaneously, but high-grade VUR usually requires surgical intervention.

• **Obstructive primary megaureter.** An aperistaltic distal ureteral segment leads to obstruction and dilatation of the more proximal ureter, analogous to Hirschsprung disease. The number of ganglion cells in the distal ureter is reduced, though it is uncertain whether this causes the obstruction.

The configuration of the ureterovesical junction (UVJ) is otherwise normal. Obstructive primary megaureter is more common on the left and is more often seen in boys. It is often encountered in the setting of UTI. The dilated ureter tapers to a short segment of normal or narrow caliber; this can be identified on US, CT, MRI, intravenous pyelogram, and retrograde studies. VCUG is normal unless the megaureter also refluxes. Megaureter is diagnosed if the diameter of the dilated segment is at least 7 mm; the length of the narrowed segment ranges from 0.5 to 4 cm. Nuclear scintigraphy is employed to assess the degree of obstruction. Circular and longitudinal muscle fibers may develop, leading to spontaneous resolution, but in other cases surgical reimplantation is necessary.

• **UVJ obstruction.** Both congenital and acquired disorders may cause UVJ obstruction. Ureteroceles (ectopic or orthotopic) often obstruct. Ureteroceles are typically encountered in the setting of complete duplication of the urinary tract, but they also develop in otherwise normal patients. Simple ectopic ureters may also obstruct. Renal calculi may lodge at the UVJ, causing obstruction.

■ Additional Differential Diagnosis

• **Bladder outlet obstruction.** Anything that leads to impaired voiding may cause secondary dilatation of the ureters. Increased bladder volume/pressure and secondary changes in the bladder wall may impair ureteral drainage, leading to obstruction. These factors may also overwhelm a normal UVJ, leading to reflux. Patients with posterior urethral valves or with prune belly syndrome may develop hydroureter by either

mechanism. (Prune belly syndrome is defined by the triad of hypoplastic abdominal wall musculature, cryptorchidism, and urinary tract anomalies that may include hydroureter and hydronephrosis.) Children with neurogenic bladder dysfunction typically develop hydroureter due to high voiding pressure and secondary VUR.

■ Diagnosis

Congenital obstructing megaureter.

✓ Pearls

• An abnormally short submucosal distal ureteral tunnel is a common cause of primary vesicoureteral reflux.
• Congenital obstructing megaureter is characterized by aperistalsis of the narrowed distal ureter.

• Secondary vesicoureteral reflux results from ureteroceles, posterior urethral valves, neurogenic bladder, etc.

Suggested Readings

Berrocal T, López-Pereira P, Arjonilla A, Gutiérrez J. Anomalies of the distal ureter, bladder, and urethra in children: embryologic, radiologic, and pathologic features. Radiographics. 2002; 22(5):1139–1164

Leroy S, Vantalon S, Larakeb A, Ducou-Le-Pointe H, Bensman A. Vesicoureteral reflux in children with urinary tract infection: comparison of diagnostic accuracy of renal US criteria. Radiology. 2010; 255(3):890–898

Case 80

Rebecca Stein-Wexler

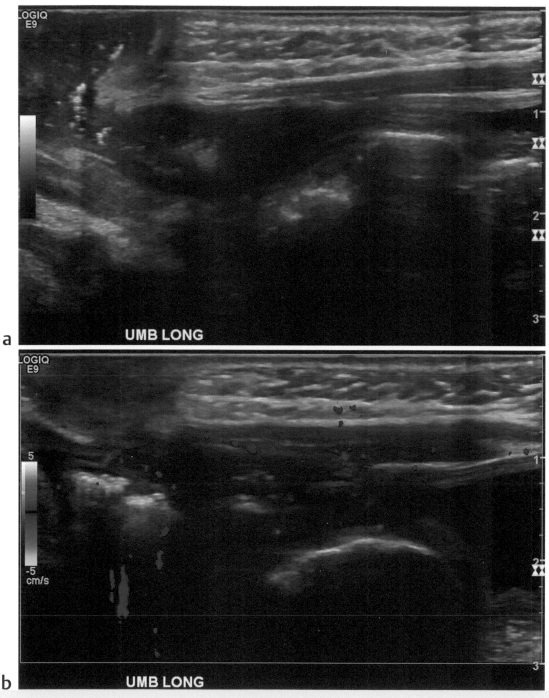

Fig. 80.1 Longitudinal US at the level of the umbilicus shows a hypodense tubular structure in continuity with the skin; there are a few echogenic foci of gas **(a)**. Longitudinal color Doppler US at the level of the bladder dome shows the hypodense structure is relatively avascular and also in continuity with the urinary bladder (bladder is at the far right side of the image) **(b)**.

■ **Clinical Presentation**

A 3-month-old with fluid draining from the umbilicus (▶Fig. 80.1).

■ Key Imaging Finding

Hypodense mass at the umbilicus.

■ Top Three Differential Diagnoses

- **Umbilical hernia.** Umbilical hernias are common in infants and young children, especially in those with low birth weight. They form if the umbilical ring does not close after separation of the umbilicus. Hernias smaller than 2 cm usually close spontaneously by the age of 5 years, but larger hernias may require surgical repair. Incarceration and strangulation are rare but more likely in older children. Umbilical hernias are usually diagnosed clinically. US shows omentum or bowel protruding through an anterior abdominal wall defect. If bowel is present within the hernia, the "gut signature" of echogenic mucosa, hypoechoic muscularis, and echogenic serosa will be evident, and peristalsis may be seen.
- **Umbilical urachal sinus.** The urachus is formed by the allantois and the cloaca and extends from the umbilicus to the bladder dome. The lumen usually becomes obliterated around gestational week 12, resulting in a fibrous cord that connects the bladder with the umbilicus (the median umbilical ligament). If some or all of the lumen persists, a variety of urachal anomalies result. Of these, the most common periumbilical anomaly is the umbilical urachal sinus. This consists of a blind-ending dilatation of the umbilical end of the urachus.

Patients usually present before age 3 months with intermittent discharge of cloudy, serous, or bloody fluid from the umbilicus. Infection is common. US shows a blind-ending soft-tissue mass that may contain fluid. Sinogram shows a blind-ending tract extending from the umbilicus.
- **Patent urachus.** Patent urachus typically presents in the newborn period. In this condition, the entire urachus remains open, from the anterosuperior bladder to the umbilicus. Clear fluid (urine) usually leaks from the umbilicus, although patients may be asymptomatic. Posterior urethral valves or other bladder outlet obstruction is present in about one-third of cases. US shows a tubular soft-tissue mass extending from the umbilicus to the bladder. It contains a variable amount of fluid. Diagnosis may also be made by cystogram or fistulogram. Other anomalies of the urachus that are seen with a normal-appearing umbilicus are urachal cyst (usually in the lower one-third of the urachus) and vesicourachal diverticulum arising cephalad from the bladder (the most common urachal remnant). Although urachal adenocarcinoma may develop in adults with urachal anomalies, this is exceedingly rare.

■ Diagnosis

Patent urachus.

✓ Pearls

- Small umbilical hernias usually close spontaneously.
- The fluid that drains from a urachal sinus is usually cloudy, serous, or bloody, whereas fluid draining from a patent urachus is usually clear.

- Incidence of urethral obstruction is increased in patients with patent urachus.

Suggested Readings

Gleason JM, Bowlin PR, Bagli DJ, et al. A comprehensive review of pediatric urachal anomalies and predictive analysis for adult urachal adenocarcinoma. J Urol. 2015; 193(2):632–636

Graf JL, Caty MG, Martin DJ, Glick PL. Pediatric hernias. Semin Ultrasound CT MR. 2002; 23(2):197–200

Parada Villavicencio C, Adam SZ, Nikolaidis P, Yaghmai V, Miller FH. Imaging of the urachus: anomalies, complications, mimics. Radiographics. 2016; 36(7):2049–2063

Yu JS, Kim KW, Lee HJ, Lee YJ, Yoon CS, Kim MJ. Urachal remnant diseases: spectrum of CT and US findings. Radiographics. 2001; 21(2):451–461

Case 81

Rebecca Stein-Wexler

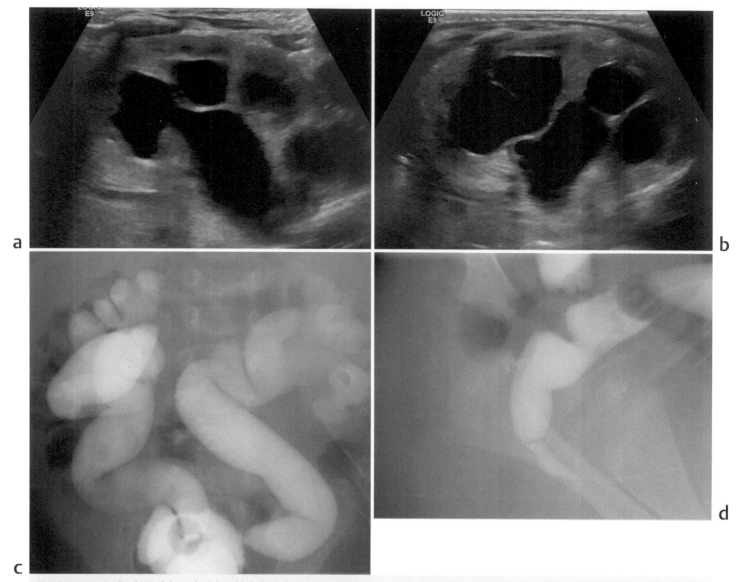

Fig. 81.1 Longitudinal US of the right **(a)** and left **(b)** kidneys shows bilateral severe hydronephrosis along with echogenic parenchyma. VCUG through a suprapubic catheter shows very severe bilateral vesicoureteral reflux with ballooned calyces and tortuous, dilated ureters; the bladder appears trabeculated **(c)**. Voiding image shows a dilated posterior urethra with a transverse lucency at the junction with the anterior urethra **(d)**.

■ **Clinical Presentation**

A 2-week-old boy with prenatal hydronephrosis (▶Fig. 81.1).

■ Key Imaging Finding

Urethral malformation.

■ Top Three Differential Diagnoses

- **Posterior urethral valves (PUV).** PUVs occur in up to 1 in 5,000 live births and only in boys. They develop from Wolffian duct tissue and consist of a membrane of smooth muscle, connective tissue, and epithelium at the junction between the posterior and anterior urethra at the level of the verumontanum. Hydronephrosis, bladder dilatation, and oligohydramnios at prenatal US usually lead to diagnosis. Vesicoureteral reflux (VUR) occurs in about 50% of patients. PUV may be identified postnatally in boys presenting with a weak urinary stream, UTI, or sepsis. US evaluates the degree of hydronephrosis and renal parenchymal dysplasia, along with hydroureter, bladder wall thickening/diverticula, and sometimes posterior urethral dilatation. VCUG is important for demonstrating VUR and the presence of an abrupt change in caliber at the junction between the posterior and anterior urethra. Surgical valve ablation treats the obstruction, but prognosis is poor if there has been significant renal damage due to VUR or obstruction.
- **Prune belly syndrome.** This syndrome is characterized by the triad of hypoplastic abdominal wall musculature, cryptorchidism, and urinary tract anomalies that may include hydroureter, hydronephrosis, and an abnormal urethra. It is basically limited to boys. Either abnormal rectus muscle development or chronic pressure causes the abdominal wall to appear lax and wrinkled. Patients with urethral atresia or severe PUVs usually die soon after birth. Those without urethral obstruction have functional impairment of bladder emptying and typically survive only to develop chronic upper urinary tract disease. Connective tissue replaces the smooth muscle in the bladder wall, leading to thickening and rarely trabeculation. US shows a large, elongated bladder, along with hydronephrosis and tortuous, severe hydroureter. VCUG demonstrates a large, irregular bladder, and, in about 80%, VUR. The prostatic urethra typically dilates with voiding, tapering at the membranous urethra. There may be urethral diverticula.
- **Urogenital sinus (UGS)/cloaca.** If the urorectal septum fails to divide the cloaca, either UGS or cloaca results. Both occur only in girls. With UGS, the urethra does not form, and there is a single exit chamber for the vagina and the bladder. Newborns have two perineal openings—the UGS and the anus. Hydrometrocolpos is common due to associated vaginal atresia. With cloaca, a single perineal opening drains a common chamber that empties the bladder, vagina, and rectum. The pelvic bones and spinal cord are often abnormal. Prenatal MRI is useful for differentiating UGS from cloaca, as with UGS the bladder contains simple fluid, whereas with cloaca there will also be high-T1 meconium within the bladder. Postnatal radiographs may show a pelvic soft-tissue mass with either. However, with cloaca, meconium within the common channel may calcify due to exposure to urine, and clumps of calcified meconium may be seen. With both conditions, MRI and genitogram delineate anatomy, which is quite variable. The kidneys may be abnormal and should also be imaged.

■ Diagnosis

Posterior urethral valves.

✓ Pearls

- In patients with posterior urethral valves, kidneys usually show hydronephrosis and/or parenchymal dysplasia.
- Prenatal US shows hydronephrosis, bladder dilatation, and oligohydramnios in patients with posterior urethral valves.

- Prune belly syndrome is characterized by lax abdominal musculature, cryptorchidism, and urinary tract abnormalities.
- Patients with cloaca—a common channel draining vagina, bladder, and rectum—often have spinal cord abnormalities.

Suggested Readings

Berrocal T, López-Pereira P, Arjonilla A, Gutiérrez J. Anomalies of the distal ureter, bladder, and urethra in children: embryologic, radiologic, and pathologic features. Radiographics. 2002; 22(5):1139–1164

Epelman M, Daneman A, Donnelly LF, Averill LW, Chauvin NA. Neonatal imaging evaluation of common prenatally diagnosed genitourinary abnormalities. Semin Ultrasound CT MR. 2014; 35(6):528–554

Case 82

Rebecca Stein-Wexler

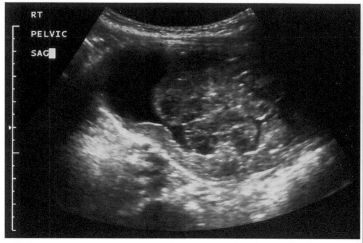

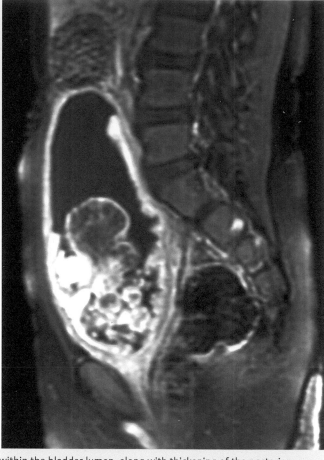

Fig. 82.1 Sagittal pelvic US demonstrates a heterogeneous, lobulated mass within the bladder lumen, along with thickening of the posterior bladder wall **(a)**. Sagittal T1-W fat-suppressed gadolinium-enhanced MRI shows the lobulated mass confined to the bladder; the bladder wall is thickened **(b)**.

■ Clinical Presentation

A 4-year-old boy with hematuria (▶Fig. 82.1).

■ Key Imaging Finding

Mass within the urinary bladder.

■ Top Three Differential Diagnoses

• **Rhabdomyosarcoma (RMS).** RMS usually involves the soft tissues of the extremities or head and neck. About 5% involve the bladder or prostate; the vagina and paratesticular tissues are affected less often. Bladder RMS is most common in boys, with mean age around 4 years. Incidence is increased in patients with congenital brain anomalies, neurofibromatosis, and nephroblastomatosis. The tumor is often polypoid and grapelike, in which case it may be described as "botryoid." Occasionally it appears infiltrative. Cell type is much more often embryonal than alveolar. The tumor is typically large and lobulated, in which case it may be difficult to determine whether it has arisen within the urinary bladder or whether it has invaded the bladder from the prostate or vagina. Smaller solitary lesions may resemble an inflammatory pseudotumor or a collapsed ureterocele. RMS usually appears as lobulated soft tissue on US or CT. On MRI, it is hypointense on T1 and hyperintense on T2; it enhances heterogeneously. RMS usually does not calcify.

• **Papillary urothelial neoplasm of low malignant potential (PUNLMP).** This common pediatric tumor is usually solitary and exophytic. The lesion usually measures 1–2 cm and occurs at the posterolateral bladder wall or ureteric orifice. Although it does not metastasize, about one-third of cases recur after resection.

• **Inflammatory pseudotumor.** This rare inflammatory condition consists of non-neoplastic proliferation of myofibroblastic spindle cells and inflammatory cells. It is more common in adults than in children, with age 7 years being the mean age in children. Etiology is unknown, but it may develop in response to infection or inflammation. It may occur anywhere in the body. In the bladder, the lesion often appears aggressive and may be mistaken for malignancy on imaging studies. It may show a classic ring-like enhancement pattern, with lack of central enhancement due to necrosis. The lesion may be polypoid or cause focal bladder wall thickening. The bladder dome is involved most often, and the trigone is typically spared.

■ Additional Differential Diagnosis

• **Plexiform neurofibroma.** Pediatric bladder neurofibromas are rare and usually associated with neurofibromatosis type 1. They develop from nerve plexuses at the bladder base. Ropey nodular thickening of the nerves results in nodular bladder wall thickening. Adjacent genitourinary structures may be affected.

■ Diagnosis

Rhabdomyosarcoma.

✓ Pearls

• Genitourinary rhabdomyosarcoma usually affects the bladder and is most common in boys.
• Bladder rhabdomyosarcoma typically has a botryoid (grapelike) appearance and is usually embryonal.

• Papillary urothelial neoplasm of low malignant potential usually occurs at the posterolateral bladder wall or ureteric orifice.

Suggested Readings

Agrons GA, Wagner BJ, Lonergan GJ, Dickey GE, Kaufman MS. From the archives of the AFIP. Genitourinary rhabdomyosarcoma in children: radiologic-pathologic correlation. Radiographics. 1997; 17(4):919–937

Fernbach SK, Feinstein KA. Abnormalities of the bladder in children: imaging findings. AJR Am J Roentgenol. 1994; 162(5):1143–1150

Shelmerdine SC, Lorenzo AJ, Gupta AA, et al. Pearls and pitfalls in diagnosing pediatric urinary bladder masses. Radiographics 2017; 13: 1872–1891

Case 83

Rebecca Stein-Wexler

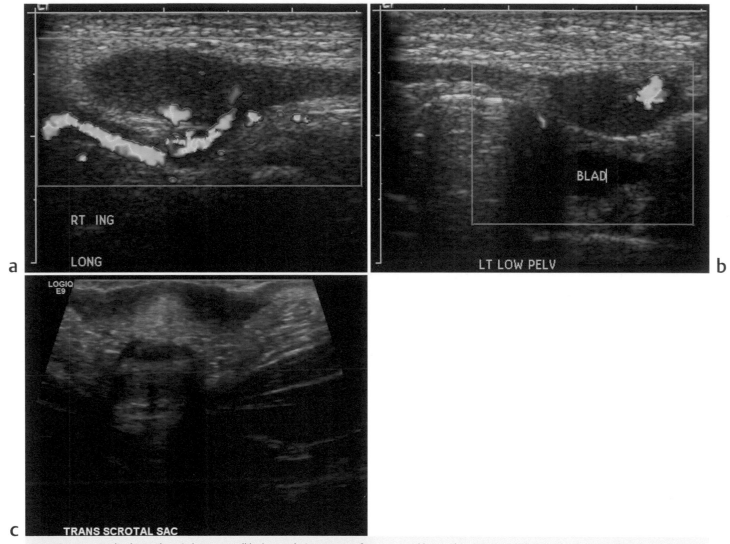

Fig. 83.1 Longitudinal Doppler US shows a cordlike hypoechoic extension from an ovoid hypoechoic structure, along with a large vessel that terminates at the junction between these structures (**a**). Longitudinal Doppler US of the left pelvis shows a hypoechoic ovoid mass anterior to the collapsed urinary bladder; a ropelike structure extends from this mass (**b**). Transverse scrotal US shows absence of testicular tissue (**c**).

■ Clinical Presentation

A 6-month-old boy with nonpalpable testes (► Fig. 83.1).

■ Key Imaging Finding

Empty scrotum.

■ Top Three Differential Diagnoses

- **Inguinal testes.** A congenital defect in the regulatory or anatomical process of testicular descent leads to cryptorchidism. Since the final descent of the testis from the inguinal canal occurs between 25 and 30 weeks of gestation, this condition is extremely common in premature infants. It is also more common in boys with hypospadias, posterior urethral valves, prune belly syndrome, gastroschisis, and myelomeningocele. Some boys with cerebral palsy develop cryptorchidism during childhood if their hyperactive cremasteric muscle prevents normal elongation of the spermatic cord. Cryptorchid testes are exposed to abnormally high temperatures, which combined with other factors increases the risk of infertility and testicular cancer in men whose cryptorchidism is not reduced in early childhood. Most cryptorchid testes are palpable in the inguinal canal. The role imaging plays in the workup of patients with a nonpalpable testis is controversial. Both US and MRI may fail to identify a testis, and a lymph node or gubernacular structure may be incorrectly diagnosed as a cryptorchid testis. Accurate identification of the testis requires demonstration of the spermatic cord and/or echogenic mediastinum testis. The

cryptorchid testis is often relatively small and may be hypo- or isoechoic when compared to the normally positioned testis.
- **Intra-abdominal testes.** Intra-abdominal testes may be positioned anywhere from the kidneys to the inguinal canal. US is relatively insensitive for diagnosis of intrapelvic or intra-abdominal testes. Such testes are more readily identified at MRI: hypointense on T1 and hyperintense on T2. However, an intra-abdominal testis may be missed on MRI. Definitive diagnosis therefore generally rests on surgical exploration—as does treatment.
- **Absent testes.** The combination of ambiguous genitalia with undescended testes suggests a disorder of sexual development, such as XY female with congenital adrenal hyperplasia. In addition, the combination of hypospadias and cryptorchidism may be associated with prenatal and postnatal androgen disruption. The severity of hypospadias correlates with the severity of cryptorchidism. US should be performed in patients with dysmorphic genitalia to evaluate for the presence of uterus and ovaries, versus intra-abdominal testes. The structures are differentiated by the presence of the mediastinum testis in the testis and the presence of small follicles in the ovary. MRI assists with challenging cases.

■ Diagnosis

Cryptorchid testes (inguinal on the right, intra-abdominal on the left).

✓ Pearls

- Accurate identification of the testis requires demonstration of the echogenic mediastinum testis and/or spermatic cord.
- Cryptorchid testes are usually located in the inguinal canal, but they may be intrapelvic or intra-abdominal.
- MRI is more accurate than US at identification of intra-abdominal testes, but the diagnosis generally rests on exploratory surgery.

- The presence of ambiguous genitalia or hypospadias combined with empty scrotum raises concern for disorders of sexual development, addressed by pelvic US to evaluate for uterus, ovaries, and/or testes.

Suggested Readings

Delaney LR, Karmazyn B. Ultrasound of the pediatric scrotum. Semin Ultrasound CT MR. 2013; 34(3):248–256

Tasian GE, Copp HL, Baskin LS. Diagnostic imaging in cryptorchidism: utility, indications, and effectiveness. J Pediatr Surg. 2011; 46(12):2406–2413

Case 84

Rebecca Stein-Wexler

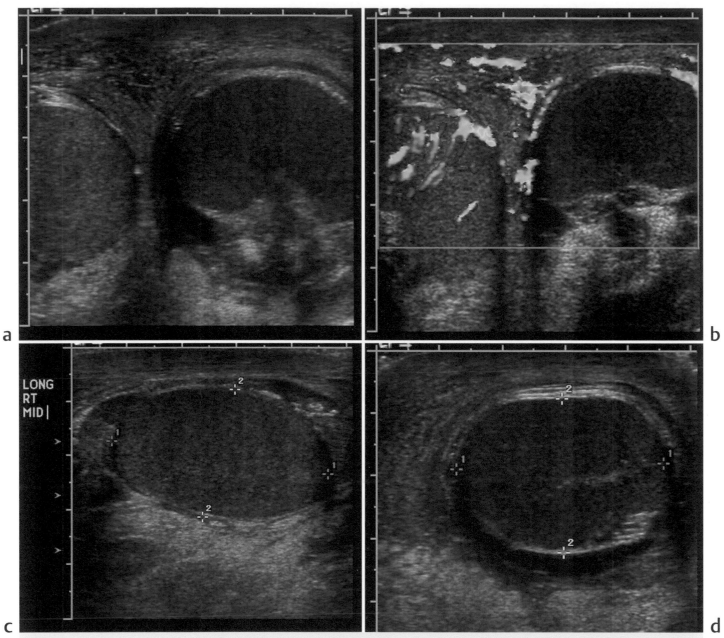

Fig. 84.1 Transverse scrotal US shows the left testis is hypoechoic **(a)**. With application of color Doppler, blood flow is identified only in the right testis and the left testicular capsule **(b)**. Longitudinal US of the right testis shows an ovoid, homogeneous testis **(c)**. Longitudinal US of the left testis shows the testis appears rounder than the right, and it is heterogeneously hypoechoic, with a few tiny cystic areas; there is also a small hydrocele **(d)**.

■ Clinical Presentation

A 14-year-old boy with sudden onset of left scrotal pain (▶Fig. 84.1).

■ Key Clinical Finding

Testicular pain.

■ Top Three Differential Diagnoses

- **Torsion of the appendix testis.** The appendix testis is located at the superior pole of the testis. Torsion of this structure is most common in prepubescent boys. Presentation is similar to testicular torsion, but onset of pain may be more gradual. The clinical findings of a tender nodule superior to the testis and corresponding "blue dot" help differentiate. The characteristic US finding is a pedunculated avascular oval nodule that is larger than 6 mm. Adjacent inflammation and hydrocele are common.
- **Testicular torsion.** Torsion is most common in adolescents and newborns. Most adolescents have intravaginal torsion, due to absence of part of the posterior tunica vaginalis ("bell clapper" deformity). Infarction occurs within 6 to 12 hours of torsion. Extravaginal torsion is common only in neonates, who usually present with testicular infarction. The torsed testis has a high transverse lie, and the cremasteric reflex may be absent. Within several hours, the testis becomes enlarged and hypoechoic; if heterogeneous, torsion is likely irreversible. Color Doppler flow is typically absent, but in early stages it may be increased or only mildly decreased. Flow may increase after detorsion. Paratesticular tissues, including the epididymis and testicular capsule, are also sometimes hyperemic. The resistive index may be increased. The spermatic cord may appear coiled. Both testes must be evaluated at US.
- **Epididymitis/epididymo-orchitis (EEO).** EEO is most common in sexually active adolescents. Younger boys often have a urogenital anomaly. Boys with mumps may have isolated orchitis. The cremasteric reflex is present, and elevation of the testis relieves pain. At US, the epididymis is often large and hypoechoic, but if hemorrhagic may be heterogeneous with hyperechoic foci. Color Doppler shows epididymal hyperemia and—unlike testicular torsion—a low resistive index. Abscess and infarction are unusual complications.

■ Additional Differential Diagnoses

- **Inguinal hernia.** Inguinal hernias are very common in newborns and especially common in premature infants. Most are diagnosed clinically as an asymptomatic bulge in the groin, scrotum, or labia. Older children may present with indolent, aching pain or sometimes with acute pain. The hernia is more obvious with Valsalva maneuvers, such as crying. US shows bowel and/or omentum in the inguinal canal and sometimes scrotum. Aperistaltic bowel is worrisome for strangulation. In the setting of inguinal hernia, scrotal soft-tissue hyperemia suggests incarceration.
- **Testicular trauma.** Testicular trauma is common, but injury is relatively rare. Hematoma and hydrocele may be identified as variable echogenicity material between the layers of the tunica vaginalis (hematocele) or in the testis, epididymis, or scrotal wall (hematoma). Rupture—a surgical emergency—is identified at US as extrusion of parenchyma through a defect in the echogenic tunica albuginea. The testis is often distorted and heterogeneous. Testicular fracture may be identified at US as a linear hypoechoic defect

■ Diagnosis

Torsion of the left testis.

✓ Pearls

- With epididymitis/epididymo-orchitis, the epididymis is enlarged and may be hypoechoic or heterogeneous.
- The resistive index is decreased with epididymitis/epididymo-orchitis, whereas it is increased with testicular torsion.
- Color Doppler flow may be increased in early testicular torsion or after detorsion.
- Enlargement of the appendix testis greater than 6 mm may indicate torsion.

Suggested Readings

Delaney LR, Karmazyn B. Ultrasound of the pediatric scrotum. Semin Ultrasound CT MR. 2013; 34(3):248–256

Yusuf GT, Sidhu PS. A review of ultrasound imaging in scrotal emergencies. J Ultrasound. 2013; 16(4):171–178

Case 85

Leslie E. Grissom

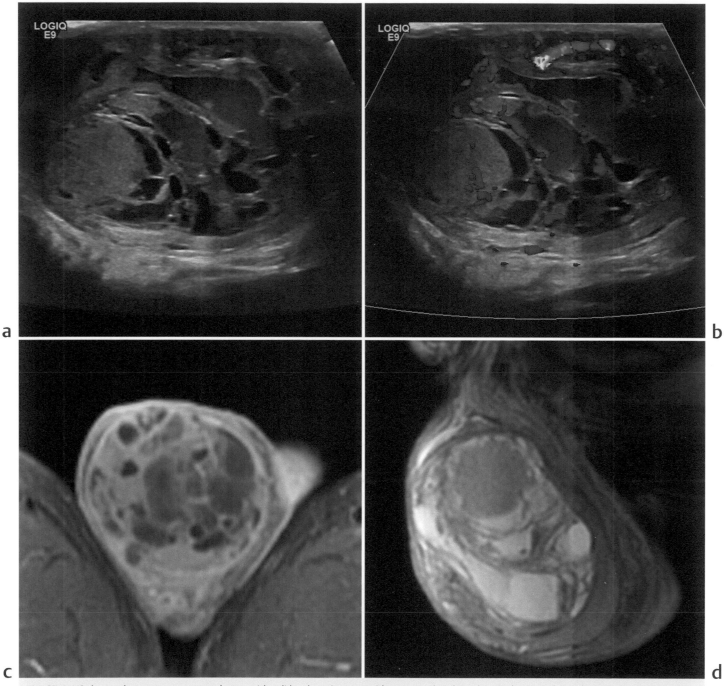

Fig. 85.1 US shows a heterogeneous scrotal mass with solid and cystic areas, with no normal ipsilateral testicular tissue (**a**). Color Doppler US shows the mass is hyperemic (**b**). Axial T1-W contrast-enhanced MRI shows that some of the solid tissue enhances, but multiple necrotic/cystic areas do not (**c**). The mass is heterogeneous on sagittal T2-W MRI, with multiple fluid spaces. The fascia of the scrotal wall also appears thickened and is probably involved (**d**).

■ **Clinical Presentation**

A 16-year-old boy with a painless scrotal mass (▶Fig. 85.1).

■ Key Imaging Finding

Painless scrotal mass.

■ Top Three Differential Diagnoses

- **Germ cell tumor.** Testicular tumors are rare in children, and most are malignant. Germ cell tumors account for about 75% of testicular tumors in childhood, and stromal tumors account for the rest. Mature teratomas and most stromal tumors are benign; the others are malignant. In prepubertal children, yolk sac tumors (also called endodermal sinus tumor) and teratomas are the most common. In postpubertal boys, the most common type is mixed germ cell tumor (MGCT). MGCTs include varying combinations of germ cell elements, including seminoma in 30% of cases. (Seminoma is also the tumor that occurs in adults with cryptorchid testes.) Embryonal cell carcinoma is much less common than MGCT, and choriocarcinoma is rare, although it may be a component of MGCTs. Many of these tumors secrete tumor markers or hormones, including alpha-fetoprotein in yolk sac tumors, beta-human chorionic gonadotropin (beta-HCG) in choriocarcinoma, and estrogens or androgens in the stromal tumors. These tumors all have a similar US appearance: mixed cystic and solid with hyperemia. MRI is helpful because of its large field of view and its potential to characterize tissue type.

- **Rhabdomyosarcoma.** This is the most common paratesticular tumor. Its US appearance resembles germ cell tumor, and it may be so large that it is difficult to appreciate the extratesticular origin.

- **Trauma.** Trauma can produce a complex scrotal hematoma that mimics germ cell tumor. Cystic areas typically have mobile debris within them. Flow may be seen in the septations of an organizing hematoma.

■ Additional Differential Diagnoses

- **Inguinal hernia.** Bowel loops in the scrotum may appear complex. They typically show peristalsis and flow within the bowel wall, as long as they are not incarcerated. It is important to interrogate the inguinal canal to determine whether what appears to be a scrotal mass is actually a hernia.

- **Metastatic lymphoma and leukemia.** Testicular leukemia/lymphoma usually occurs in the setting of widespread metastatic disease. The testes may serve as a tumor sanctuary and site of relapse. The tumors may be nodular or have a more solid, uniform hypoechoic appearance, similar to seminoma. They may appear hyperemic. Involvement is often bilateral and may include the epididymis.

■ Diagnosis

Embryonal cell carcinoma.

✓ Pearls

- Germ cell tumors in older children are more likely to be malignant.
- Stromal tumors (Leydig and Sertoli) produce hormones causing virilization or gynecomastia.

- Seminoma, the most common testicular tumor in adults, is the tumor that may occur in cryptorchid testes.
- Rhabdomyosarcoma is the most common paratesticular tumor.

Suggested Readings

Cassidy FH, Ishioka KM, McMahon CJ, et al. MR imaging of scrotal tumors and pseudotumors. Radiographics. 2010; 30(3):665–683

Sohaib SA, Koh DM, Husband JE. The role of imaging in the diagnosis, staging, and management of testicular cancer. AJR Am J Roentgenol. 2008; 191(2):387–395

Sung EK, Setty BN, Castro-Aragon I. Sonography of the pediatric scrotum: emphasis on the Ts: torsion, trauma, and tumors. AJR Am J Roentgenol. 2012; 198(5):996–1003

Case 86

Ellen Cheang

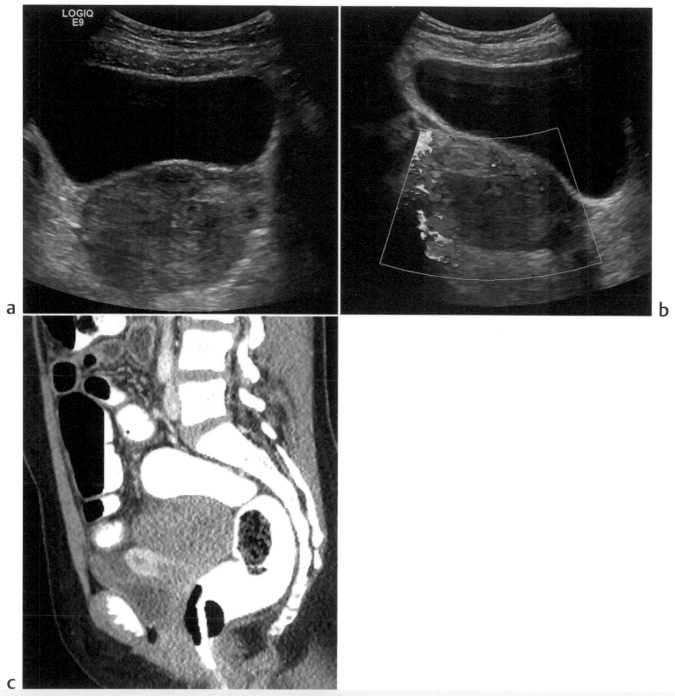

Fig. 86.1 Transverse pelvic US reveals a heterogeneous, hypoechoic mass posterior to a small, prepubescent uterus; a normal-appearing right ovary was also seen (not shown) **(a)**. Sagittal color Doppler US shows no blood flow within this mass **(b)**. Contrast-enhanced sagittal reformatted CT shows a midline pelvic mass superior and posterior to the uterus **(c)**.

■ **Clinical Presentation**

A 10-year-old girl with right lower quadrant pain (▶ Fig. 86.1).

■ **Key Imaging Finding**

Painful pelvic mass.

■ **Top Three Differential Diagnoses**

• **Perforated appendicitis.** Appendicitis is the most common pediatric surgical emergency in the United States. Although CT offers greater than 90% sensitivity and specificity for diagnosis, US is the initial modality of choice due to concern for radiation exposure. US shows a noncompressible, blind-ending, tubular structure arising from the cecum, greater than 6 mm in diameter. Possible associated findings include a shadowing appendicolith, echogenic periappendiceal fat, free fluid, and hyperemia of the appendiceal wall. CT is useful for equivocal cases and to assess complications. If perforation has occurred, a heterogeneous, inflammatory soft tissue mass (early) or a thick-walled fluid collection (late) may be seen in the right lower quadrant, cul-de-sac, or elsewhere. Resultant small bowel obstruction is common.

• **Ovarian torsion.** Ovarian torsion is a common gynecological surgical emergency, often encountered around puberty but also seen in infants. Symptoms are nonspecific. Although patients classically present with sharp, acute pain, pain may be chronic and intermittent. Adnexal mobility and/or the presence of a large cyst or mass (typically teratoma) predispose the pediatric ovary to torsion. US appearance varies. Unilateral painful ovarian enlargement (at least 3 times larger than the other side) is the most constant finding. The ovary may be heterogeneous, with multiple peripheral follicles due to edema and venous congestion ("string of pearls"). Midline or other abnormal location of the ovary is suggestive. The affected ovary may lack blood flow on color Doppler US. However, normal blood flow in the adnexa does not exclude torsion, as the ovary has a dual blood supply and torsion may be incomplete or intermittent. Torsion in neonates usually occurs prenatally in an ovary enlarged by a cyst larger than 4–5 cm. The appearance therefore reflects hemorrhagic necrosis: a fluid–fluid level, retracting clot, or reticular pattern within a large cyst.

• **Ectopic pregnancy.** Ectopic pregnancy is caused by implantation of the conceptus outside the endometrial canal, usually within the fallopian tube. Patients present with pain and/or vaginal bleeding, usually in the first trimester. US is diagnostic if there is a complex adnexal mass, echogenic free fluid, and no intrauterine gestation sac in the setting of a positive beta-human chorionic gonadotropin (beta-HCG). The classic thick, hyperechoic rim with peripheral flow in a "ring of fire" pattern may be seen. US findings must be correlated with beta-HCG levels.

■ **Additional Differential Diagnosis**

• **Pelvic inflammatory disease (PID)/tubo-ovarian abscess.** The diagnosis of PID is made in the appropriate clinical setting of fever, pelvic pain, and vaginal discharge in a sexually active teen. Tubo-ovarian abscess appears as a distended, serpiginous, tubular, fluid-filled structure with layering debris and/or a complex solid and cystic adnexal mass with scattered internal echogenicity and increased vascularity.

■ **Diagnosis**

Ovarian torsion.

✓ **Pearls**

• A single enlarged, edematous ovary with multiple peripheral cysts suggests ovarian torsion in adolescents.
• Torsion may be incomplete or intermittent, so the presence of adnexal blood flow does not exclude torsion.

• Ectopic pregnancy must be considered if no intrauterine gestation is seen in a patient with a positive beta-HCG.

Suggested Readings

Callahan MJ, Rodriguez DP, Taylor GA. CT of appendicitis in children. Radiology. 2002; 224(2):325–332
Kaakaji Y, Nghiem HV, Nodell C, Winter TC. Sonography of obstetric and gynecologic emergencies: part II, gynecologic emergencies. AJR Am J Roentgenol. 2000; 174(3):651–656

Levine D. Ectopic pregnancy. Radiology. 2007; 245(2):385–397
Sintim-Damoa A, Majmudar AS, Cohen HL, et al. Pediatric ovarian torsion: spectrum of imaging findings. Radiographics 2017; 37:1892–1908.

Case 87

Fabienne Joseph and Rebecca Stein-Wexler

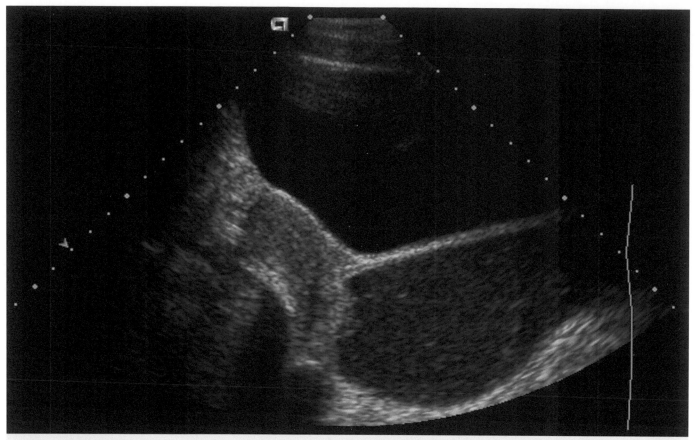

Fig. 87.1 Longitudinal transabdominal US shows a retrovesical cystic mass that contains low-level echoes. The normal uterus is located cephalad to it.

■ Clinical Presentation

A 14-year-old girl with suprapubic pain and delayed menses (▶Fig. 87.1).

■ Key Imaging Finding

Cystic pelvic mass.

■ Top Three Differential Diagnoses

- **Ovarian cyst.** Ovarian cysts constitute almost 50% of adnexal lesions and are the most common abdominal mass in newborn girls. They usually occur in neonates or post menarche. Functional cysts are rare between years 1 and 8, when about one-fourth of ovarian masses are malignant. Cysts are often simple, appearing anechoic on US or as simple fluid on MRI. They appear more complex if hemorrhagic: US may show a lacy appearance, and MRI signal varies depending on hemorrhage stage. There should be no nodular or central enhancement. Cysts up to 3 cm in diameter are considered physiological, whereas larger cysts are considered functional. Cysts larger than 5 cm are at increased risk for torsion. Ovarian neoplasms are addressed elsewhere in this book and, if cystic, are usually of the germ cell subtype.
- **Hemato/hydrometrocolpos.** Imperforate hymen or—less often—vaginal septum/atresia leads to accumulation of fluid. If the fluid is confined to the vagina, it is termed "colpos," whereas if it also fills the uterine cavity it is termed "metrocolpos." In newborns, the fluid is usually mucus ("hydro"), whereas in perimenarchal girls, it is usually hemorrhage ("hemato"). Thus the newborn will usually have hydrocolpos or hydrometrocolpos, whereas the older girl will usually have hematocolpos or hematometrocolpos. Identification of the uterine cervix protruding into the cephalad aspect of the fluid collection assists with diagnosing these conditions.
- **Enteric duplication cysts.** These rare congenital malformations are most often found near the esophagus or distal ileum but may occur anywhere along the gastrointestinal tract. Only 5% involve the rectum. The cysts are usually round. If tubular, they are more likely to communicate with the bowel lumen. They occur on the mesenteric side of bowel. Most present with obstruction, but they may perforate, torse, or—if they contain gastric mucosa—bleed. At US, they show the "gut signature," formed by central echogenic mucosa and peripheral hypoechoic muscularis, and may demonstrate peristalsis.

■ Additional Differential Diagnoses

- **Sacrococcygeal teratoma (SCT).** These congenital lesions are the most common type of teratoma in children. They may be internal, external, or combined. Although usually solid, they may be completely cystic. SCTs in neonates are usually benign, but by age 2 months 50% are malignant. As they are intimately related to the coccyx, the coccyx must be resected to prevent recurrence.
- **Anterior sacral meningocele.** Meninges rarely herniate through a congenital defect in the anterior aspect of the sacrum. Patients may be asymptomatic or present with neurological impairment, infection, or complications due to mass effect.

■ Diagnosis

Hematocolpos.

✓ Pearls

- Most pediatric ovarian cysts are benign, especially in neonates and post menarche.
- Hydro/hematometrocolpos presents in neonates or at puberty and is usually caused by imperforate hymen.
- Duplication cysts are most common near the ileocecal junction or at the esophagus; only 5% are rectal.
- Sacrococcygeal teratomas usually wrap around the coccyx, whereas anterior sacral meningoceles are near the sacrum.

Suggested Readings

Pai DR, Ladino-Torres MF. Magnetic resonance imaging of pediatric pelvic masses. Magn Reson Imaging Clin N Am. 2013; 21(4):751–772

Rao P. Neonatal gastrointestinal imaging. Eur J Radiol. 2006; 60(2):171–186

Part 4

Musculoskeletal Imaging

4

Case 90

Rebecca Stein-Wexler

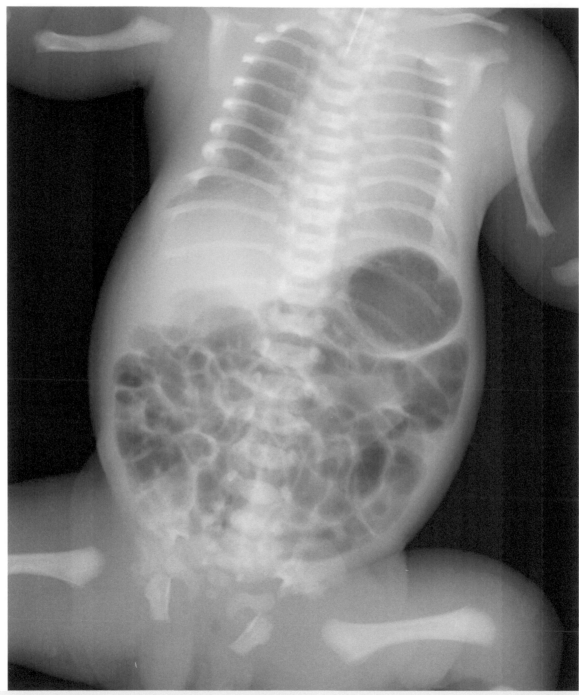

Fig. 90.1 Frontal radiograph shows unusually short ribs. The iliac wings are flared, and the acetabula have a trident configuration. The spine is normal, but humeri and femora are short and thick. The cardiothymic silhouette appears enlarged.

■ Clinical Presentation

A newborn with an abnormal prenatal US (▶Fig. 90.1).

■ Key Imaging Finding

Short rib skeletal dysplasia.

■ Top Three Differential Diagnoses

- **Asphyxiating thoracic dystrophy (Jeune syndrome).** In this syndrome, the thorax is long and bell-shaped, with short, horizontal ribs that flare anteriorly. This configuration results in early respiratory compromise. Dysplastic acetabula resembling an upside-down trident are often seen. There is associated mild acromelic (distal) limb shortening, but long bones are not bowed. A normal spine and trident acetabula help differentiate this condition from thanatophoric dysplasia.
- **Ellis–van Creveld syndrome (chondroectodermal dysplasia).** Hair, nail, and teeth abnormalities are clinical hallmarks of this syndrome. There is progressive mesomelic (middle—tibial and radial) and acromelic (distal) limb shortening. The fibulae are markedly shortened. Radiographic features also include short ribs, fused capitate and hamate, cone-shaped epiphyses, and postaxial polydactyly. The femoral heads ossify prematurely, and the pelvis is abnormal, with flared iliac wings and a trident acetabulum. Congenital heart disease, typically atrial septal defect or atrioventricular cushion defect, is the major cause of morbidity.
- **Short rib polydactyly.** In this condition, the ribs are extremely short. Polydactyly may be either preaxial or postaxial. The pelvis and spine appear fairly normal, and long bones are normal. However, there may be cleft palate, hypoplastic epiglottis, cystic kidneys, and fetal hydrops.

■ Additional Differential Diagnoses

- **Thanatophoric dysplasia.** Thanatophoric dysplasia is the most common lethal skeletal dysplasia and is uniformly fatal in the neonatal period. The ribs are very short, and as a result the thorax is narrow. Lung hypoplasia causes respiratory failure. Patients with this disproportionate dwarfism have severe platyspondyly but wide intervertebral disks, leading to normal trunk length. The head is disproportionately large, and some patients have cloverleaf skull. Iliac bones are small. There is rhizomelic (proximal) limb shortening. Long bones are bowed and short. The femurs have a characteristic "telephone receiver" appearance.
- **Holt–Oram syndrome.** Like Ellis–van Creveld syndrome, this condition is characterized by cardiac disease (usually an atrial or ventricular septal defect) and limb abnormalities. However, the ribs are normal. The thumb is usually duplicated, hypoplastic, or triphalangeal. The radius is often hypoplastic, and there may be other anomalies of the shoulder and upper extremity.

■ Diagnosis

Ellis–van Creveld syndrome.

✓ Pearls

- Jeune syndrome (asphyxiating thoracic dysplasia) demonstrates a bell-shaped thorax, trident acetabula, and normal spine.
- Patients with Ellis–van Creveld syndrome have cardiac disease as well as progressive limb shortening, short ribs, and postaxial polydactyly.
- Bones in patients with short rib polydactyly are otherwise normal.

Suggested Readings

Glass RB, Norton KI, Mitre SA, Kang E. Pediatric ribs: a spectrum of abnormalities. Radiographics. 2002; 22(1):87–104

Miller E, Blaser S, Shannon P, Widjaja E. Brain and bone abnormalities of thanatophoric dwarfism. AJR Am J Roentgenol. 2009; 192(1):48–51

Panda A, Gamanagatti S, Jana M, Gupta AK. Skeletal dysplasias: a radiographic approach and review of common non-lethal skeletal dysplasias. World J Radiol. 2014; 6(10):808–825

Parnell SE, Phillips GS. Neonatal skeletal dysplasias. Pediatr Radiol. 2012; 42 Suppl 1:S150–S157

Case 91

Rebecca Stein-Wexler

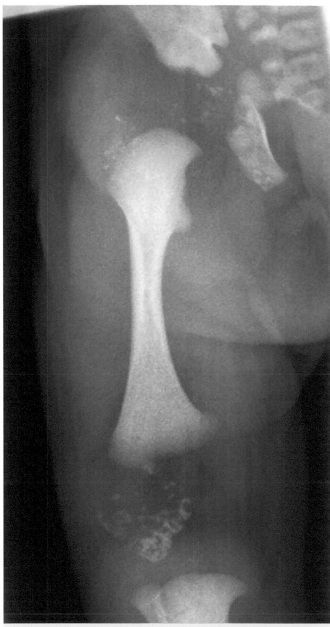

Fig. 91.1 There are stippled densities at the epiphyses and apophyses. (This image is provided courtesy of Leslie E. Grissom, Nemours/Alfred I. duPont Hospital for Children.)

■ Clinical Presentation

A 1-day-old with abnormal prenatal US (▶ Fig. 91.1).

■ Key Imaging Finding

Abnormal epiphyses.

■ Top Three Differential Diagnoses

- **Spondyloepiphyseal dysplasia (SED).** SED "congenita" manifests at birth with absent calcaneal, knee, and pubic bone ossification, pear-shaped vertebrae, and short, broad iliac wings. Severe platyspondyly develops, with thin intervertebral disks. SED "tarda" usually manifests at age 5 to 10 years with platyspondyly (including hump-shaped posterior vertebral bodies), small pelvis, and mildly to moderately small, irregular epiphyses.
- **Chondrodysplasia punctata.** There are two common subtypes, both characterized by stippled epiphyses at birth. The autosomal-recessive form shows symmetrical rhizomelic shortening, stippling in the large joints, and sometimes stippling of laryngeal and tracheal cartilage. Coronal clefts are

seen in vertebrae. The hands and feet are normal. The X-linked dominant type, "Conradi–Hünermann," shows occasional and asymmetrical limb shortening and involvement of the hands and feet as well as the large joints. The larynx and trachea are normal, but vertebral bodies and endplates are stippled, leading to eventual kyphoscoliosis. Stippling resolves over time, and the patients have a normal life span. Mental retardation is a feature of the lethal form but not Conradi–Hünermann syndrome.
- **Spondyloepimetaphyseal dysplasia.** This dysplasia resembles multiple epiphyseal dysplasia, but there is concomitant metaphyseal involvement.

■ Additional Differential Diagnoses

- **Multiple epiphyseal dysplasia.** This genetically heterogeneous disorder presents after age 2 to 4 years. Bilateral and symmetrical delayed and fragmented epiphyses of long bones and distal extremities are characteristic. Pronounced wedging of distal tibial epiphysis may trigger the diagnosis. The spine resembles Scheuermann disease, with endplate irregularities, slight anterior wedging, and numerous Schmorl nodes.
- **Morquio syndrome.** A mucopolysaccharidosis, Morquio syndrome is characterized by delayed ossification of femoral heads, irregular epiphyses, and secondary metaphyseal widening. Other bones are involved as well—notably the spine, where there is platyspondyly with anterior beaking of the mid portion of vertebral bodies. The bases of the second through fifth metacarpals are pointed and clustered together. Ribs have a paddle appearance.

■ Diagnosis

Chondrodysplasia punctata.

✓ Pearls

- Spondyloepiphyseal dysplasia tarda manifests during childhood with mild to moderately small, irregular epiphyses and platyspondyly with hump-shaped posterior vertebral bodies.
- A wedged, slightly small distal tibial epiphysis is a clue to the diagnosis of multiple epiphyseal dysplasia.
- With Morquio syndrome, ossification of the femoral heads is delayed, and there are multiple irregular epiphyses; as with Hurler syndrome, there is anterior vertebral body beaking.
- The autosomal-recessive type of chondrodysplasia punctata has stippled epiphyses of large joints and less involvement of the axial skeleton, whereas with Conradi–Hünermann syndrome the spine, hands, and feet may be affected as well.

Suggested Readings

Panda A, Gamanagatti S, Jana M, Gupta AK. Skeletal dysplasias: a radiographic approach and review of common non-lethal skeletal dysplasias. World J Radiol. 2014; 6(10):808–825

Parnell SE, Phillips GS. Neonatal skeletal dysplasias. Pediatr Radiol. 2012; 42 Suppl 1:S150–S157

Case 92

Myles Mitsunaga

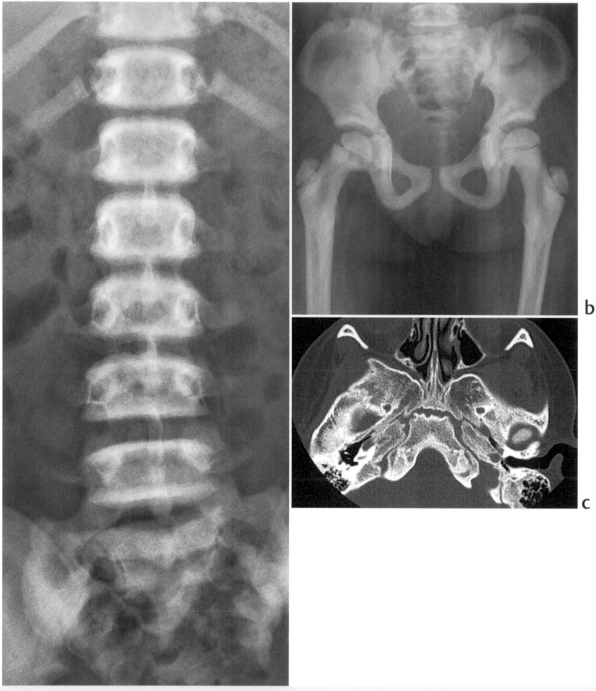

Fig. 92.1 Radiograph of the lumbar spine shows a "picture frame" appearance of the vertebral bodies **(a)**. The pelvis and femurs show a "bone-within-bone" appearance" **(b)**. Axial CT through the skull base shows generalized increased bone density **(c)**.

■ Clinical Presentation

A 6-year-old girl with diffuse bone pain (▶ Fig. 92.1).

■ Key Imaging Finding

Dense bones.

■ Top Three Differential Diagnoses

- **Osteopetrosis.** Osteopetrosis refers to a rare, heterogeneous group of heritable diseases. All have increased predominantly medullary bone density and sclerosis, due to impaired osteoclast differentiation/function. Patients often present with fractures, as the bones are relatively inelastic. The skull may have a "hair-on-end" appearance in older patients. Vertebral bodies have a "sandwich" appearance, with a sharp transition between the sclerotic endplates and the relatively lucent center (unlike the "rugger jersey" spine of renal osteodystrophy, which has an ill-defined transition). A "bone-within-bone" appearance may be seen at the pelvis and long bones. Characteristic radiolucent bands may alternate with areas of increased density in the metaphyses. The appendicular skeleton may also be diffusely dense, with flaring at the metaphyses of long bones ("Erlenmeyer flask" deformity). Marrow crowding leads to extramedullary hematopoiesis and splenomegaly. If children are not treated with bone marrow transplantation, overwhelming infection and other complications of bone marrow suppression generally prove fatal. However, patients with adult-onset disease have normal life expectancy.

- **Osteopoikilosis.** Also known as "spotted bones," osteopoikilosis is a diagnosis of exclusion. Existing in hereditary and sporadic forms, osteopoikilosis is caused by defective endochondral bone formation in the long and flat bones. Radiographs show multiple round, oval, or lenticular sclerotic foci in a periarticular distribution within the epiphyseal and metaphyseal regions. It is usually benign and asymptomatic. However, giant cell tumor, chondrosarcoma, osteosarcoma, and spinal stenosis have been reported. Osteopoikilosis must be differentiated from osteoblastic metastases and other sclerosing dysplasias.

- **Melorheostosis.** This sporadic mesenchymal disorder is characterized by cortical and medullary hyperostosis along a sclerotome, leading to undulating longitudinal sclerosis that resembles dripping candle wax. The axial skeleton is generally spared. Melorheostosis is often asymptomatic in childhood.

■ Additional Differential Diagnoses

- **Metastatic disease.** Medulloblastoma, neuroblastoma, and lymphoma may present with sclerotic osseous metastases. Skeletal metastases from other pediatric tumors are typically lytic.

- **Fluorosis.** This metabolic disorder is caused by ingestion or inhalation of large amounts of fluoride, causing increased bone turnover, impaired collagen synthesis, and irregular osteoid deposition. Fumes from household coal-burning stoves along with high fluoride levels in water may lead to this disorder. Classic X-ray appearance includes increased bone density, blurred trabeculae, periosteal bone formation, and ossification of attachments of tendons, ligaments, and muscles. Patients may develop areas of osteopenia.

■ Diagnosis

Osteopetrosis.

✓ Pearls

- Osteopetrosis is an inherited disorder characterized by diffuse sclerosis or "bone-within-bone" appearance, increased risk for fractures, and—in its most severe form—bone marrow failure.
- Osteopoikilosis is characterized by multiple sclerotic lesions in a periarticular distribution.

- Fluorosis results from ingestion or inhalation of large amounts of fluoride, with radiographs showing coarse trabeculae and diffuse sclerosis, predominantly within the axial skeleton.

Suggested Readings

Di Primio G. Benign spotted bones: a diagnostic dilemma. CMAJ. 2011; 183(4):456–459

Stark Z, Savarirayan R. Osteopetrosis. Orphanet J Rare Dis. 2009; 4:5

Wang Y, Yin Y, Gilula LA, Wilson AJ. Endemic fluorosis of the skeleton: radiographic features in 127 patients. AJR Am J Roentgenol. 1994; 162(1):93–98

Case 93

Robert J. Wood and Sandra L. Wootton-Gorges

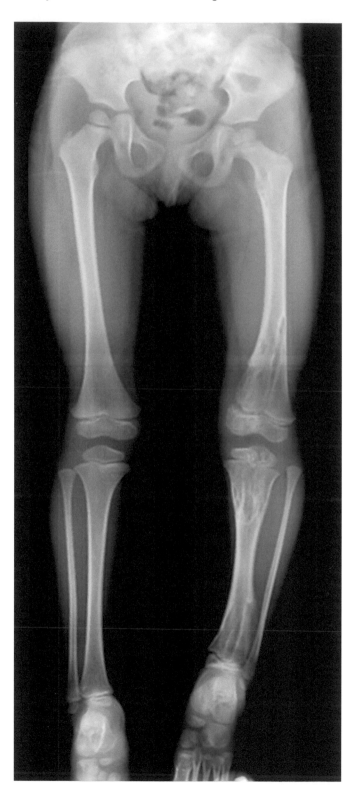

Fig. 93.1 The left leg is shorter than the right. There are multiple predominantly metaphyseal columnar, expansile, geographic lucencies. (This image is provided courtesy of Leslie E. Grissom, Nemours/Alfred I. duPont Hospital for Children.)

■ Clinical Presentation

A 15-year-old boy with asymmetrical short stature (▶ Fig. 93.1).

■ Key Imaging Finding

Multifocal osseous deformities.

■ Top Three Differential Diagnoses

- **Ollier disease.** Ollier disease is a relatively rare nonhereditary enchondromatosis, characterized by intraosseous cartilaginous benign enchondromas located near the growth plate. Unilateral limb-length discrepancy and extremity bowing are common clinical findings. The enchondromas are usually distributed asymmetrically. The affected metaphysis and epiphysis may fuse prematurely, with resultant limb shortening. Radiographically, enchondromas appear as geographic, columnar radiolucent defects extending from the metaphysis into the diaphysis of the affected bone. Phalanges and metacarpals are involved most often. About 50% of enchondromas calcify with typical chondroid "snowflake" or "ring and arc" patterns. About 40% of patients with Ollier disease eventually develop chondrosarcoma. Patients may develop other tumors as well.
- **Maffucci syndrome.** This extremely rare enchondromatosis presents with multiple enchondromas associated with soft-tissue venous malformations and potentially also lymphatic malformations. Clinical presentation is similar to that of Ollier disease but is distinguished by dermal raised bluish-red areas with obvious blood vessels and surrounding pallor. In addition to the enchondromas, calcifications within the soft-tissue venous malformations are a radiographic hallmark of this disease. In up to half of cases, enchondromas eventually transform into chondrosarcoma. The incidence of liver, pancreas, ovary, brain, and other tumors is increased.
- **Polyostotic fibrous dysplasia.** Fibrous dysplasia is characterized by abnormal fibrous tissue that replaces normal bone. It may be monostotic or polyostotic, and may appear as a geographic lucency, as "ground glass" opacity, or as sclerosis. Osseous deformities may result, including "shepherd's crook" configuration of the proximal femur. McCune–Albright syndrome is polyostotic fibrous dysplasia associated with such endocrine abnormalities as precocious puberty.

■ Diagnosis

Ollier disease.

✓ Pearls

- Enchondromatosis is characterized by asymmetrical distribution of radiolucent metaphyseal lesions.
- Enchondromas originate in the metaphyses and may extend to the diaphysis as bone grows.
- Chondroid calcifications are seen in about 50% of enchondromas.
- Degeneration to chondrosarcoma is more common in Maffucci syndrome than in Ollier syndrome.

Suggested Readings

Foreman KL, Kransdorf MJ, O'Connor MI, Krishna M. AIRP best cases in radiologic-pathologic correlation: Maffucci syndrome. Radiographics. 2013; 33(3):861–868

Kumar A, Jain VK, Bharadwaj M, Arya RK. Ollier disease: pathogenesis, diagnosis and management. Orthopedics. 2015; 38(6):e497–e506

Silve C, Jüppner H. Ollier disease. Orphanet J Rare Dis. 2006; 1:37

Vlychou M, Athanasou NA. Radiological and pathological diagnosis of paediatric bone tumours and tumour-like lesions. Pathology. 2008; 40(2):196–216

Case 94

Arvind Sonik

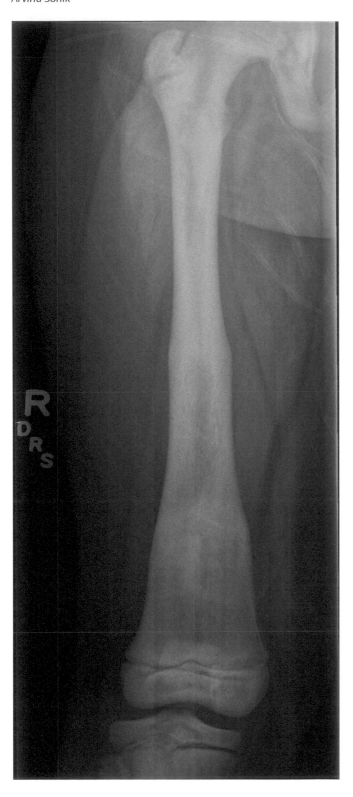

Fig. 94.1 There is expansion of the distal metadiaphysis with loss of normal contour, resulting in Erlenmeyer flask deformity. The bone is sclerotic.

■ **Clinical Presentation**

An 8-year-old girl with leg pain (▶Fig. 94.1).

■ Key Imaging Finding

Erlenmeyer flask deformity.

■ Top Three Differential Diagnoses

- **Multiple hereditary exostoses.** Osteochondromatosis is an autosomal-dominant dysplasia. As with solitary lesions, the cortex of the lesions is continuous with the underlying bone. Lesions that cause Erlenmeyer flask deformity tend to be sessile rather than pedunculated. Complications include growth disturbance, pain due to compression of neurovascular bundles, and—rarely—malignant transformation.
- **Fibrous dysplasia.** Fibrous dysplasia may be monostotic or polyostotic. Lesions typically arise in the central part of the bone and are expansile; they rarely involve the epiphysis. Density varies depending on the amount of osseous and fibrous tissue, but the classic lesion has a ground glass matrix and thin

cortex. Pathological fracture is the most common complication. The polyostotic form is more aggressive and often affects one side of the body. Associated disorders include McCune–Albright (precocious puberty and café au lait spots) and Mazabraud (intramuscular myxomas) syndromes.
- **Hemoglobinopathy.** The most common hemoglobinopathies include sickle cell disease and the thalassemias. Bony changes in these conditions are due to marrow hyperplasia and vascular occlusion. Marrow hyperplasia causes osteopenia, hair-on-end appearance of the skull, and remodeling. Vascular occlusion may cause avascular necrosis, bone infarcts, and dactylitis. Physeal involvement may lead to growth disturbance.

■ Additional Differential Diagnoses

- **Osteopetrosis.** Osteopetrosis is an inherited disorder caused by failure of osteoclast function. As a result, primary spongiosa accumulates in the medullary space. In addition to Erlenmeyer flask deformity, findings include increased bone density, encroachment on the medullary space, bone-in-bone appearance, and alternating dense and lucent metaphyseal bands. Complications include fractures, anemia, and thrombocytopenia.
- **Gaucher disease.** Gaucher disease is a rare, inherited metabolic disorder caused by deficiency of a lysosomal enzyme. The deficiency leads to accumulation of glucosylceramide in reticuloendothelial cells, which infiltrate marrow spaces. Radiographs demonstrate osteopenia, medullary expansion, and remodeling. Complications include bone infarcts, avascular necrosis, and pathological fractures. MRI may be useful to determine the extent of marrow infiltration. Infiltrating cells have signal similar to hematopoietic marrow.

■ Diagnosis

Osteopetrosis.

✓ Pearls

- Sessile lesions associated with multiple hereditary exostoses may cause Erlenmeyer flask deformity.
- Fibrous dysplasia may be monostotic or polyostotic; the classic lesion has a ground glass matrix and thin cortex.
- Hemoglobinopathies (sickle cell and thalassemias) result in marrow hyperplasia, expansion, and infarcts.
- Osteopetrosis results from osteoclast failure, leading to dense but fragile bones.

Suggested Readings

Ihde LL, Forrester DM, Gottsegen CJ, et al. Sclerosing bone dysplasias: review and differentiation from other causes of osteosclerosis. Radiographics. 2011; 31(7):1865–1882

Katz R, Booth T, Hargunani R, Wylie P, Holloway B. Radiological aspects of Gaucher disease. Skeletal Radiol. 2011; 40(12):1505–1513

Khanna G, Bennett DL. Pediatric bone lesions: beyond the plain radiographic evaluation. Semin Roentgenol. 2012; 47(1):90–99

States LJ. Imaging of metabolic bone disease and marrow disorders in children. Radiol Clin North Am. 2001; 39(4):749–772

Case 95

Stephen Henrichon

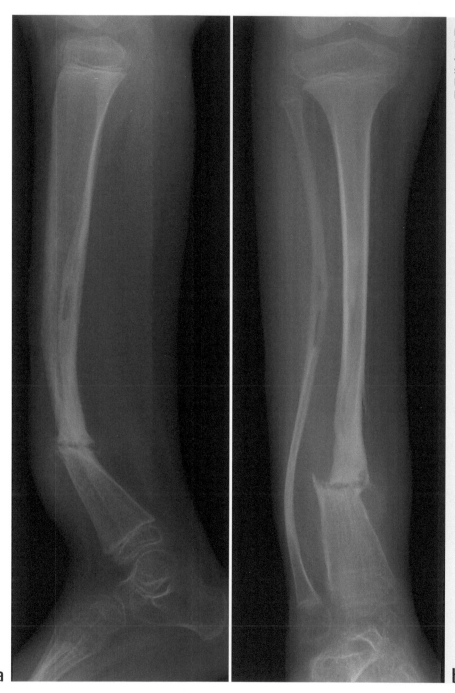

Fig. 95.1 Lateral radiograph demonstrates bowing, irregular mixed lucent and sclerotic bone density, and a transverse distal tibial lucency that has smooth, sclerotic margins (a). Frontal radiograph shows bowing of the fibula and nonunion at the distal tibial lucency (b).

■ Clinical Presentation

A 10-year-old boy with a deformed lower leg (▶Fig. 95.1).

■ Key Imaging Finding

Pseudarthrosis.

■ Top Three Differential Diagnoses

- **Posttraumatic deformity.** Nonunion is most common in fractures that were initially not recognized and/or inadequately reduced. The lateral condyle of the elbow is most often affected, sometimes leading to angular deformity. The patient should have a clinical history of traumatic fracture. In Salter–Harris fractures, lateral bowing may ensue if medial growth is halted and lateral growth continues. Radiographs will show normal bone adjacent to the pseudarthrosis, rather than the smooth, tapered margins commonly seen with either neurofibromatosis type 1 (NF1) or non-NF1 congenital pseudarthrosis.
- **NF1.** Tibial pseudarthrosis develops in up to 10% of patients with NF1, and about 50% of cases of tibial pseudarthrosis are associated with NF1. The fibula is affected less often than the tibia. Other bones may be affected as well. Pseudarthrosis usually occurs at the junction between the middle and distal thirds of the diaphysis. Considered congenital, it is usually diagnosed by age 2 years and may be apparent at birth. More often, dysplastic bone is bowed at birth, usually anterolaterally; bowing progresses, leading to pathological fracture as the child bears weight. If the abnormal bone fails to heal, pseudarthrosis results. Hamartomatous fibrous proliferation is found at the site of pseudarthrosis. The pseudarthrosis appears as a transverse defect with smooth, sclerotic margins. Unlike in posttraumatic pseudarthrosis, the adjacent tibia may appear thin,

sclerotic, tapered, or cystic. Serial imaging shows no evidence of callus formation. MRI shows hypointense periosteum intact across the pseudarthrosis. Treatment is challenging, and residual deformity is common. Satisfactory healing is more likely if patients are older at presentation. Other relatively common osseous manifestations of NF1 include calvarial defects, dysmorphic vertebrae, scoliosis and kyphosis, and thin, ribbon-like ribs. Nonossifying fibromas are often numerous. NF1 is diagnosed on the basis of the presence of at least two of the following diagnostic criteria: at least six café au lait large macules, neurofibromas, axillary/groin freckling, optic pathway gliomas, Lisch nodules, bony dysplasia, and/or a first-degree affected relative.
- **Non-neurofibromatosis (non-NF1) congenital pseudarthrosis.** Fifty percent of cases of pseudarthrosis are not associated with NF1. As with NF1, patients may present at birth with apex anterolateral tibial bowing or with a bony defect due to pseudarthrosis. Some present as infants, when an area of weak bone fractures and does not heal, resulting in pseudarthrosis. The appearance is indistinguishable from pseudarthrosis in patients with NF1. A thorough systemic and familial evaluation is necessary to determine the presence of NF1 diagnostic criteria (see above).

■ Diagnosis

Tibial pseudarthrosis in a patient with neurofibromatosis type 1.

✓ Pearls

- Congenital pseudarthrosis in patients with or without neurofibromatosis type 1 typically develops in an area of bowed, dysplastic bone.
- Fifty percent of congenital pseudarthroses are associated with neurofibromatosis type 1.

- The presence or absence of associated diagnostic criteria is important for determining whether a pseudarthrosis is isolated or associated with neurofibromatosis type 1, since the radiographic appearance is similar.
- Posttraumatic pseudarthrosis is most common at the lateral condyle of the elbow.

Suggested Readings

Feldman DS, Jordan C, Fonseca L. Orthopaedic manifestations of neurofibromatosis type 1. J Am Acad Orthop Surg. 2010; 18(6):346–357

Pannier S. Congenital pseudarthrosis of the tibia. Orthop Traumatol Surg Res. 2011; 97(7):750–761

Patel NB, Stacy GS. Musculoskeletal manifestations of neurofibromatosis type 1. AJR Am J Roentgenol. 2012; 199(1):W99–W106

Case 96

Karen M. Ayotte

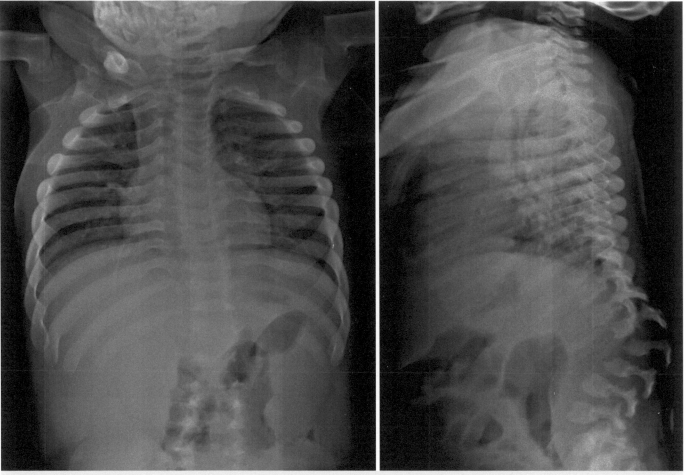

a

b

Fig. 96.1 Frontal radiograph shows broad, paddlelike ribs and thick proximal humeri **(a)**. The lateral spine radiograph shows mild concavity of the posterior vertebral bodies (vertebral scalloping), most pronounced from L2 to L5 **(b)**. L2 is hypoplastic, resulting in focal kyphosis. There is anterior beaking of multiple vertebral bodies.

■ Clinical Presentation
....

A child with hepatosplenomegaly and coarse facial features
(▶Fig. 96.1).

■ Key Imaging Finding

Posterior vertebral body scalloping.

■ Top Three Differential Diagnoses

- **Dural ectasia.** Dural ectasia refers to enlargement or widening of the dural sac. Common causes include connective tissue disorders, such as Marfan and Ehlers–Danlos syndromes, and neurofibromatosis (NF). The weak dura transmits pressure along the posterior aspect of the vertebral bodies, with resultant posterior vertebral body scalloping. In patients with NF, masses such as neurofibromas and thoracic meningoceles may also cause posterior vertebral body scalloping. Patients with Marfan and Ehlers–Danlos syndromes are prone to connective tissue abnormalities elsewhere, such as aneurysms. NF patients may have cutaneous and neurological manifestations of the disease.
- **Mucopolysaccharidosis (MPS).** These inherited disorders are caused by deficiencies in lysosomal enzymes necessary to break down certain complex carbohydrates. This leads to excessive accumulation and deposition of lysosomal glycosaminoglycans. Patients often present with short stature, craniofacial abnormalities, and in some cases mental retardation. There are multiple variants of MPS, with Hurler and Morquio

syndromes being the most common. Both syndromes are associated with diffuse posterior vertebral scalloping, but the mechanism is not established. Those with Hurler syndrome also demonstrate anterior beaking of the inferior aspect of the vertebral body, while patients with Morquio syndrome have anterior beaking in the midportion of the vertebral body. An enlarged, **J**-shaped sella is classically seen with Hurler syndrome.
- **Skeletal dysplasia/achondroplasia.** Achondroplasia is a common skeletal dysplasia, with autosomal-dominant inheritance. Radiographic findings include a large skull with narrow foramen magnum, spinal stenosis, squared iliac wings, progressively decreasing interpediculate distance in the lumbar spine, flat acetabula, short metacarpals, and short ribs. Posterior vertebral body scalloping is common and believed to be an adaptive response to congenital spinal stenosis. Posterior scalloping is also associated with metatropic dwarfism and osteogenesis imperfecta.

■ Additional Differential Diagnoses

- **Spinal tumor.** Intrathecal tumors may cause increased pressure within the spinal canal, leading to compensatory posterior vertebral body scalloping. The level of the vertebral scalloping typically corresponds to the location of the tumor. Common primary spinal cord tumors include ependymoma (most common primary cord tumor in adults) and astrocytoma (most common spinal cord tumor in children). Lipomas, dermoids/

epidermoids, and perineural cysts may also lead to mass effect and vertebral body scalloping.
- **Normal variant.** When mild and not associated with other skeletal abnormalities, posterior vertebral body scalloping may be a normal variant. Patients are typically followed after other causes are excluded.

■ Diagnosis

Mucopolysaccharidosis (Hurler syndrome).

✓ Pearls

- Dural ectasia with posterior vertebral body scalloping occurs in connective tissue disorders and neurofibromatosis.
- Mucopolysaccharidoses (Hurler and Morquio syndromes) show posterior scalloping and anterior beaking of the vertebral body.

- Intrathecal tumors may show focal posterior vertebral scalloping (and wide interpediculate distance).
- Mild posterior vertebral body scalloping may be a normal developmental variant.

Suggested Readings

Lachman R, Martin KW, Castro S, Basto MA, Adams A, Teles EL. Radiologic and neuroradiologic findings in the mucopolysaccharidoses. J Pediatr Rehabil Med. 2010; 3(2):109–118

Wakely SL. The posterior vertebral scalloping sign. Radiology. 2006; 239(2):607–609

Case 97

Rebecca Stein-Wexler

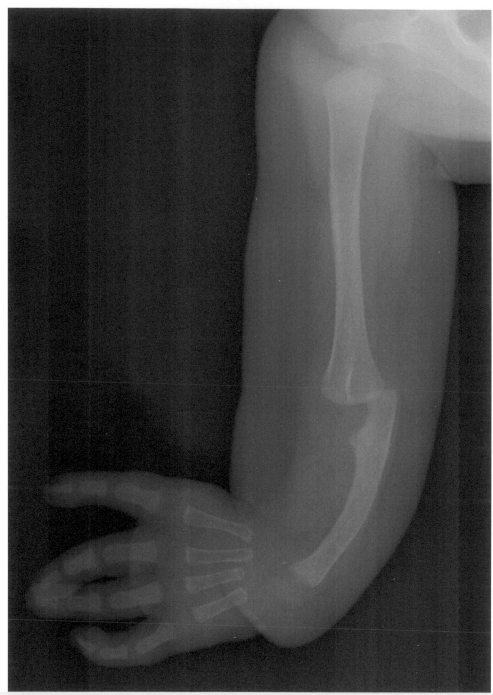

Fig. 97.1 Frontal radiograph of the upper extremity shows no ossified radius. The ulna is short, thick, bowed, and sclerotic, and it appears subluxated. There are only four rays, with the thumb and first metacarpal absent.

■ Clinical Presentation

A 1-year-old with a deformed hand (▶ Fig. 97.1).

■ Key Imaging Finding

Limb deficiency.

■ Top Three Differential Diagnoses

- **Longitudinal deficiency of the fibula.** In this condition, the fibula may be partly or completely absent, or it may simply be mildly hypoplastic. The anomaly is often accompanied by proximal focal femoral deficiency, coxa vara, clubfoot, and absent lateral rays. The remainder of the skeleton is usually normal. Perhaps counterintuitively, femoral abnormalities are more common with a hypoplastic fibula than with one that is completely absent. A cartilaginous fibular anlage is often present, which tethers growth of the tibia. If the hip and/or femur is clearly abnormal as well, the diagnosis may be made in utero. If the fibula is absent or markedly hypoplastic, X-ray diagnosis is straightforward. The tibia is often bowed, short, and thick. However, subtle cases are diagnosed by an abnormally high distal fibular physis (above the proximal tibial physis). Treatment is directed at establishing a usable weight-bearing lower extremity and often involves amputation. Longitudinal deficiency of the tibia is much less common than that of the fibula.
- **Longitudinal deficiency of the radius.** This sporadic condition usually consists of complete absence of the radius. However, the deficiency may be more limited and is occasionally manifested only by absence or hypoplasia of the thumb. One-third of patients are otherwise normal, but one-third have a syndrome, such as thrombocytopenia-absent radius (TAR), **V**ertebral anomalies, **A**nal atresia, **C**ardiac defects, **T**racheo-**E**sophageal fistula, **R**enal anomalies, with or without **L**imb malformations (VACTERL), or Holt–Oram syndrome. One-third have nonsyndromic-associated bone anomalies, with the likelihood of this increasing with the severity of deficiency. The radius is partly or (more often) completely absent, and the thumb is hypoplastic or absent. The ulna is short and bowed. If the radius is partially present, it may be fused with the ulna, and the radial head is often congenitally dislocated. The hand may be at a right angle to the forearm (radial clubhand).
- **Proximal focal femoral deficiency (PFFD).** This nonhereditary malformation ranges from mild dysgenesis of the proximal femur to near-complete absence of the entire bone. Usually isolated and unilateral, it may be part of caudal regression syndrome. The tibia and fibula may be hypoplastic as well. The condition is classified according to the presence of the femoral head, connection between the femoral head and the shaft (bony, cartilaginous, or absent), and extent of acetabular dysplasia. US and MRI assess nonossified structures.

■ Additional Differential Diagnosis

- **Longitudinal deficiency of the ulna.** At least part of the ulna is usually present in this disorder, which is more common in boys, usually on the right, and infrequently bilateral. Anomalies of the hand, wrist, and elbow bones are more severe than with radial deficiency. Carpal bones and digits are often missing or fused. Clubhand alignment is uncommon. Remote bony anomalies are common, including scoliosis, phocomelia, and PFFD. Other organ systems are usually normal. X-rays usually show a hypoplastic ulna, with ossification sometimes delayed until age 2 years. The radius appears bowed and short. The radial head may be normal, dislocated, or fused to the humerus. The rays are often deficient or fused.

■ Diagnosis

Longitudinal deficiency of the radius with clubhand.

✓ Pearls

- Mild cases of fibular longitudinal deficiency are diagnosed by an unusually high distal fibular physis.
- One-third of patients with longitudinal deficiency of the radius have an accompanying syndrome.
- US and MRI are useful for evaluating nonossified cartilaginous structures in proximal focal femoral deficiency.

Suggested Readings

Birch JG, Lincoln TL, Mack PW, et al. Congenital fibular deficiency: a review of 30 years' experience at one institution. J Bone Joint Surg Am. 2011; 93:1144–1151

Stein-Wexler R. The elbow and forearm: congenital and developmental conditions. In Stein-Wexler R, Wootton-Gorges SL, Ozonoff MB, eds. Pediatric Orthopedic Imaging. Berlin/Heidelberg: Springer; 2015:159–186

Case 98

Rebecca Stein-Wexler

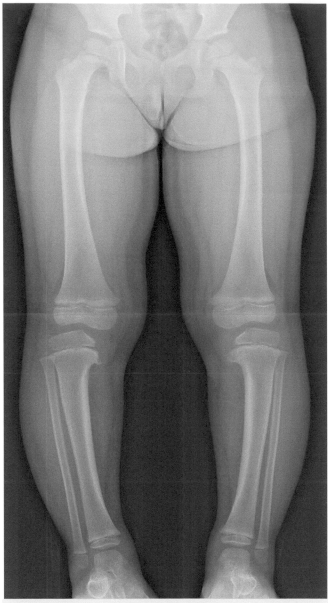

Fig. 98.1 Standing view of both lower extremities shows mild genu varus. The proximal medial tibial metaphyses are beaked and mildly depressed, and there is sclerosis and thickening of the medial tibial cortices.

■ Clinical Presentation

A 3-year-old girl with bowed legs (▶ Fig. 98.1).

■ Key Imaging Finding

Genu varum.

■ Top Three Differential Diagnoses

- **Physiological bowing.** Tibial bowing is a common normal developmental finding until age 2 years, but it does increase the risk of developing pathological tibia vara. It results from either intrauterine molding or delayed transition to normal mild genu valgus. Measurement depends on the tibiofemoral angle, which is the angle subtended by lines drawn longitudinally to the diaphyses. In infants, up to 16 to 20 degrees of varus angulation at the knee is normal, but by about age 3 years this should change to 10-degree valgus. Images show prominent but nonfragmented medial proximal tibial beaks. Distal femoral and proximal tibial medial epiphyses are wedge-shaped. Medial cortical thickening of femurs and tibias resolves as the bones straighten.
- **Blount disease (tibia vara).** Obesity or early walking stresses the posteromedial proximal tibial metaphysis, leading to deformity of the epiphysis and physeal damage due to shearing stress. Like developmental bowing, this condition is more common in African-Americans. Infantile Blount disease presents before age 4 years, whereas juvenile and adolescent forms manifest in older children, likely constituting later presentations of the same disease. Infantile Blount disease is defined by a tibial metaphyseal/diaphyseal angle of at least 16

degrees. Early cases show only metaphyseal beaking, but as disease progresses the metaphysis becomes more irregular, depressed, and possibly fragmented. The tibia may subluxate laterally. Conservative treatment with orthoses is effective in mild cases of infantile Blount disease. Severe or delayed disease may be treated with realignment wedge osteotomy. MRI is primarily employed to evaluate for formation of a medial physeal bar, which, if present, mandates more complex surgery.
- **Rickets.** Cartilage accumulates due to deficient growth plate cartilage and osteoid mineralization, leading to growth failure and osseous deformity. Nutritional vitamin D deficiency and X-linked hypophosphatemia are the most common underlying metabolic abnormalities. The growth plate widens due to disorganized, excessive cartilage. The metaphyses and metaphyseal equivalents of rapidly growing bones are most severely affected: wrist, knees, and anterior ribs. Insufficiency fractures, periosteal new bone, and bowing are seen in the diaphyses. Lower extremity bowing develops as children begin to stand. In addition to bowing, X-rays show physeal widening and metaphyseal flaring, cupping, and fraying.

■ Additional Differential Diagnosis

- **Syndromic bowing.** Metaphyseal chondrodysplasia, osteogenesis imperfecta, neurofibromatosis, and other syndromes may cause genu varum due to a variety of mechanisms.

■ Diagnosis

Blount disease.

✓ Pearls

- Genu varus up to 16 to 20 degrees is normal in children younger than 2 years of age.
- Pathological tibia vara shows excess bowing in children younger than 2 years or bowing that persists beyond age 2 years.
- In Blount disease, metaphyseal beaking progresses to irregularity and sometimes fragmentation with lateral subluxation of the tibia.

- Rickets, commonly due to nutritional vitamin D deficiency or X-linked hypophosphatemia, shows physeal widening and metaphyseal cupping and fraying along with insufficiency fractures and diaphyseal bowing.

Suggested Readings

Cheema JI, Grissom LE, Harcke HT. Radiographic characteristics of lower-extremity bowing in children. Radiographics. 2003; 23(4):871–880

Ho-Fung V, Jaimes C, Delgado J, Davidson RS, Jaramillo D. MRI evaluation of the knee in children with infantile Blount disease: tibial and extra-tibial findings. Pediatr Radiol. 2013; 43(10):1316–1326

Shore RM, Chesney RW. Rickets: part I. Pediatr Radiol. 2013; 43(2):140–151

Shore RM, Chesney RW. Rickets: part II. Pediatr Radiol. 2013; 43(2):152–172

Case 99

Robert J. Wood and Sandra L. Wootton- Gorges

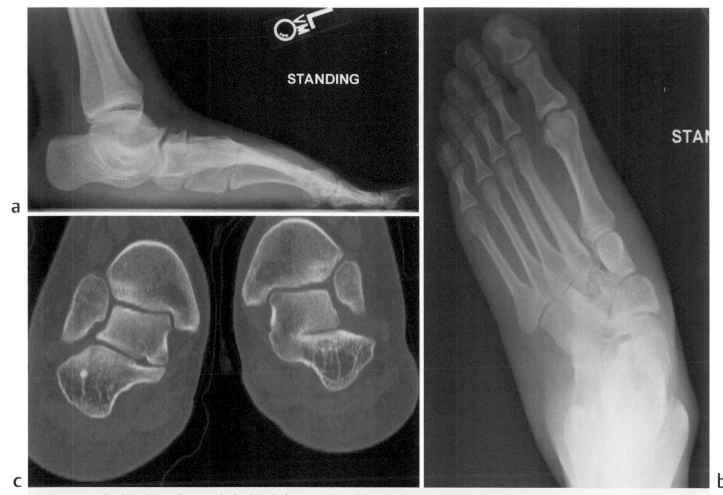

Fig. 99.1 Standing lateral view shows a talar beak and sclerosis at the middle subtalar joint as well as pes planus; nonvisualization of the subtalar joint results in the continuous "C" sign **(a)**. Standing frontal view shows hindfoot valgus **(b)**. Coronal reformatted CT shows left subtalar bony coalition **(c)**.

■ **Clinical Presentation**

A 16-year-old with painful flat foot deformity (▶ Fig. 99.1).

■ Key Imaging Finding

Tarsal coalition.

■ Top Three Differential Diagnoses

• **Talocalcaneal coalition.** Talocalcaneal (or subtalar) and calcaneonavicular are the most common tarsal coalitions. They result from failure of segmentation of the hindfoot bony anlage during development. Fusion between the talus and calcaneus may be osseous (*synostosis*), cartilaginous (*synchondrosis*), or fibrous (*syndesmosis*). Talocalcaneal coalition is bilateral in about half of cases, and boys are affected more often than girls. Patients usually present around age 12 to 16 years, classically complaining of painful flatfoot. Some patients have pes cavus, however, and many are asymptomatic. X-ray findings include a distal talar beak and continuous "C" sign (a continuous arc formed by the medial outline of the talar dome and postero-inferior aspect of the sustentaculum tali) on the lateral view. There is narrowing or obliteration of the subtalar joint on the Harris–Beath view. CT and MRI (especially coronal) provide more precise evaluation of the extent of coalition. MRI is especially useful for defining fibrous or cartilaginous coalition.

• **Calcaneonavicular coalition.** This fusion connects the calcaneus and navicular. Patients usually present at age 8 to 12 years, with symptoms similar to those for talocalcaneal coalition. Normal feet have no articulation between the calcaneus and the navicular, but in cases of coalition the anterior process of the calcaneus is elongated, providing an articulation with the inferolateral aspect of the navicular. The elongated anterior process results in the "anteater" sign, evident on the lateral view. The coalition itself is best seen on the oblique view. Radiographic findings on this view range from osseous apposition with a narrow articulation and marginal sclerosis (for fibrocartilaginous coalitions) to a solid bony bar connecting the calcaneus and navicular. Sagittal MRI facilitates detailed analysis of this coalition.

• **Talonavicular coalition.** This unusual coalition connects the talus and navicular. It may be bilateral in 25% and if symptomatic usually presents before age 10 years.

■ Additional Differential Diagnosis

• **Other coalitions.** Other or multiple coalitions are rare. They are often associated with congenital abnormalities such as longitudinal deficiency of the fibula or Apert syndrome.

■ Diagnosis

Talocalcaneal coalition.

✓ Pearls

• Talocalcaneal and calcaneonavicular coalitions are most common.
• Talocalcaneal coalition may show a talar beak and continuous "C" on the lateral view, with narrowing or fusion of the subtalar joint on the Harris–Beath view.

• Calcaneonavicular coalition may show an elongated anterior calcaneal process on the lateral view, and an osseous or fibrocartilaginous calcaneonavicular articulation on the oblique view.
• CT and MRI allow more precise evaluation of type of coalition—fibrous, cartilaginous, osseous, or combined.

Suggested Readings

Iyer RS, Thapa MM. MR imaging of the paediatric foot and ankle. Pediatr Radiol. 2013; 43 Suppl 1:S107–S119

Lawrence DA, Rolen MF, Haims AH, Zayour Z, Moukaddam HA. Tarsal coalitions: radiographic, CT and MR imaging findings. HSS J. 2014; 10(2):153–166

Mosca VS. Subtalar coalition in pediatrics. Foot Ankle Clin. 2015; 20(2):265–281

Case 100

Wonsuk Kim

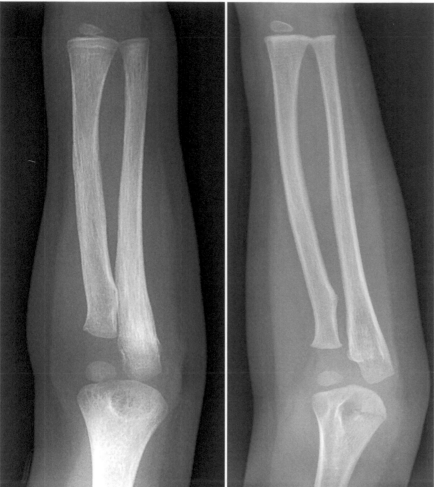

Fig. 100.1 There is subtle, ill-defined lucency in the metaphyses, most striking at the distal radius and ulna; the bone is osteopenic (a). Normal metaphyses for comparison, with supracondylar fracture (b).

a

b

■ Clinical Presentation

A 2-year-old boy with a complex medical history (▶Fig. 100.1).

■ Key Imaging Finding

Lucent metaphyses.

■ Top Three Differential Diagnoses

- **Leukemia.** Acute leukemia is the most common pediatric malignancy, and acute lymphocytic leukemia comprises the majority of cases. Radiographic abnormalities are seen in up to two-thirds of patients at diagnosis. Metaphyseal lucencies are the most common finding and occur at sites of fastest growth, such as the knees, ankles, and wrists. Other findings include periosteal reaction, focal osteolytic lesions, osteopenia, and fractures. Compression fractures of the spine are common.
- **Osteomyelitis.** Acute osteomyelitis is a significant cause of bone pathology in children, especially those younger than 5 years. Most cases are due to hematogenous spread and involve the metaphyses. Scintigraphy and MRI are more sensi-

tive than radiographs for early diagnosis. After about 10 days, radiographic findings such as ill-defined metaphyseal lucencies and periosteal bone formation may be seen.
- **Neuroblastoma.** Neuroblastoma commonly metastasizes to bone. Children with skeletal metastases may complain of bone pain and arthritis-like symptoms. Radiographic appearance resembles that of other small round blue cell tumors, such as Ewing sarcoma and leukemia. There may be periosteal reaction, one or more lytic foci, lucent horizontal metaphyseal lines, and pathological fractures. MRI, positron emission tomographic CT (PET-CT), and metaiodobenzylguanidine (MIBG) scans help assess for metastases.

■ Additional Differential Diagnoses

- **TORSCH.** TORSCH (toxoplasmosis, rubella, syphilis, cytomegalovirus [CMV], herpes) infections are acquired transplacentally and often affect the metaphyses. Syphilis and others may cause symmetrical lucent metaphyseal bands adjacent to a subphyseal dense band. Wimberger sign—symmetrical focal destruction of the medial proximal tibial metaphyses—is seen in about 50% of cases of congenital syphilis as well. Rubella classically leads to a "celery stalk" appearance with longitudinally arrayed linear striations extending from the epiphyses into the metaphyses. Other TORSCH infections may cause similar findings.

- **Rickets.** Rickets is caused by vitamin D deficiency and leads to decreased mineralization of physeal cartilage. X-ray findings of physeal widening, loss of the zone of provisional calcification, metaphyseal fraying, and metaphyseal cupping are most evident at the fastest growing long bones (wrist and knee).
- **Scurvy.** This lethal but treatable disease is caused by vitamin C deficiency. Radiographic findings include prominent zones of provisional calcification in the metaphyses ("white lines" of Frankel) with subjacent lines of demineralization ("scurvy lines") and physeal widening.

■ Diagnosis

Osseous acute lymphocytic leukemia.

✓ Pearls

- Metaphyseal lucent bands are commonly seen with leukemia.
- TORSCH infections may manifest metaphyseal lucency with a "celery-stalk" appearance.

- Bony metastases are common in neuroblastoma and may show periosteal reaction, metaphyseal lucencies, lucent foci in other locations as well, and pathological fractures.

Suggested Readings

Blickman JG, van Die CE, de Rooy JW. Current imaging concepts in pediatric osteomyelitis. Eur Radiol. 2004; 14 Suppl 4:L55–L64

Mostoufi-Moab S, Halton J. Bone morbidity in childhood leukemia: epidemiology, mechanisms, diagnosis, and treatment. Curr Osteoporos Rep. 2014; 12(3):300–312

Ranson M. Imaging of pediatric musculoskeletal infection. Semin Musculoskelet Radiol. 2009; 13(3):277–299

Case 101

Rebecca Stein-Wexler

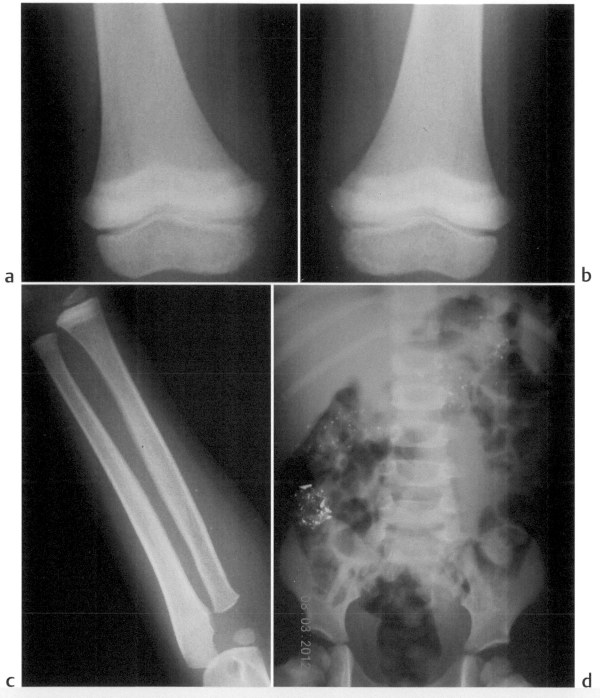

Fig. 101.1 Both knees show wide, sclerotic metaphyseal bands **(a,b)**. Similar bands of sclerosis are seen at the distal radius and ulna, but not at the proximal ends of these bones **(c)**. Supine abdomen radiograph shows flecks of dense material in the colon **(d)**.

■ **Clinical Presentation**

A 2-year-old with abdominal pain (▶Fig. 101.1).

■ Key Imaging Finding

Dense metaphyses.

■ Top Three Differential Diagnoses

- **Physiological dense metaphyses.** In healthy young children age 2 to 6 years, increased metaphyseal density may be seen during periods of prolonged exposure to sunlight, especially common after winter. The exact mechanism is unknown, but this phenomenon may result from overproduction of endogenous vitamin D. Clues to diagnosis are that (1) at the knee the proximal end of the fibula appears normal, with no dense band, and (2) the dense band is no more dense than the diaphyseal or metaphyseal cortex.
- **Lead toxicity (plumbism).** Lead toxicity is most common between ages 1 and 3 years. It results from inhalation of lead dust or ingestion of contaminated water or fragments of lead paint. When serum lead levels exceed 50 µg/dL, excess lead impairs osteoclast function, leading to failure of bone resorption in the zone of provisional calcification. Bilateral, symmetrical, dense metaphyseal bands develop—typically denser than the cortex of the adjacent metaphysis or diaphysis. Such a band at the proximal end of the fibula is useful for diagnosis, since density in this area does not increase even with physiological dense metaphyses. If high lead levels persist, growth deformity, such as Erlenmeyer flask deformity, may develop. Other heavy metals have a similar effect. Although radiological findings are suggestive, diagnosis rests on laboratory tests.
- **Treated leukemia.** After treatment for leukemia, the metaphyses may appear dense. However, children with leukemia more often demonstrate lucent metaphyses.

■ Additional Differential Diagnoses

- **Healing rickets.** Although patients with active rickets have frayed, flared, cupped metaphyses with widening of the physis, healing bone shows dense juxtaphyseal metaphyseal bands. This is most pronounced in the metaphyses or metaphyseal equivalents of rapidly growing bones: the wrists, knees, and anterior ribs.
- **Bisphosphonate therapy.** Bisphosphonates treat patients with osteoporosis, usually due to osteogenesis imperfecta, steroid treatment, and neuromuscular disorders. These drugs increase bone density by inhibiting osteoclast-mediated bone resorption. Cyclical therapy leads to thin dense metaphyseal lines that parallel the physis in long bones ("zebra stripes") and a "bone-within-bone" appearance of the spine and flat bones.
- **Syphilis.** In utero infection with *Treponema pallidum* may lead to bone abnormalities that manifest during the first 2 months of life. A dense sclerotic band may be positioned between the physis and the abnormally lucent metaphysis. About 50% of patients demonstrate the Wimberger sign, focal osteolysis of the medial proximal tibial metaphysis. Pathological fractures and periosteal new bone formation may be present as well. Patients may have a rash, hepatosplenomegaly, anemia, ascites, and nephrotic syndrome.

■ Diagnosis

Lead toxicity.

✓ Pearls

- Physiological dense metaphyses appear no denser than adjacent cortex and spare the proximal fibula.
- Although active rickets is characterized by wide, frayed metaphysis, during the treatment phase the metaphyses may appear dense.
- If lead levels exceed 50 µg/dL, dense metaphyseal bands may develop.
- Infants with syphilis may show a dense band between the physis and the abnormally lucent metaphysis.

Suggested Readings

Raber SA. The dense metaphyseal band sign. Radiology. 1999; 211(3):773–774
States LJ. Imaging of metabolic bone disease and marrow disorders in children. Radiol Clin North Am. 2001; 39(4):749–772

Case 102

Rebecca Stein-Wexler

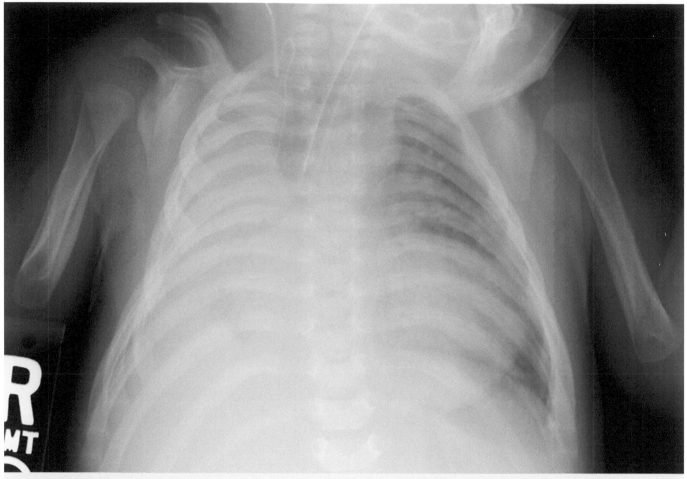

Fig. 102.1 Thick, smooth periosteal thickening affects the diaphyses and distal metaphyses of both humeri, as well as the clavicles and ribs (note vascular catheter and low endotracheal tube).

■ Clinical Presentation

A 3-month-old with cyanotic heart disease (▶Fig. 102.1).

▪ Key Imaging Finding

Periosteal thickening.

▪ Top Three Differential Diagnoses

- **Physiological periostitis of infancy.** In up to half of all infants between ages 1 and 6 months, rapid growth and relatively loose, thick periosteum may lead to periosteal thickening. Both the upper and lower extremities may be affected, and findings are typically symmetrical. The tibia is most commonly involved. Initially, a faint, amorphous line parallels the cortex; with time, the new bone thickens and becomes denser. This is eventually absorbed into the cortex, contributing to transverse bone growth. Unlike pathological periosteal thickening, physiological periostitis spares the metaphysis and is relatively thin (<2 mm).
- **Trauma.** Periosteal new bone formation may manifest as early as 7 to 10 days after injury, becoming progressively denser

and thicker until it is incorporated into adjacent bone, beginning about 2 months post injury. There may be no associated fracture in cases of stress reaction, or with nonaccidental trauma. Unlike physiological periostitis of infancy, periosteal new bone formation resulting from trauma may involve the metaphysis.
- **Infection.** MRI may show periosteal elevation by day 2, and by about days 7 to 10 lamellar periosteal thickening may be radiographically evident. Chronic osteomyelitis may show thick, ossified periosteal reaction ("involucrum").

▪ Additional Differential Diagnoses

- **Neoplasm.** Slow-growing tumors are often associated with solid periosteal reaction, whereas aggressive lesions classically show a lamellated, spiculated, or interrupted (Codman triangle) periosteal reaction.
- **Prostaglandin therapy.** Children with cyanotic heart disease who are treated with prostaglandins may develop diffuse, symmetrical periosteal new bone formation as early as 6 days but more often 30 to 40 days from treatment onset. Remodeling eventually occurs.

- **Caffey disease (infantile cortical hyperostosis).** This rare, self-limited disease usually affects infants younger than 5 months. Painful, often asymmetrical periosteal inflammation leads to lamellar periosteal thickening and eventual remodeling. The mandible is classically involved, but many bones may be affected.

▪ Diagnosis

Periosteal thickening due to prostaglandin therapy.

✓ Pearls

- Physiological periostitis is typically symmetrical, measures less than 2 mm, and spares the metaphysis.
- With nonaccidental trauma and stress reaction, periosteal new bone formation may be the only sign of injury.

- The periosteal thickening in infants treated with prostaglandins is usually symmetrical, whereas with Caffey disease it is often asymmetrical.

Suggested Readings

Kwon DS, Spevak MR, Fletcher K, Kleinman PK. Physiologic subperiosteal new bone formation: prevalence, distribution, and thickness in neonates and infants. AJR Am J Roentgenol. 2002; 179(4):985–988

Poznanski AK, Fernbach SK, Berry TE. Bone changes from prostaglandin therapy. Skeletal Radiol. 1985; 14(1):20–25

Wenaden AE, Szyszko TA, Saifuddin A. Imaging of periosteal reactions associated with focal lesions of bone. Clin Radiol. 2005; 60(4):439–456

Case 103

Wonsuk Kim

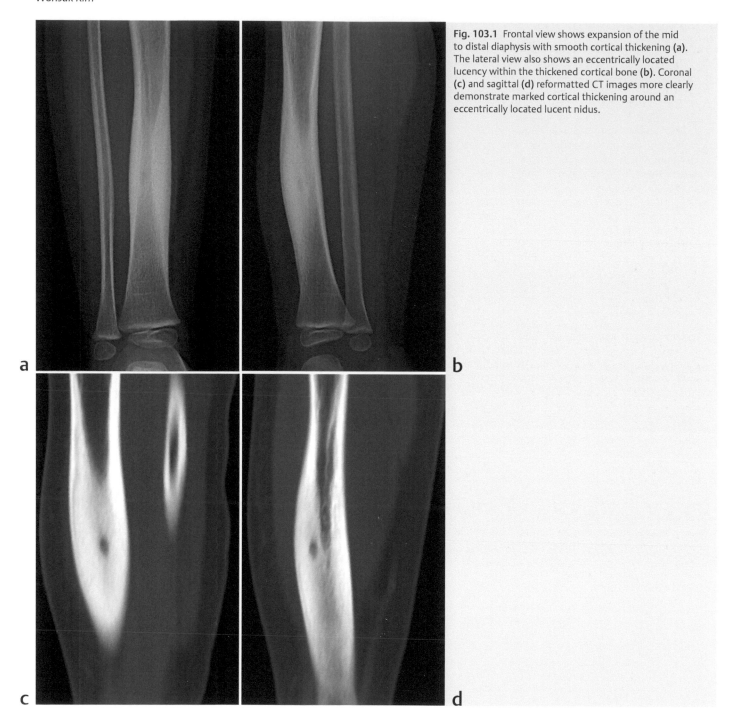

Fig. 103.1 Frontal view shows expansion of the mid to distal diaphysis with smooth cortical thickening **(a)**. The lateral view also shows an eccentrically located lucency within the thickened cortical bone **(b)**. Coronal **(c)** and sagittal **(d)** reformatted CT images more clearly demonstrate marked cortical thickening around an eccentrically located lucent nidus.

■ **Clinical Presentation**

A child with pain in the lower leg (▶ Fig. 103.1).

■ Key Imaging Finding

Cortical thickening.

■ Top Three Differential Diagnoses

- **Stress fracture.** Children and adolescents are prone to stress (fatigue) fractures, which occur when normal bone is subjected to abnormal activity. The most common etiology of fatigue fractures is chronic and repetitive workload. The tibia and fibula are most often affected in children, but the femur, tarsals, and metatarsals may be involved. Radiographs are relatively insensitive and detect 15% of fractures in the acute setting. Manifestations vary with age and type of load. Tibial/fibular toddler fractures, associated with onset of ambulation, may show a slight linear lucency and, as they heal, periosteal reaction and eventual smooth cortical thickening, whereas tarsal fractures manifest as a band of sclerosis due to callus. MRI is more sensitive and specific and demonstrates marrow edema and a hypointense fracture line. Scintigraphy is sensitive but nonspecific.
- **Osteoid osteoma.** Osteoid osteoma typically presents in patients under age 20 years, about twice as often in males. Classic presentation is pain at night, relieved by salicylates. These diaphyseal or metaphyseal lesions are typically eccentric. More than half of these lesions occur in the tibia or femur, with most others in the spine, hands, or feet. X-rays show a lucent nidus, typically less than 1 cm in diameter and surrounded by a rim of sclerosis. MRI shows the lesion, along with bone marrow and soft-tissue edema. The goal of treatment is removal or destruction of the nidus, performed surgically or by image-guided percutaneous thermoablation.
- **Chronic osteomyelitis.** Chronic osteomyelitis is sometimes characterized by sequestra (necrotic bone in an area of inflammation) and involucra (periosteal new bone formation around dead bone). The radiographic appearance is of diffuse cortical thickening, sometimes with a lucent central lesion. One-third of cases occur in patients younger than 2 years, with a 2:1 male predominance. Over 75% of cases involve the long bones, especially the faster growing bones and metaphyses. MRI and scintigraphy may be helpful. Other findings that suggest infection include marrow edema, subperiosteal fluid, and a sinus tract, with relatively little soft-tissue involvement. Tissue biopsy is often necessary for confirmation.

■ Additional Differential Diagnosis

- **Osteoblastoma.** Osteoblastoma is a rare, benign tumor that is most common in the flat bones or the vertebrae (posterior elements) and less common in the extremities. Though a distinct entity, it may mimic the appearance of a large osteoid osteoma (but osteoblastoma is larger). It may be blastic, lytic, or mixed, and well defined, exophytic, or aggressive. On histological analysis, there is osteoid and pure woven bone production, occasionally with focal osteoblastic rimming.

■ Diagnosis

Osteoid osteoma.

✓ Pearls

- Radiographs are relatively insensitive for stress fractures but may show subtle periosteal reaction.
- Osteoid osteoma is an eccentrically located benign lesion with a lucent nidus surrounded by sclerosis.
- MRI findings in chronic osteomyelitis may include sequestra and involucra, marrow edema, subperiosteal fluid, and a sinus tract, with relatively little involvement of surrounding soft tissues.
- Osteoblastoma is a rare, benign tumor that may appear blastic, lytic, or mixed.

Suggested Readings

Blickman JG, van Die CE, de Rooy JW. Current imaging concepts in pediatric osteomyelitis. Eur Radiol. 2004; 14 Suppl 4:L55–L64

Jaimes C, Jimenez M, Shabshin N, Laor T, Jaramillo D. Taking the stress out of evaluating stress injuries in children. Radiographics. 2012; 32(2):537–555

Levine SM, Lambiase RE, Petchprapa CN. Cortical lesions of the tibia: characteristic appearances at conventional radiography. Radiographics. 2003; 23(1):157–177

Case 104

Stephen Henrichon

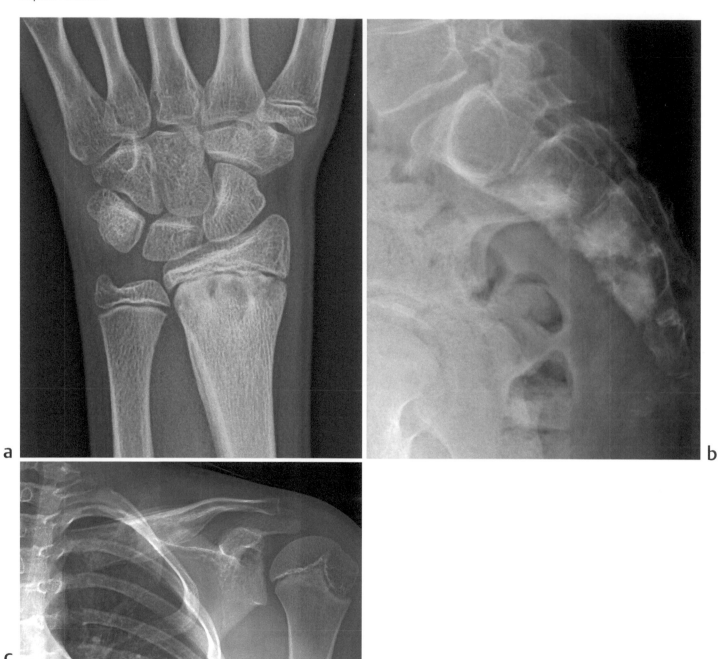

a

b

c

Fig. 104.1 There is patchy sclerosis and lucency at the distal radial metaphysis **(a)**. Multiple sacral segments demonstrate ill-defined sclerotic foci **(b)**. The clavicle appears heterogeneous, and there is lamellated periosteal thickening **(c)**.

■ Clinical Presentation

A 13-year-old girl with recurrent bone pain (▶Fig. 104.1).

■ Key Imaging Finding

Multiple sclerotic lesions.

■ Top Three Differential Diagnoses

- **Chronic recurrent multifocal osteomyelitis (CRMO).** CRMO is a nonbacterial inflammatory disorder that presents in early adolescence with pain and swelling. Early findings include multiple lytic lesions, often at the medial clavicle (not typical of bacterial osteomyelitis), metaphyses of long bones, spine, pelvis, mandible, and hands/feet. Lesions are initially lytic but become sclerotic. Adjacent joints are commonly involved. MRI initially shows high T2 signal in the marrow and surrounding tissue. Mature lesions are hypointense on T1- and T2-W MRI corresponding to sclerosis. Diffuse enhancement may be present.
- **Metastatic disease.** Most pediatric bone metastases are lytic, but medulloblastoma, neuroblastoma, osteosarcoma, and rarely lymphoma may appear sclerotic. Langerhans cell histiocytosis may occasionally appear sclerotic. Metastases from neuroblastoma, retinoblastoma, Ewing sarcoma, and rhabdomyosarcoma are usually lytic. Lesions may have sharp or ill-defined margins and may expand bone. Pathological fractures are common. Periosteal reaction is not typical except in neuroblastoma and retinoblastoma. Nuclear medicine bone scan optimally assesses skeletal distribution. Active lesions usually show increased radiotracer uptake, but large, lytic lesions may demonstrate photopenia. Whole body MRI is used in some centers.
- **Chronic osteomyelitis.** Bacterial osteomyelitis spreads hematogenously and is uncommonly multifocal. Metaphyseal involvement is typical. The acute phase is characterized by osteopenia, periostitis, and progressive osteolysis. However, indolent, unsuccessfully treated, or otherwise progressive cases may lead to chronic osteomyelitis. Radiographs of chronic osteomyelitis show heterogeneous sclerosis and thick periosteal reaction. There may be infarcted bone in the medullary cavity ("sequestrum") and a draining tract ("cloaca"). MRI generally shows less soft-tissue inflammation than is seen in acute osteomyelitis.

■ Additional Differential Diagnoses

- **Tuberculosis (TB).** TB spreads hematogenously to bones and joints, most often to the spine, hips, knees, and elbows. It manifests in the spine as "TB spondylitis," also known as Pott disease (usually low thoracic and lumbar, resulting in kyphosis). Multilevel involvement is typical, and intervertebral disks are often affected in children. Painless paraspinal abscesses are very common. Calcifications within an abscess suggest TB. Lytic lesions may be seen on X-ray, whereas MRI shows marrow and (in the spine) intervertebral disk edema as well as enhancement. Fifty percent of patients have concomitant pulmonary disease.
- **Melorheostosis.** This nonfamilial mesenchymal dysplasia appears as "dripping candle wax" sclerosis, along one or several bones in one sclerotome of an extremity. A painless condition, melorheostosis develops in early childhood and is diagnosed in about half of patients by age 20 years.

■ Diagnosis

Chronic recurrent multifocal osteomyelitis.

✓ Pearls

- Chronic recurrent multifocal osteomyelitis resembles osteomyelitis but is nonbacterial; it commonly involves the clavicle.
- Most skeletal metastases in children are lytic, but medulloblastoma, neuroblastoma, osteosarcoma, lymphoma, and Langerhans cell histiocytosis may appear sclerotic.
- Chronic osteomyelitis may demonstrate a sequestrum and/or cloaca.

Suggested Readings

Iyer RS, Thapa MM, Chew FS. Chronic recurrent multifocal osteomyelitis: review. Review AJR Am J Roentgenol. 2011; 196(6) Suppl:S87–S91

Jaramillo D. Infection: musculoskeletal. Pediatr Radiol. 2011; 41 Suppl 1: S127–S134

Khanna G, Sato TS, Ferguson P. Imaging of chronic recurrent multifocal osteomyelitis. Radiographics. 2009; 29(4):1159–1177

Case 105

Rebecca Stein-Wexler

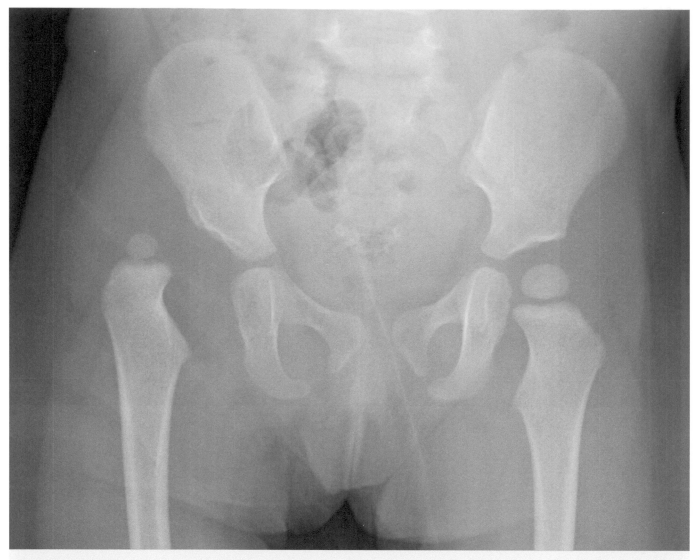

Fig. 105.1 Frontal pelvic radiograph with hips neutral shows the right femoral head projects superolateral to a shallow, irregular acetabulum, whereas the left is normal.

■ Clinical Presentation

A 1-year-old with limited abduction of the right hip (▶Fig. 105.1).

■ Key Imaging Finding

Dislocated hip.

■ Top Three Differential Diagnoses

- **Developmental dysplasia of the hip (DDH).** DDH is most common in infants who are female, firstborn, and/or with breech presentation or a family history of DDH or joint laxity. The Barlow maneuver attempts to displace the femoral head by pistoning the flexed hip. The Ortolani maneuver attempts to reduce a displaced hip by flexion and abduction. US is used for diagnosis until age 6 months, when ossification of the femoral head causes too much acoustic shadowing. The coronal view best depicts acetabular contour, with an "alpha angle" of 60 degrees or more considered normal. Transverse flexion views best depict femoral head motion within the acetabulum. In older children, the acetabulum and femoral head position are assessed on X-rays. Pavlik harness treatment is usually successful. Occasionally casting is needed. Refractory DDH may be treated with acetabuloplasty to improve acetabular angle and coverage, along with femoral osteotomy to improve the position of the femoral head. Limited CT or MRI is then employed to assess hip position.

- **Neuromuscular disorder.** The hip may subluxate and eventually dislocate in patients with cerebral palsy (CP) and other spastic neuromuscular conditions. With hyperactive adductor and iliopsoas muscles leading to persistent hip adduction, the acetabulum becomes oblique and shallow. Severe subluxation is common by age 7 years in patients with spastic CP. However, lateral coverage of the femoral head may be reduced for other reasons, such as disparity in size between a small acetabulum and a large femoral head, pelvic obliquity, adduction contracture, or femoral neck valgus/anteversion.

- **Trauma.** A traumatic hemarthrosis may lead to posterolateral subluxation or rarely dislocation of the hip. In cases where the femoral head has not ossified, a Salter I fracture with lateral displacement of the distal fragment may mimic femoral head dislocation. This may be seen with nonaccidental trauma. Severe trauma, such as motor vehicle collision, may cause posterior dislocation of the femoral head.

■ Additional Differential Diagnosis

- **Teratologic hip dysplasia.** The incidence of hip dysplasia is increased with many skeletal dysplasias and syndromes. For example, as many as 5% of ambulatory children with trisomy 21 have recurrent hip subluxation or dislocation. Patients with Ehlers–Danlos syndrome and Larsen syndrome also have an increased incidence of hip dislocation.

■ Diagnosis

Developmental dysplasia of the hip.

✓ Pearls

- Developmental dysplasia of the hip is most common in girls and first-borns, and in those with breech presentation and/or a family history of ligamentous laxity.
- Hip US is most useful until age 6 months.
- Patients with spastic cerebral palsy have increased incidence of hip dislocation due to persistent hip adduction.

- Before the femoral head ossifies, Salter I fracture of the proximal femoral physis with lateral displacement of the metaphysis, which may occur with nonaccidental trauma, mimics developmental dysplasia of the hip.

Suggested Readings

Grissom LE. The pelvis and hip: congenital and developmental conditions. In Stein-Wexler R, Wootton-Gorges SL, Ozonoff MB, eds. Pediatric Orthopedic Imaging. Berlin/Heidelberg: Springer; 2015:273–318

Hägglund G, Lauge-Pedersen H, Wagner P. Characteristics of children with hip displacement in cerebral palsy. BMC Musculoskelet Disord. 2007; 8:101

Harcke HT. The role of ultrasound in diagnosis and management of developmental dysplasia of the hip. Pediatr Radiol. 1995; 25(3):225–227

Case 106

Rebecca Stein-Wexler

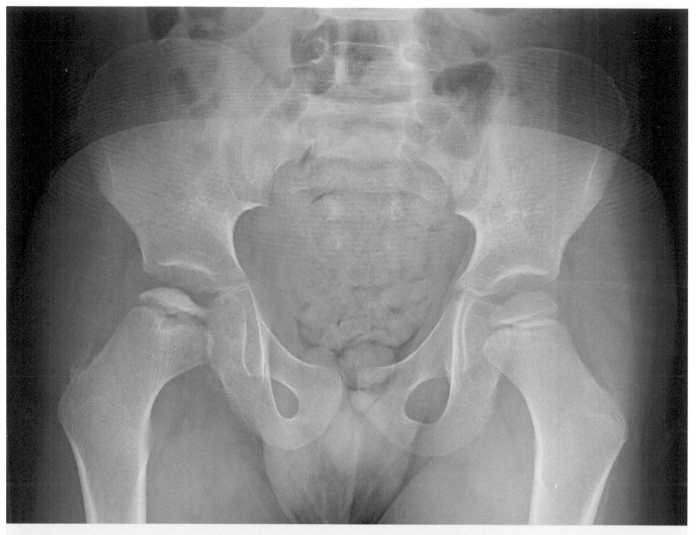

Fig. 106.1 Frontal radiograph of the pelvis shows the right femoral head is dense, small, and irregular.

■ Clinical Presentation

A 5-year-old boy with a limp (▶Fig. 106.1).

■ Key Imaging Finding

Avascular necrosis (AVN) of the femoral head.

■ Top Three Differential Diagnoses

• **Legg–Calvé–Perthes.** This condition is most common between ages 4 and 9 years, especially in boys. About 10% of cases are bilateral. Patients typically have no history of trauma and present with a limp and decreased range of motion. AVN of the femoral head results from impaired epiphyseal blood supply across the physis. MRI allows earliest detection, demonstrating linear hypointensity on coronal T1-W sequences. In more advanced cases, T2-W MRI allows assessment of articular cartilage. Initial radiographs may show widening of the hip joint, subchondral lucency, and diminished height of the femoral head. The epiphysis then becomes denser, flattened, and fragmented. The paraphyseal metaphysis may become cystic. In the reparative stage, normal bone replaces sclerotic bone, and the femoral head appears smoother and less heterogeneous. Femoral head contour as well as congruence between the femoral head and the acetabulum determine long-term prognosis.

• **Traumatic injury.** Traumatic injury to the fragile blood vessels that traverse the physis may cause femoral head ischemia and subsequent AVN. This may result from a specific episode of trauma or from reduction of a dislocated hip. In the latter setting, risk for AVN may be proportional to the degree of flexion and abduction.

• **Sickle cell disease.** Sickled erythrocytes occlude vessels, and subsequent hypoxemia further increases vascular distortion, exacerbating ischemia. The femoral and humeral heads are commonly involved, along with the vertebral endplates and the diametaphyseal region of the long bones.

■ Additional Differential Diagnoses

• **Corticosteroid use.** Corticosteroid use predisposes to AVN due to a variety of mechanisms, including demineralization and occlusion of small vessels by fat emboli. Risk is greatest with high doses and relatively short-duration treatment. Corticosteroid-induced AVN is more likely to be bilateral.

• **Gaucher disease.** This manifests as inability to clear glucosylceramide from the reticuloendothelial system. Resultant increased pressure occludes interosseous sinusoids, causing infarction. Additional radiographic findings include osteopenia, medullary expansion, and bony remodeling (Erlenmeyer flask).

• **Meyer dysplasia.** Meyer dysplasia affects the proximal femoral epiphyses, which appear irregular and small. It occurs between ages 2 and 4 years, especially in boys. Meyer dysplasia is painless and often bilateral. The radiographic appearance mimics AVN. The epiphyses of patients with epiphyseal dysplasia and spondyloepiphyseal dysplasia may also resemble AVN.

■ Diagnosis

Legg–Calvé–Perthes disease.

✓ Pearls

• MRI is more sensitive than radiography for detecting early avascular necrosis.

• Legg–Calvé–Perthes disease results in avascular necrosis in the absence of trauma; it is more common in boys and is usually unilateral.

• Trauma may cause avascular necrosis by disrupting blood supply to the femoral head.

• Sickle cell disease may cause avascular necrosis due to vascular occlusion; corticosteroid use predisposes to bilateral avascular necrosis.

Suggested Readings

Dillman JR, Hernandez RJ. MRI of Legg-Calve-Perthes disease. AJR Am J Roentgenol. 2009; 193(5):1394–1407

Dwek JR. The hip: MR imaging of uniquely pediatric disorders. Magn Reson Imaging Clin N Am. 2009; 17(3):509–520, vi

Mankin HJ. Nontraumatic necrosis of bone (osteonecrosis). N Engl J Med. 1992; 326(22):1473–1479

Case 107

Robert J. Wood and Sandra L. Wootton-Gorges

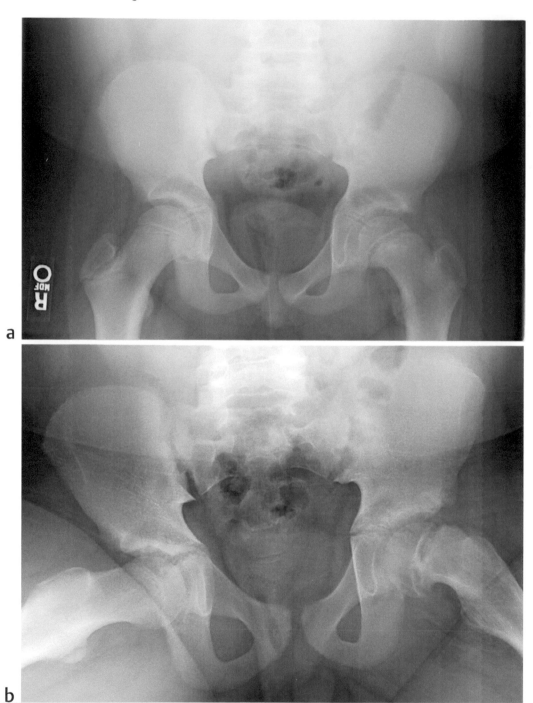

Fig. 107.1 Frontal view with hips neutral shows a normal right hip and, on the left, physeal widening along with subtle relative decreased height of the femoral head. The entire femoral head is positioned medial to Klein line (a). The frog lateral view shows the left femoral head projects posteromedial to the femoral neck. The "ice cream scoop" of the femoral head is offset from the "cone" of the femoral neck (b).

■ Clinical Presentation

A 12-year-old boy with limp and hip pain (▶Fig. 107.1).

■ Key Imaging Finding

Physeal widening.

■ Top Three Differential Diagnoses

- **Salter–Harris type I fracture.** This relatively uncommon fracture results from a shearing force that parallels the growth plate. It is most often seen in children younger than 5 years of age. Although transient displacement is common, the fracture usually reduces spontaneously before imaging, making diagnosis difficult. Comparison with the contralateral side may be helpful.
- **Slipped capital femoral epiphysis (SCFE).** This Salter–Harris I shearing fracture of the capital femoral physis is the most common hip problem of adolescence. It is more common in boys, in African-Americans, and in overweight patients with mildly delayed skeletal maturation. Children with endocrinopathies, especially those with hypothyroidism or undergoing growth hormone therapy, are more likely to develop SCFE. SCFE is bilateral at presentation in about 10%, but up to one-third will eventually develop SCFE in the contralateral hip. Patients present with limp and hip or knee pain. Those with "stable" SCFE can walk, whereas those with "unstable" SCFE cannot. The frontal neutral view shows physeal widening, a relatively short-appearing femoral head (due to rotation), and no femoral head projecting lateral to Klein line (drawn along the lateral femoral neck). The frog lateral view shows posteromedial offset of the femoral head with respect to the femoral neck. Sclerotic reactive bone, with posteromedial buttressing at the femoral neck, may be seen in subacute cases. Complications include chondrolysis, premature arthritis, pistol-grip deformity resulting in femoroacetabular impingement, and limb-length discrepancy due to premature physeal closure.
- **Rickets.** Rickets causes deficient resorption of the zone of provisional calcification. The disease results from lack of calcium absorption or overexcretion of phosphate. Patients may manifest bowing deformity or increased risk of fractures, including SCFE. X-rays may show fraying and cupping of the long bone metaphyses (most prominent at the knees and wrists), physeal widening, osteopenia with coarse trabeculae, bowing deformity, and insufficiency fractures. Flared and irregular anterior rib ends may result in the "rachitic rosary." The metaphyseal fraying resolves with treatment, and metaphyses become unusually dense.

■ Additional Differential Diagnosis

- **Osteomyelitis.** *Staphylococcus aureus* is the most common pathogen for bone infection. From age 18 months until skeletal maturity, the metaphysis is most often affected due to localized sluggish blood flow. Radiographs may demonstrate cortical fraying and periosteal reaction, moth-eaten lucency of the bone, and associated soft-tissue swelling. Sometimes the physis becomes widened. MRI shows low T1 and high T2 signal within bone when radiographs are still normal.

■ Diagnosis

Slipped capital femoral epiphysis.

✓ Pearls

- Slipped capital femoral epiphysis is a Salter I fracture of the capital femoral physis.
- Offset of the femoral head with respect to the neck is best diagnosed on a frog lateral view.
- Rickets demonstrates metaphyseal fraying and cupping, along with bowing deformity and insufficiency fractures.
- Osteomyelitis most often affects the metaphysis and demonstrates periostitis, moth-eaten lucency, and soft-tissue swelling.

Suggested Readings

Aronsson DD, Loder RT, Breur GJ, Weinstein SL. Slipped capital femoral epiphysis: current concepts. J Am Acad Orthop Surg. 2006; 14(12):666–679

Gill KG. Pediatric hip: pearls and pitfalls. Semin Musculoskelet Radiol. 2013; 17(3):328–338

Jarrett DY, Matheney T, Kleinman PK. Imaging SCFE: diagnosis, treatment and complications. Pediatr Radiol. 2013; 43 Suppl 1:S71–S82

Case 108

Wonsuk Kim

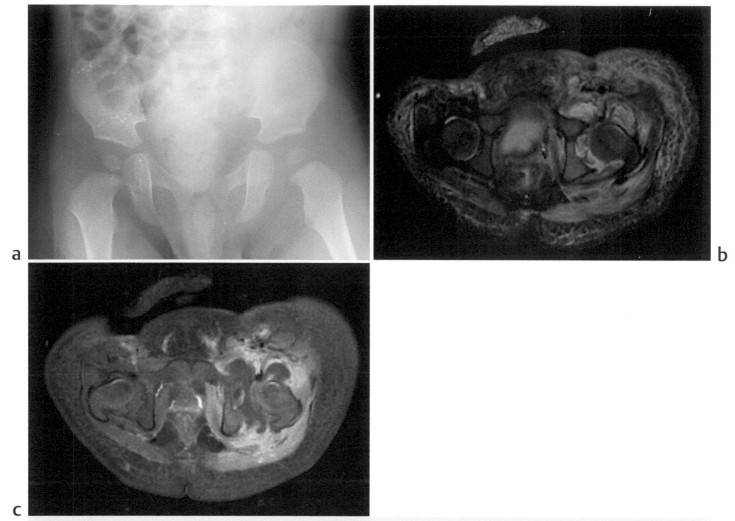

Fig. 108.1 Radiograph shows asymmetrical soft-tissue fullness of the left hip with widening of the joint space **(a)**. Axial short tau inversion recovery (STIR) image shows a joint effusion and edema in the surrounding musculature **(b)**. T1-W fat-saturated gadolinium-enhanced image shows a loculated effusion, extensive synovial enhancement, enhancement of the surrounding musculature/soft tissues, and possible disruption of the articular bony cortex **(c)**.

■ **Clinical Presentation**

A 2-year-old boy with hip pain (▶ Fig. 108.1).

■ Key Imaging Finding

Hip effusion.

■ Top Three Differential Diagnoses

- **Toxic synovitis.** Toxic synovitis is the most common atraumatic cause of hip pain in young children. Most patients are between 3 and 8 years old, and many cases are preceded by an upper respiratory infection. Joint fluid is present, better demonstrated with US than radiography. Treatment is supportive, and symptoms should resolve within 2 weeks. Avascular necrosis may develop in 1% to 2% of cases.
- **Septic arthritis.** This usually affects the hip or knee of young children. Common causative organisms are Gram-positive cocci, especially *Staphylococcus aureus* and various *Streptococci*. Septic arthritis is an orthopedic emergency, as delay in diagnosis may lead to articular cartilage destruction,

osteonecrosis, impaired growth, and deformity. US is useful for diagnosing joint effusions prior to arthrocentesis. MRI findings of bone marrow edema, soft tissue edema, and decreased femoral head enhancement are more prevalent in septic arthritis than toxic synovitis. Contrast-enhanced MRI demonstrates drainable fluid collections and appropriate sites for bone biopsy. Osteomyelitis may accompany septic arthritis.
- **Trauma.** Joint effusions in the setting of trauma often result from fracture. However, patients with septic arthritis or toxic synovitis may present with a history of trauma, so these diagnoses must also be entertained.

■ Additional Differential Diagnoses

- **Juvenile idiopathic arthritis (JIA).** JIA is a clinical diagnosis with varied manifestations. It encompasses all arthritides of unknown origin in patients younger than 16 years that last more than 6 weeks. Depending on disease stage, X-rays may show joint effusion, soft-tissue swelling, osteopenia, joint space narrowing, and erosions. MRI may show synovial thickening, joint effusion, marrow edema, erosions, and cartilage thinning.
- **Hemophilia.** Hemophilia may be associated with recurrent bleeding into the joints with subsequent development of arthropathy. Arthropathy typically develops in the first and second decades. The knee, ankle, elbow, and shoulder are most commonly affected. Radiographic findings in the acute phase include hemorrhagic joint effusion (hemarthrosis). On

MRI, the hypertrophied synovial membrane appears dark on all sequences secondary to susceptibility artifact from hemosiderin. Erosions may eventually develop.
- **Pigmented villonodular synovitis (PVNS).** PVNS represents the diffuse, intra-articular form of a spectrum of benign proliferative disorders that may affect the synovium, bursae, and tendon sheaths. PVNS occurs most often in the knee (80%), followed by hip, ankle, shoulder, and elbow. Peak presentation is in the third and fourth decades. Malignant transformation is rare. Radiographs may be normal or show periarticular soft-tissue swelling. Chronic findings include erosions on both sides of the joint. MRI may show diffuse or nodular thickening of the synovium, with susceptibility artifact from hemosiderin deposition.

■ Diagnosis

Septic arthritis with myositis and secondary osteomyelitis.

✓ Pearls

- Toxic synovitis is the most common atraumatic cause of hip pain in young children.
- Septic arthritis is a surgical emergency, as bacterial enzymes rapidly destroy joint cartilage.

- Trauma commonly precedes the onset of other causes of hip pain and may be a concomitant diagnosis.

Suggested Readings

Damasio MB, Malattia C, Martini A, Tomà P. Synovial and inflammatory diseases in childhood: role of new imaging modalities in the assessment of patients with juvenile idiopathic arthritis. Pediatr Radiol. 2010; 40(6):985–998

Jaramillo D, Dormans JP, Delgado J, Laor T, St Geme JW III. Hematogenous osteomyelitis in infants and children: imaging of a changing disease. Radiology. 2017; 283(3):629–643

Llauger J, Palmer J, Rosón N, Bagué S, Camins A, Cremades R. Nonseptic monoarthritis: imaging features with clinical and histopathologic correlation. Radiographics. 2000; 20 Spec No:S263–S278

Case 109

Rebecca Stein-Wexler

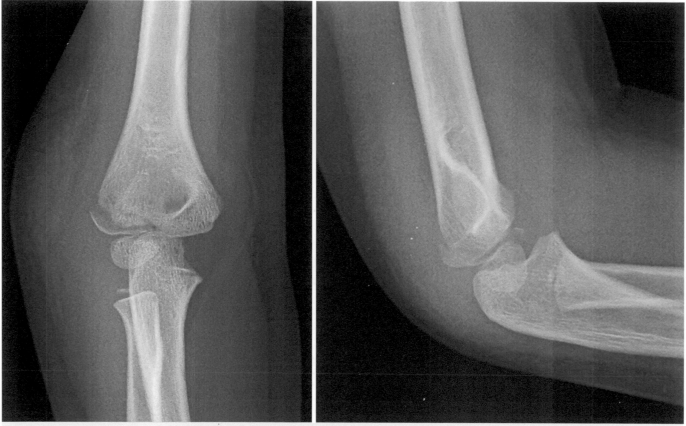

Fig. 109.1 Frontal elbow radiograph shows marked lateral soft-tissue swelling along with lucency paralleling the lateral portion of the distal humeral physis (a). Lateral view shows the lucency as well as elevation of anterior and posterior fat pads (b).

■ **Clinical Presentation**

A 4-year-old boy with elbow pain after falling on an outstretched hand (▶Fig. 109.1).

■ Key Imaging Finding

Fractured distal humerus.

■ Top Three Differential Diagnoses

- **Supracondylar fracture.** Falling onto an outstretched hand commonly causes this fracture. Incidence peaks at 5 to 9 years. The fracture line extends all the way across the metaphysis, unlike lateral condylar fracture (below). Treatment depends on the extent of posterior displacement of the distal fragment. Effusion is common, indicated by elevated posterior and anterior fat pads. If there is an effusion but no visible fracture in the setting of elbow trauma, occult supracondylar fracture is likely. The anterior humeral line, drawn on a well-positioned lateral view along the anterior cortex of the humerus, should intersect the posterior or middle third of the capitellum. Posterior positioning of the capitellum suggests an occult fracture.
- **Lateral condylar fracture.** This is most common between ages 4 and 10 years and results from varus force to the extended, supinated elbow. It involves the lateral aspect of the metaphysis (Salter II) and may extend into the epiphysis (Salter IV). If it involves the trochlear groove, it is considered unstable. Since the epiphyses are not ossified in young children, fracture severity may be underestimated. Traction from forearm extensors often displaces the fragment distally, which may mandate surgery. These fractures heal slowly. Nonunion and cubitus varus are common complications. Sometimes very subtle, this fracture may appear as a very thin lucent line paralleling the distal lateral physis, or a tiny flake of bone lateral to the metaphysis. Lateral soft-tissue swelling is an important clue.
- **Medial epicondylar fracture.** These fractures typically occur in children age 8 to 15 years, as a result of valgus strain to the elbow. The medial epicondyle fails due to excessive strain from the ulnar collateral ligament. In about half of cases, the radius and ulna are posteriorly dislocated. A displaced fragment may damage the ulnar nerve. Guidelines for surgical reduction and fixation vary, but in general this is performed for displacement greater than 15 mm. It is essential to bear in mind the sequence and timing of the trochlear and medial epicondylar ossification centers, since a displaced medial epicondyle may be mistaken for the trochlea. The CRITOL (capitellum, radial head, internal [medial] epicondyle, trochlea, olecranon, lateral epicondyle) mnemonic is helpful.

■ Additional Differential Diagnosis

- **Complete distal humeral physeal fracture and displacement.** This fracture through all the physes of the distal humerus (medial epicondyle, trochlea, capitellum, and lateral epicondyle) usually occurs in children younger than 2 years of age. The distal block of humeral cartilage is usually displaced in a posteromedial direction. Since the earliest apophysis to ossify—the capitellum—may do so as late as 12 months, in very young children this fracture resembles elbow dislocation without fracture. However, the latter is quite rare in this age group, and the displacement is generally posterolateral.

■ Diagnosis

Lateral condylar fracture of the humerus.

✓ Pearls

- The degree of posterior displacement of a supracondylar fracture determines need for surgery.
- Since lateral condylar fractures may traverse nonossified cartilaginous epiphyses, their extent may be underestimated on radiographs.
- It is important not to mistake a displaced medial epicondyle for the trochlear ossification center.
- The direction of displacement of the radius and ulna help differentiate complete distal humeral physeal fracture/displacement from elbow dislocation.

Suggested Readings

Ip D, Tsang WL. Medial humeral epicondylar fracture in children and adolescents. J Orthop Surg (Hong Kong). 2007; 15(2):170–173

Iyer RS, Thapa MM, Khanna PC, Chew FS. Pediatric bone imaging: imaging elbow trauma in children: a review of acute and chronic injuries. AJR Am J Roentgenol. 2012; 198(5):1053–1068

Uhl M. The elbow and forearm: acquired disorders. In Stein-Wexler R, Wootton-Gorges SL, Ozonoff MB, eds. Pediatric Orthopedic Imaging. Berlin/Heidelberg: Springer; 2015:187–221

Case 110

Aleksandar Kitich

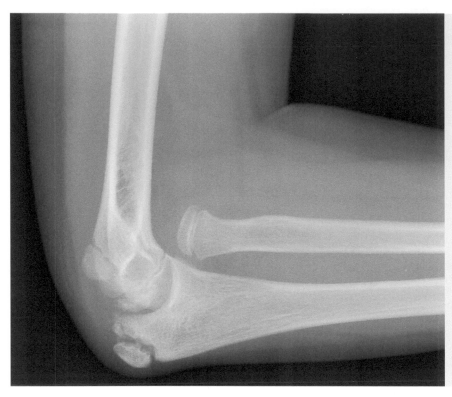

Fig. 110.1 Lateral view of the elbow shows the radial head is positioned anterior to an imaginary radiocapitellar line. The radial head contour is convex, and the radial neck is slightly narrowed.

■ Clinical Presentation

A 10-year-old boy with elbow pain after falling on an out-stretched hand (▶Fig. 110.1).

■ Key Imaging Finding

Radial head dislocation.

■ Top Three Differential Diagnoses

- **Nursemaid elbow.** Radial head subluxation is the most common elbow injury between ages 1 and 4 years. It is caused by sudden pull on an extended, pronated forearm. Ligamentous laxity and immature bone contours make it possible for the radial head to slip out of the annular ligament and subluxate. The annular ligament rarely becomes entrapped between the radial head and capitellum, preventing spontaneous reduction. The patient often holds the elbow fixed in flexion. Radial head subluxation is a clinical diagnosis, with radiographs sometimes performed to exclude fracture. Supinating the forearm to obtain the AP (anteroposterior) image may inadvertently reduce the radial head. The position of the radial head is evaluated by drawing a line along the center of the radial neck; this should also pass through the center of the capitellum (radiocapitellar line). Disruption of this line indicates radial head subluxation or dislocation. The radiocapitellar line must be carefully evaluated on all views.
- **Traumatic radial head dislocation.** Isolated radial head dislocation is very rare in older children, and usually there is injury to the ulna as well. It is therefore essential to image the entire forearm if radial head dislocation is identified, especially in the older child. Plastic bowing deformity of the ulna is the most common accompanying injury, but there may be an ulnar fracture, as in the Monteggia complex. These fractures are most often proximal and may be very subtle. In most cases, the radial head is dislocated anteriorly. The most common mechanism of injury is a fall on an outstretched hand.
- **Congenital radial head dislocation.** Congenital radial head dislocation is rare and often bilateral. The diagnosis is made when patients present with elbow deformity, pain, or limited range of motion. Dislocation may be an isolated abnormality or a feature of Apert, Ehlers–Danlos, Klinefelter, and other syndromes. Posterior dislocation is most commonly reported, occurring in two-thirds of patients. In addition to radial head dislocation, radiographs may show a hypoplastic capitellum, foreshortened ulna relative to the radius, dome-shaped radial head with a narrow neck, and defective trochlea.

■ Additional Differential Diagnosis

- **Madelung deformity.** This rare distal radial deformity results from premature closure of the medial volar aspect of the distal radial physis. This results in dorsal and radial bowing of the growing radius. The radius may be foreshortened, with a large gap between the capitellum and the dysplastic radial head, simulating radial head dislocation. Patients present with forearm deformity and decreased grip strength.

■ Diagnosis

Congenital anterior radial head dislocation.

✓ Pearls

- Radial head dislocation is best recognized on the lateral radiograph where the radiocapitellar line (drawn along the center of the radial neck) fails to pass through the center of the capitellum.
- X-rays of nursemaid elbow are often normal, as it is reduced during supination for proper positioning.
- Congenital radial head dislocation is often bilateral and associated with a hypoplastic capitellum, convex radial head, and narrow radial neck.

Suggested Readings

Ali S, Kaplan S, Kaufman T, Fenerty S, Kozin S, Zlotolow DA. Madelung deformity and Madelung-type deformities: a review of the clinical and radiological characteristics. Pediatr Radiol. 2015; 45(12):1856–1863

Gupta V, Kundu Z, Sangwan S, Lamba D. Isolated post-traumatic radial head dislocation, a rare and easily missed injury: a case report. Malays Orthop J. 2013; 7(1):74–78

Iyer RS, Thapa MM, Khanna PC, Chew FS. Pediatric bone imaging: imaging elbow trauma in children: a review of acute and chronic injuries. AJR Am J Roentgenol. 2012; 198(5):1053–1068

Kaas L, Struijs PA. Congenital radial head dislocation with a progressive cubitus valgus: a case report. Strateg Trauma Limb Reconstr. 2012; 7(1):39–44

Case 111

Myles Mitsunaga

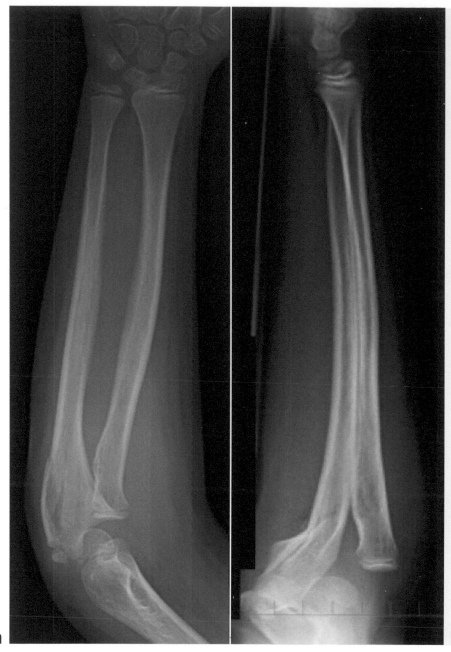

a

b

Fig. 111.1 Frontal (a) and lateral (b) views of the forearm show an angulated fracture of the proximal ulna, along with lateral and slight anterior dislocation of the radial head.

■ Clinical Presentation

A 7-year-old boy with pain, swelling, and deformity of the elbow after falling on an outstretched arm (►Fig. 111.1).

■ Key Imaging Finding

Fractures of the forearm.

■ Top Three Differential Diagnoses

- **Buckle fractures of distal radius and ulna.** These extremely common fractures result from a fall on an outstretched hand (FOOSH), typically accidental in younger children and sports related in older children. Buckle fractures usually involve the dorsal cortex and are inherently stable, healing without incident. Bicortical fractures are more likely to require reduction, especially if there is rotational malalignment.
- **Radial neck fracture.** Most radial neck fractures result from axial overloading of the lateral elbow after a FOOSH. Alternatively, if the radial head is trapped on the posterior capitellum during reduction of elbow dislocation, transphyseal fracture of the radial neck may occur. Standard views show a joint effusion and usually the fracture, but sometimes a radiocapitellar (Greenspan) view is needed. Casting is sufficient for angulation less than 30 degrees, while closed reduction is indicated for more angulation. Failed closed reduction

leads to open surgery, with increased risk of nonunion, avascular necrosis, and loss of motion. Radial head fractures are rare in children.
- **Monteggia fracture-dislocation.** Most Monteggia injuries result from a FOOSH in pronation, leading to proximal ulnar fracture or plastic deformation combined with radial head dislocation. Peak incidence is in children age 4 to 10 years. The radiocapitellar line (drawn along the center of the radial shaft and through the capitellum) fails to bisect the radial head. A proximal ulnar buckle fracture (most common) may be treated by closed reduction, but open reduction is generally needed if the fracture is comminuted or longitudinal/oblique. If a Monteggia injury is not reduced, chronic radiocapitellar instability may ensue, along with nonunion or malunion of the ulnar fracture. This may then cause ulnar shortening, pain, and limited pronation–supination.

■ Additional Differential Diagnoses

- **Olecranon fracture.** Olecranon fractures usually result from direct force to the proximal ulna. Sometimes quite subtle, they are often oblique or transverse. Above-elbow casting suffices for minimally displaced fractures, but those with more than 3-mm displacement are typically reduced and fixed with a tension band.
- **Galeazzi fracture-dislocation.** Usually a result of a FOOSH with hyperpronation, this injury consists of fracture of the

distal radius and dislocation of the distal radioulnar joint. The peak incidence is at age 9 to 12 years. A true lateral radiograph is important for determining the direction and degree of radial fracture displacement, whereas separation of the distal radioulnar joint is evident on a frontal view. Most injuries in children are treated with an above-elbow cast, with open reduction and fixation if there is pronounced distal radial angulation and/or foreshortening.

■ Diagnosis

Monteggia fracture-dislocation.

✓ Pearls

- A displaced fracture of the radius or ulna is often associated with fracture or dislocation of the other bone.
- A direct force to a single bone (the olecranon, e.g.) may result in a fracture of only that bone.

- A Monteggia injury is a proximal ulnar shaft fracture with a dislocated radial head.
- A Galeazzi injury is a fracture of the radial shaft with dislocation of the distal radioulnar joint.

Suggested Readings

Little KJ. Elbow fractures and dislocations. Orthop Clin North Am. 2014; 45(3):327–340

Rehim SA, Maynard MA, Sebastin SJ, Chung KC. Monteggia fracture dislocations: a historical review. J Hand Surg Am. 2014; 39(7):1384–1394

Rodríguez-Merchán EC. Pediatric fractures of the forearm. Clin Orthop Relat Res. 2005(432):65–72

Case 112

Rebecca Stein-Wexler

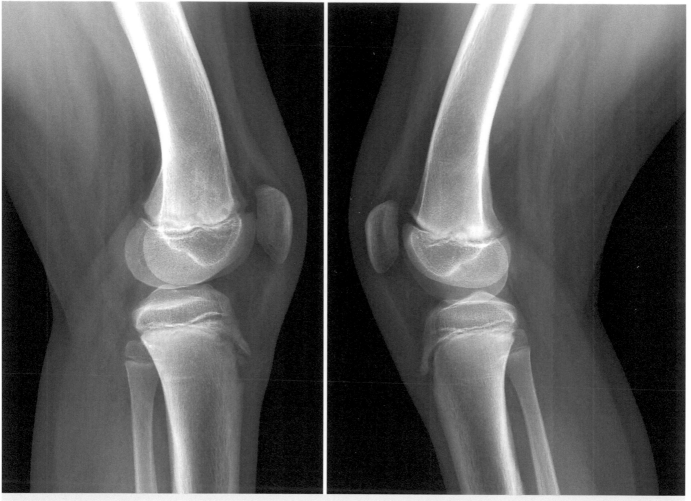

Fig. 112.1 There is fragmentation of the tibial tuberosity, and the infrapatellar tendon is thick and ill-defined (**a**). Normal for comparison (**b**).

■ **Clinical Presentation**

A 14-year-old male athlete with unilateral knee pain (▶Fig. 112.1).

■ Key Imaging Finding

Infrapatellar soft-tissue swelling.

■ Top Three Differential Diagnoses

- **Osgood–Schlatter disease.** This traction "apophysitis" typically occurs in adolescent boys during growth spurts. Patella alta and valgus alignment at the knee predispose to the condition. Repetitive tensile force causes microfracture and avulsion of tibial tuberosity cartilage. If the tibial tuberosity has ossified, X-rays show one or more adjacent ossific densities, soft-tissue swelling, and edema of the distal patellar tendon and Hoffa's fat pad. If the fracture goes through cartilage only, ossific fragments will be seen after 3 to 4 weeks. Up to 50% of cases are bilateral. This benign, self-limited disorder heals with nonsteroidal anti-inflammatory drugs (NSAIDs) and physical therapy.
- **Sinding-Larsen–Johansson disease.** Repetitive microtrauma causes this inferior patellar pole traction injury, usually in children age 10 to 14 years who are approaching skeletal maturity. Radiographs show at least one bone fragment near the lower pole of the patella and possibly patella alta. MRI shows abnormal signal in the lower pole of the patella, thickening of the patellar tendon, and edema in Hoffa's fat pad. Most lesions heal with NSAIDs and physical therapy.
- **Patellar sleeve fracture.** This acute avulsion injury affects children between ages 8 and 12 years after forceful contraction of the quadriceps muscle. Fracture of the cartilaginous lower pole of the patella results in a high-riding patella. The only radiographic evidence of this fracture may be a tiny sliver of bone at a variable distance from the patella's lower pole. MRI delineates the full extent of injury.

■ Additional Differential Diagnoses

- **Proximal tibial transverse metaphyseal fracture.** This common and sometimes subtle fracture is often sustained in young children age 2 to 5 years while jumping on a trampoline. Slight cortical buckling and/or a subtle transverse lucency suggest the diagnosis.
- **Tibial tuberosity fracture.** The tibial tuberosity is prone to fracture during adolescence, as the physeal cartilage in this area matures to bone. Active knee extension and vigorous quadriceps contraction (jumping) cause this uncommon injury. This fracture is more common in those with prior Osgood–Schlatter disease. The avulsed bone is typically either displaced cephalad or hinged upward. Surgical fixation is usually needed.

■ Diagnosis

Osgood–Schlatter disease.

✓ Pearls

- Osgood–Schlatter disease shows patellar tendon thickening, edema in Hoffa's fat pad, and variable fragments adjacent to the tibial tuberosity.
- As children approach skeletal maturity, repetitive microtrauma may cause avulsion of the lower pole of the patella, or Sinding-Larsen–Johansson disease.
- The tiny infrapatellar sliver of bone that may be seen with patellar sleeve fractures greatly underestimates extent of disease, and MRI is generally needed for accurate diagnosis.

Suggested Readings

Kjellin I. The lower extremity: acquired disorders. In Stein-Wexler R, Wootton-Gorges SL, Ozonoff MB, eds. Pediatric Orthopedic Imaging. Berlin/Heidelberg: Springer; 2015:435–461

Merrow AC, Reiter MP, Zbojniewicz AM, Laor T. Avulsion fractures of the pediatric knee. Pediatr Radiol. 2014; 44(11):1436–1445, quiz 1433–1436

Sanchez R, Strouse PJ. The knee: MR imaging of uniquely pediatric disorders. Magn Reson Imaging Clin N Am. 2009; 17(3):521–537, vii

Case 113

Aleksandar Kitich

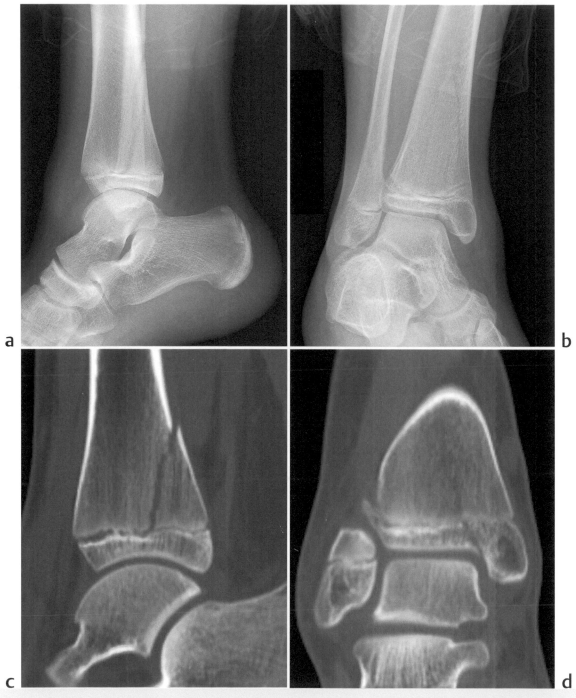

Fig. 113.1 Lateral radiograph of the ankle shows an oblique fracture through the dorsal aspect of the distal tibial metaphysis, extending to the physis; there is slight widening of the anterior physis **(a)**. Oblique view shows the epiphyseal component of the fracture **(b)**. Sagittal reformatted CT better demonstrates the physeal widening **(c)**. Coronal reformat shows the epiphyseal fracture **(d)**.

■ Clinical Presentation

A 13-year-old boy fell off a trampoline (▶ Fig. 113.1).

■ **Key Imaging Finding**

Ankle fracture.

■ **Top Three Differential Diagnoses**

• **Salter–Harris II fracture.** The Salter–Harris classification is based on involvement of the epiphysis and metaphysis (the physis is always involved). Type I involves only the physis. Type II extends from the physis to the metaphysis and is the most common ankle fracture, usually after age 10 years. Type III involves the epiphysis and physis, whereas type IV involves the metaphysis, physis, and epiphysis. Type V, a crush injury of the physis, is least common. Physeal fractures are particularly important due to the possibility of growth arrest and resultant limb shortening or angular deformity, more likely with types III to V. Growth arrest is almost universal with type V injuries.

• **Juvenile Tillaux fracture.** The juvenile Tillaux fracture occurs at age 12 to 15 years, as the physis closes. This Salter–Harris III fracture involves the smooth anterolateral physis and extends vertically into the epiphysis. There is no metaphyseal component. Most of these fractures are attributed to forceful abduction and external rotation, resulting in avulsion of a bone fragment by the strong anteroinferior tibiofibular ligament. Reduction is necessary if displacement exceeds 2 mm.

• **Triplane fracture.** This fracture also occurs in children age 12 to 15 years. During this time, the distal tibial epiphysis undergoes asymmetrical closure, with the central portion closing first and the anterolateral corner closing last. The transverse component of this fracture involves the unclosed anterolateral portion of the physis. The dorsal aspect of the tibial metaphysis is fractured in the coronal plane, and the epiphysis is fractured in the sagittal plane; both fractures are in continuity with the physeal fracture. The fibula is often fractured as well. The fracture is most commonly a result of external rotation of the foot. Given the complexity of the triplane fracture, it is generally imaged with CT and then managed with open reduction and internal fixation. The fracture is further categorized as a two-, three-, or four-part fracture.

■ **Additional Differential Diagnosis**

• **Pilon fracture.** This fracture is rare in children, but it is important because of the potential for both articular and physeal displacement. High-energy axial load forces the talus into the distal tibial plafond, resulting in a distal tibial comminuted intra-articular fracture. CT demonstrates multiple fragments, intra-articular extension, and variable talar and fibular involvement. In the pediatric population, open reduction and internal fixation are needed to avoid physeal bone bridge and growth arrest.

■ **Diagnosis**

Triplane fracture.

✓ **Pearls**

• Bone bridging and growth arrest are more likely in high-grade Salter–Harris fractures.
• The triplane fracture involves the metaphysis, the growth plate, and the epiphysis in three planes, unlike the Tillaux fracture, which involves two planes.

• The juvenile Tillaux fracture is a Salter–Harris III distal tibial fracture.
• The triplane fracture is distinguished from the Tillaux fracture by a coronal plane metaphyseal fracture.

Suggested Readings

Podeszwa DA, Mubarak SJ. Physeal fractures of the distal tibia and fibula (Salter-Harris Type I, II, III, and IV fractures). J Pediatr Orthop. 2012; 32 Suppl 1: S62–S68

Rosenbaum AJ, DiPreta JA, Uhl RL. Review of distal tibial epiphyseal transitional fractures. Orthopedics. 2012; 35(12):1046–1049

Schnetzler KA, Hoernschemeyer D. The pediatric triplane ankle fracture. J Am Acad Orthop Surg. 2007; 15(12):738–747

Topliss CJ, Jackson M, Atkins RM. Anatomy of pilon fractures of the distal tibia. J Bone Joint Surg Br. 2005; 87(5):692–697

Case 114

Myles Mitsunaga

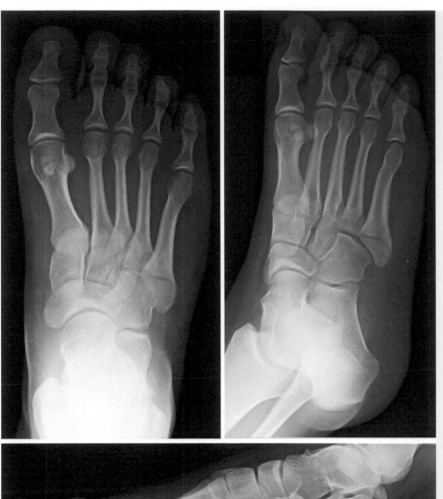

Fig. 114.1 Anteroposterior (**a**), oblique (**b**), and lateral (**c**) radiographs of the right foot show a transverse lucency at the base of the fifth metatarsal, extending to the fourth to fifth metatarsal articulation.

■ **Clinical Presentation**

A 12-year-old boy with pain over the lateral forefoot after trauma (▶Fig. 114.1).

■ Key Imaging Finding

Lucency at the base of the fifth metatarsal.

■ Top Three Differential Diagnoses

- **Normal apophysis.** The apophysis at the base of the fifth metatarsal begins to ossify around age 8 years and then fuses to the adjacent bone at approximately age 12 years in girls and age 15 years in boys. The apophysis may appear fragmented, but margins are smooth and well corticated. The dominant lucency is longitudinal to the axis of the metatarsal.
- **Apophyseal tubercle avulsion fracture.** This transverse fracture occurs at the insertion site of the peroneus brevis tendon. An apophyseal avulsion fracture is the most common fracture of the fifth metatarsal in children older than 5 years (stress-type fractures being more common in younger children).

Twisting injury with a fixed forefoot is the typical mechanism. These fractures may be intra-articular.
- **Stress fracture.** Like stress fractures elsewhere, those at the fifth metatarsal result from repetitive injury. They are rarely displaced and may not be apparent on initial radiographs. Sometimes an incomplete fracture line may be evident, usually at the proximal diaphysis. If not stabilized, this may progress to a complete fracture. Since there is often a delay in seeking treatment for these insidious injuries, radiographs are uncommonly performed acutely, and focal periosteal reaction may therefore be evident. Treatment is conservative.

■ Additional Differential Diagnoses

- **Jones fracture.** This fracture occurs at the proximal fifth metatarsal distal to the tubercle or apophysis. Most Jones fractures are transverse or oblique. They are usually treated conservatively with casting, unless they are intra-articular or located at the proximal diaphysis. Unlike tubercle fractures, they are prone to nonunion. Jones fractures are distal to apophyseal tubercle avulsion fractures and proximal to diaphyseal stress fractures.

- **Ossification center.** The os vesalianum is an uncommon accessory ossification center located lateral to the base of the fifth metatarsal, within the peroneus brevis tendon. Radiographically, accessory ossification centers have rounded, well-corticated margins and are oriented parallel to the metatarsal shaft. Avulsion fracture fragments, on the other hand, are typically jagged, non-corticated and oriented obliquely. Accessory ossification centers of the foot are rarely symptomatic.

■ Diagnosis

Avulsion fracture at the base of the fifth metatarsal.

✓ Pearls

- Avulsion fractures at the base of the fifth metatarsal are common, usually transverse or oblique, and caused by direct trauma.
- Stress fractures are diaphyseal and may not be evident on initial radiographs; they may progress to a complete fracture or

demonstrate periosteal reaction 7 to 10 days after precipitating injury.
- The developing apophysis at the base of the fifth metatarsal is differentiated from fracture by its longitudinal orientation and smoothly corticated margins.

Suggested Readings

Coskun N, Yuksel M, Cevener M, et al. Incidence of accessory ossicles and sesamoid bones in the feet: a radiographic study of the Turkish subjects. Surg Radiol Anat. 2009; 31(1):19–24

Herrera-Soto JA, Scherb M, Duffy MF, Albright JC. Fractures of the fifth metatarsal in children and adolescents. J Pediatr Orthop. 2007; 27(4):427–431

Kose O. Os vesalianum pedis misdiagnosed as fifth metatarsal avulsion fracture. Emerg Med Australas. 2009; 21(5):426

Case 115

Rebecca Stein-Wexler

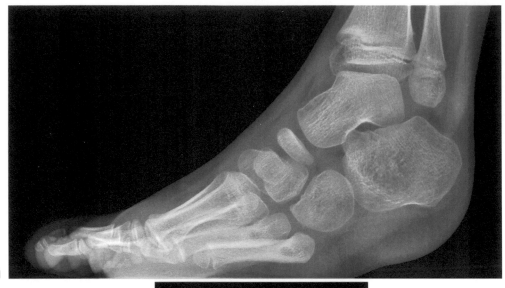

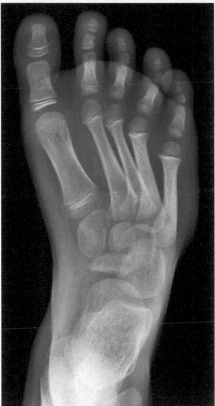

Fig. 115.1 Lateral weight-bearing view shows the talus and calcaneus are parallel and have a boxy configuration; the metatarsals appear stacked above each other in a ladderlike configuration **(a)**. The frontal weight-bearing view shows varus configuration of the calcaneus, deviated laterally to overlap with the talus; the metatarsal bases overlap more than normal **(b)**.

■ Clinical Presentation

Child with a funny gait (▶ Fig. 115.1).

■ Key Imaging Finding

Foot malalignment.

■ Top Three Differential Diagnoses

- **Planovalgus foot (flatfoot).** This familial, acquired, flexible deformity is characterized by flattening of the plantar arch. It is usually asymptomatic. The condition is very common, especially in young children. However, by age 10 years the incidence is similar to that in adults. Imaging is usually only performed if the condition is painful, to exclude other etiologies such as tarsal coalition. Ligamentous laxity allows the calcaneal position to deviate toward the midline (hindfoot valgus). The calcaneus is more horizontal than normal when viewed on a lateral weight-bearing X-ray. In addition, the Meary line, which is drawn along long axis of the talus and first metatarsal, is convex downward. With severe cases, the talus may be directed inferiorly, more parallel to the long axis of the tibia than normal. However, it articulates normally with the navicular. Planovalgus foot may develop in patients with cerebral palsy and other neuromuscular disorders, but in that case the foot is usually stiffer than with familial flatfoot.
- **Clubfoot (equinovarus).** The congenital form of this disorder may be inherited but may also result from muscle imbalance, connective tissue abnormalities, and intrauterine positioning. Older patients may develop clubfoot due to myelomeningocele, arthrogryposis, and a variety of syndromes. Patients show plantar flexion at the ankle, hindfoot varus, and forefoot inversion and adduction. On X-rays, the talus is often small and deformed. The calcaneus is usually in equinus (more parallel to the tibial long axis than normal). The calcaneus is parallel to the talus and often superimposed. The navicular is displaced medially, and the forefoot is adducted. Inversion of the foot causes the metatarsal bases to be superimposed on each other on the frontal view and leads to a ladderlike appearance on the lateral view. The lateral metatarsals may be thick and sclerotic due to abnormal weight bearing on the lateral side of the foot and stress reaction/fractures.
- **Congenital vertical talus.** This rare condition is usually bilateral and is syndromic in at least half the cases. Nonsyndromic cases may result from abnormal rotational development of the foot and/or muscle imbalance. The tibialis posterior and peroneus longus tendons are positioned more anteriorly than normal and may function as dorsiflexors, and the Achilles tendon is short. As a result, the talus is severely plantar flexed, almost paralleling the tibial long axis. Unlike with planovalgus foot, the navicular is dorsally dislocated so it lies on the talar neck. The navicular aligns normally with the tarsal bones, but the talus does not. The calcaneus is laterally deviated into severe valgus, and like the talus it is in equinus, almost parallel to the long axis of the tibia. There is marked plantar flexion, resulting in rocker-bottom deformity.

■ Diagnosis

Clubfoot deformity.

✓ Pearls

- With flatfoot deformity, the calcaneus is more horizontal than usual and deviated into valgus; in severe cases, the talar axis may align somewhat with the long axis of the tibia.
- Clubfoot is characterized by deviation of the calcaneus laterally so it is parallel to the talus, along with forefoot adduction and foot inversion so the metatarsals overlap too much on the frontal view but not enough on the lateral (ladder configuration).
- In congenital vertical talus, the talus is in equinus, and the calcaneus is deviated laterally into severe valgus.
- An important difference between flatfoot and congenital vertical talus is that with the former the talus and navicular are aligned, whereas with the latter the navicular is dorsally dislocated.

Suggested Readings

Hammer MR, Pai DR. The foot and ankle: congenital and developmental conditions. In Stein-Wexler R, Wootton-Gorges SL, Ozonoff MB, eds. Pediatric Orthopedic Imaging. Berlin/Heidelberg: Springer; 2015:463–516

Harty MP. Imaging of pediatric foot disorders. Radiol Clin North Am. 2001; 39(4):733–748

Case 116

Rebecca Stein-Wexler

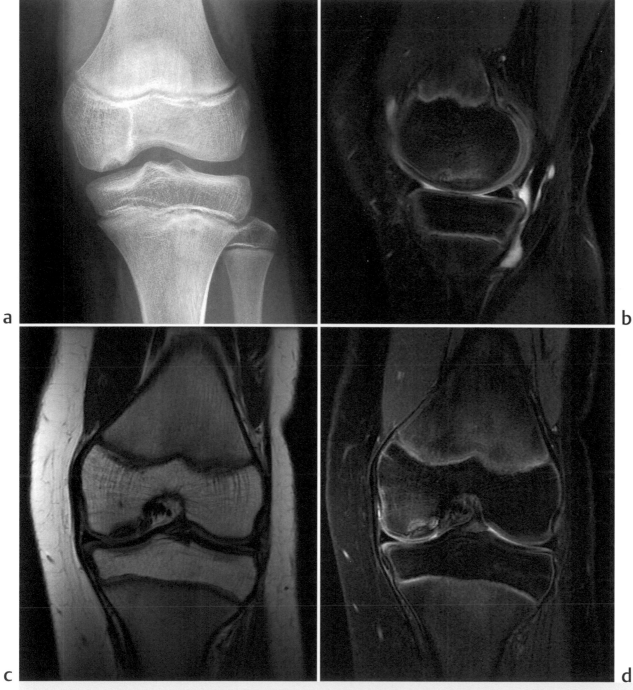

Fig. 116.1 Frontal radiograph shows a scalloped lucency at the lateral aspect of the medial femoral condyle, with surrounding sclerosis **(a)**. Sagittal PD fat-saturated image shows the lesion is centered at the weight-bearing articular surface, and there is surrounding edema **(b)**. Coronal T1-W image shows the lesion is hypointense **(c)**. Coronal PD fat-saturated image delineates an ossific fragment with underlying hyperintensity **(d)**.

■ Clinical Presentation

A 12-year-old girl complains of knee locking (▶Fig. 116.1).

■ Key Imaging Finding

Epiphyseal cortical irregularity.

■ Top Three Differential Diagnoses

- **Developmental cortical irregularity (DCI) at the knee.** DCI at the distal femoral condyles is present in up to one-third of children. This normal variant is usually posterior, on the non-weight-bearing surface, and therefore best seen on tunnel views. The posterior position is also evident on laterals. DCI resembles osteochondral lesion (OCL) on radiographs. However, the position differentiates these entities, since OCL is more anterior, on the weight-bearing surface. Also, unlike OCL, DCI never involves the intercondylar notch. On MRI, signal intensity of the overlying cartilage and adjacent marrow is normal with DCI, unlike with OCL.
- **Osteochondral lesion (OCL; osteochondritis dissecans).** This lesion consists of a subchondral fracture and an osteochondral fragment, which may be completely detached. Etiology is multifactorial, with repetitive microtrauma often playing a role. OCL is most common at the knee, where it affects children between ages 11 and 17 years. In children, the lateral aspect of the medial femoral condyle ("LAME") is affected much more often than the anteroinferior lateral femoral condyle. The lesion often extends into the intercondylar notch. X-rays show a lucent crater with irregular or sclerotic margins, and possibly a loose body. Notch, tunnel, and oblique views are useful. At MRI (especially T2-W or STIR), the following findings suggest instability: fluid signal around the lesion, multiple marginal cysts (or one large cyst > 5 mm), a hypointense subchondral rim, and/or multiple disruptions in the subchondral plate. Stable lesions usually heal spontaneously. OCL is also common at the talus, with the anteromedial talar dome affected most often. The X-ray appearance is similar to that of OCL at the knee, and similar features determine fragment stability. Anteromedial lesions are more likely to heal spontaneously than those in other locations. OCL also affects the capitellum, second or third metatarsal head (Freiberg infraction), tarsal navicular (Kohler disease), and other bones.
- **Panner disease.** This osteochondrosis differs from OCL in that it involves the entire capitellum, not just a superficial focus. It affects younger children (boys younger than 10 years) than OCL of the capitellum (male pitchers, age 10–15 years). Repetitive trauma and compression loading cause avascular necrosis. Radiographs show irregular contour and fissures that lead to fragmentation and flattening. Most lesions heal, with restoration of contours. Loose bodies do not usually occur. On MRI, the capitellum appears fragmented and T1 hypointense.

■ Additional Differential Diagnosis

- **Skeletal dysplasia.** Mild cases of multiple epiphyseal dysplasias and spondyloepiphyseal dysplasia may resemble osteochondritis dissecans, but multiple epiphyses will be involved.

■ Diagnosis

Osteochondral lesion (osteochondritis dissecans).

✓ Pearls

- Developmental cortical irregularity of the knee affects the non-weight-bearing surface and does not extend to the intercondylar notch.
- MRI features of osteochondral lesion that favor instability include a T2-hyperintense fluid rim, multiple or large marginal cysts, and multiple disruptions in the subchondral plate.
- Osteochondral lesion of the knee usually affects the lateral weight-bearing surface of the medial femoral condyle, whereas osteochondral lesion of the talus usually affects the anteromedial dome.
- Panner disease involves the entire capitellar ossification center, unlike osteochondral lesions, which involve the articular surface.

■ Suggested Readings

Kjellin I. The lower extremity: acquired disorders. In Stein-Wexler R, Wootton-Gorges SL, Ozonoff MB, eds. Pediatric Orthopedic Imaging. Berlin/Heidelberg: Springer; 2015:435–461

Prince JS. The lower extremity: congenital and developmental conditions. In Stein-Wexler R, Wootton-Gorges SL, Ozonoff MB, eds. Berlin/Heidelberg: Springer; 2015:373–433

Sanchez R., Strouse PJ. The knee: MR imaging of uniquely pediatric disorders. MRI Clin North Am. 2009; 17(3):521–537, vii

Case 117

Fabienne Joseph and Rebecca Stein-Wexler

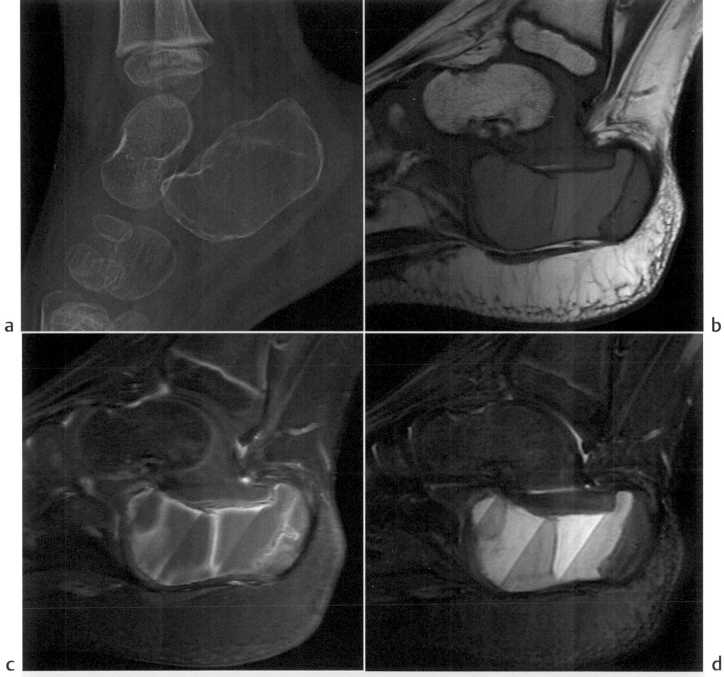

Fig. 117.1 Lateral ankle radiograph shows an expansile, lytic calcaneal lesion **(a)**. Sagittal T1-W MRI demonstrates multiple fluid–fluid levels within the lesion **(b)**. Sagittal T1-W gadolinium-enhanced fat-suppressed MRI shows septal enhancement **(c)**. Sagittal STIR image suggests some of the intralesional fluid is hemorrhagic **(d)**.

■ Clinical Presentation

A 7-year-old girl with heel pain (▶Fig. 117.1).

■ Key Imaging Finding

Benign expansile lucent bone lesion.

■ Top Three Differential Diagnoses

- **Nonossifying fibroma (NOF).** This very common cortically based non-neoplastic lesion migrates from the metaphysis to the diaphysis as the child grows. NOF is usually identified between ages 10 and 15 years and is rare before age 2 years. Eccentric and cortically based, NOFs may enlarge to involve the intramedullary region, often appearing central in thin bones such as the fibula or ulna. The lesions have a thin, sclerotic margin and no calcific matrix. Their orientation parallels the long axis of the bone. Periosteal reaction occurs only with pathological fracture. NOFs spontaneously regress as bone replaces fibrous tissue, though large lesions may require curettage and bone grafting to prevent pathological fracture.
- **Unicameral bone cyst (UBC, also known as simple bone cyst).** Also very common, the UBC is typically a unilocular fluid-filled cyst that most often occurs in the metadiaphysis of long bones—especially the proximal humerus. Typical age is 10 to 15 years. In patients older than 17 years, about half are located in the pelvis or calcaneus. The lesions are central in location and elongated; they demonstrate mild cortical expansion with a well-defined margin. In the absence of fracture, there should be no periosteal reaction. The "fallen fragment," seen in the dependent portion of the cyst after fracture, suggests the diagnosis of UBC.
- **Aneurysmal bone cyst (ABC).** ABC is a benign, eccentric, lucent bone lesion that consists of blood-filled cystic cavities. It is typically located within the juxtaphyseal metaphysis of long bones, spine, or pelvis. The lesion is often identified between ages 10 and 20 years. ABC is usually primary. However, it may develop after trauma or within a preexisting benign or malignant lesion, including giant cell tumor (GCT), osteoblastoma, chondroblastoma, fibrous dysplasia, or osteosarcoma. It has a characteristic "soap bubble" appearance, and it may cause extreme ("aneurysmal") bone expansion and severe cortical thinning. The margin is usually well defined, with a narrow zone of transition. If the lesion is rapidly expanding, periosteal reaction may appear aggressive. Fluid–fluid levels (best seen on MRI) strongly suggest the diagnosis but may be seen in other lesions, notably telangiectatic osteosarcoma and GCT. The absence of intralesional matrix and epiphyseal extension helps exclude other diagnoses. Treatment is surgical resection.

■ Additional Differential Diagnoses

- **Giant cell tumor (GCT).** GCTs do not cross the open physis and almost always occur after physeal closure, generally in patients older than 15 years. They are most common about the knee. GCTs are solitary, eccentric, and lytic. Margins are well defined but not sclerotic. Solid elements enhance at MRI. They are treated with surgical excision or, less often, radiation therapy.
- **Langerhans cell histiocytosis.** These small round cell tumors are most common in flat bones and proximal long bones of children younger than 10 years. Lesions typically initially appear permeative but later appear lytic and well defined.

■ Diagnosis

Aneurysmal bone cyst.

✓ Pearls

- Nonossifying fibromas may appear central in the ulna or fibula but in larger bones appear eccentric and cortically based.
- The "fallen fragment" is highly suggestive of unicameral bone cyst.
- Fluid–fluid levels most often indicate aneurysmal bone cyst but may be seen with other benign and malignant lesions.
- Giant cell tumors usually occur after physeal closure; they do not cross an open physis.

Suggested Readings

Khanna G, Bennett DL. Pediatric bone lesions: beyond the plain radiographic evaluation. Semin Roentgenol. 2012; 47(1):90–99

Wyers MR. Evaluation of pediatric bone lesions. Pediatr Radiol. 2010; 40(4):468–473

Case 118

Rebecca Stein-Wexler

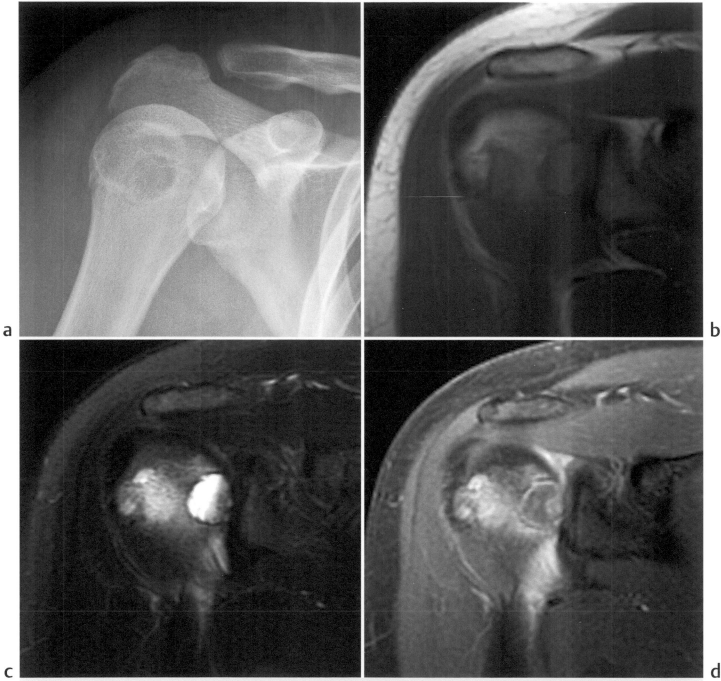

Fig. 118.1 Radiograph shows a well-circumscribed lytic lesion that crosses the physis, spanning the humeral head and the metaphysis **(a)**. Coronal T1-W image shows it is slightly hyperintense compared with muscle **(b)**. Coronal T2-W fat-suppressed image shows the lesion is predominantly hyperintense, and there is marrow edema **(c)**. Coronal T1-W gadolinium-enhanced fat-suppressed image shows the periphery of the lesion enhances, as does marrow **(d)**.

■ Clinical Presentation

A 17-year-old male with shoulder pain (▶Fig. 118.1).

■ Key Imaging Finding

Lucent epiphyseal lesion.

■ Top Three Differential Diagnoses

- **Chondroblastoma.** This benign cartilaginous tumor is most common in patients between ages 10 and 30 years. It is positioned eccentrically in the epiphysis (or apophysis) and in about half of cases extends into the metaphysis. The most common locations are the femur, humerus, and tibia. Radiographs show a lucent lesion with well-defined, sclerotic margins, sometimes with central, stippled, chondroid calcification. If calcification is present, MRI shows central T1 and T2 hypointensity, whereas purely cartilaginous tumors are T1 hypointense and T2 hyperintense. Marginal sclerosis appears as a thin (<1 mm) hypointense rim. Both marrow and soft-tissue edema are common, and if the lesion extends into the joint there may be synovitis as well. Aneurysmal bone cysts may be found within this lesion, indicated by septal enhancement.
- **Osteomyelitis.** Although osteomyelitis most often arises in the metaphysis, in infants it may spread to the epiphysis since blood vessels traverse the physis in these patients. Alternatively, young children may develop subacute primary epiphyseal osteomyelitis due to hematogenous seeding. The latter almost always affects the knee, usually the distal femoral epiphysis. Radiographs show a well-circumscribed epiphyseal lucent lesion. MRI features resemble those of osteomyelitis elsewhere.

- **Eosinophilic granuloma (EG).** This asymptomatic or painful condition is characterized by proliferating Langerhans cells that produce prostaglandin, which causes localized bone resorption. Lesions are most common in the skull, jaw, ribs, spine, and proximal long bones, but may occur in any hematopoietically active bone. Most cases are seen in children younger than 10 years of age. Multisystem involvement ("Langerhans cell histiocytosis") is rare and typically limited to much younger children. EG typically initially appears permeative but later becomes uniformly lytic, with variably sclerotic margins. Appearance on bone scan varies. MRI demonstrates the extent of marrow involvement, soft-tissue mass, and surrounding inflammation. T1 appearance varies, but lesions are usually bright on T2. EG is treated with chemotherapy, radiation therapy, and/or surgical resection.

■ Additional Differential Diagnosis

- **Giant cell tumor (GCT).** GCT arises in the metaphysis, does not cross the open physis, and is thus epiphyseal only after physeal closure. Most patients are older than 15 years, and most lesions develop after the adjacent physis has closed. GCT is most common about the knee. The tumor is solitary, eccentric, and lytic. Margins are well defined but not sclerotic. Solid elements enhance at MRI. The lesion is treated with surgical excision or, less often, radiation therapy.

■ Diagnosis

Giant cell tumor.

✓ Pearls

- Chondroblastoma is most common about the knee, where it is as an eccentric, epiphyseal lucent lesion.
- Epiphyseal osteomyelitis in infants results from transphyseal spread, whereas in older children hematogenous seeding leads to subacute primary epiphyseal osteomyelitis, usually at the knee.

- Eosinophilic granuloma most often occurs in the skull, jaw, ribs, spine, and proximal long bones.
- Giant cell tumor occurs in the metaphysis but may extend into the epiphysis after physeal closure.

Suggested Readings

Khanna G, Bennett DL. Pediatric bone lesions: beyond the plain radiographic evaluation. Semin Roentgenol. 2012; 47(1):90–99

Nichols RE, Dixon LB. Radiographic analysis of solitary bone lesions. Radiol Clin North Am. 2011; 49(6):1095–1114, v

Wootton-Gorges SL. Tumors and tumor-like conditions of bone. In Stein-Wexler R, Wootton-Gorges SL, Ozonoff MB, eds. Pediatric Orthopedic Imaging. Berlin/Heidelberg: Springer; 2015:315–326

Wyers MR. Evaluation of pediatric bone lesions. Pediatr Radiol. 2010; 40(4):468–473

Case 119

James S. Chalfant

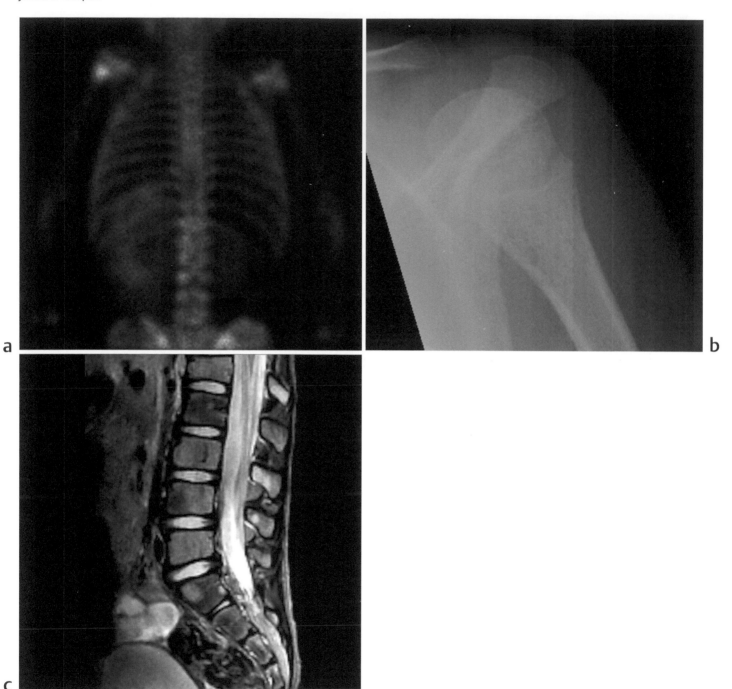

Fig. 119.1 Technetium-99m bone scan shows increased uptake at the left proximal humerus and patchy uptake throughout the thoracolumbar spine; there is increased uptake in the left upper quadrant as well **(a)**. Radiograph of the left shoulder shows a lytic metaphyseal lesion **(b)**. T2-W sagittal MRI of the lumbosacral spine shows multilevel involvement, with high-T2 lesions affecting vertebral bodies as well as spinous processes **(c)**.

■ Clinical Presentation

A 4-year-old girl with multifocal bone pain (▶Fig. 119.1).

■ Key Imaging Finding

Multiple lytic lesions.

■ Top Three Differential Diagnoses

- **Langerhans cell histiocytosis.** Langerhans cell histiocytosis affects both flat and long bones and has a very variable appearance. Most often, the lesions are intramedullary and lytic, with little sclerosis. Periosteal reaction, if present, usually appears lamellated and benign. A bony sequestrum may be present. MRI may demonstrate a soft-tissue mass. Lesions show variable signal intensity on T1, increased signal intensity on T2, and florid enhancement. Vertebra plana (wafer-thin vertebrae) may be seen.
- **Neuroblastoma metastases.** Neuroblastoma is the most common pediatric malignancy to metastasize to bone, and over half of patients have osseous metastases at diagnosis. Bone metastases are typically widespread. Radiographs may reveal multiple lytic lesions favoring the metaphysis. MRI plays a role in determining the extent of marrow involvement, which is often extensive (hypointense on T1 and hyperintense on T2).

Metaiodobenzylguanidine (MIBG) scintigraphy is highly sensitive and specific for detecting metastatic disease. Ninety percent of cases are diagnosed before the age of 5 years. The primary is usually adrenal but may be anywhere along the sympathetic chain. Very rarely the imaging workup fails to identify a primary tumor.
- **Leukemia/lymphoma.** Multifocal bone lymphoma/leukemia is usually secondary and most often involves the spine or pelvis, whereas primary bone lymphoma is usually unifocal at the metaphyses of long bones. Secondary bone lymphoma is almost always permeative or purely lytic, with no periosteal reaction. There may be a soft-tissue mass. Bone marrow involvement is hypointense on T1 and hyperintense on T2; it shows gadolinium enhancement. Most osseous lymphoma is non-Hodgkin lymphoma. If more than 25% of the marrow is involved on biopsy, the disease is termed leukemia.

■ Additional Differential Diagnoses

- **Fibrous dysplasia.** Polyostotic fibrous dysplasia may involve any bone but is often unilateral and monomelic. In the long bones, it is typically metadiaphyseal. Lesions are intramedullary, expansile, and well defined with variable but classically ground glass matrix. There is no periosteal reaction or soft-tissue mass.
- **Chronic recurrent multifocal osteomyelitis.** This autoimmune/inflammatory, noninfectious disorder is characterized

by a relapsing, remitting course. Lesions occur anywhere in the skeleton but commonly involve the medial third of the clavicle and long bone metaphyses adjacent to the growth plate (lower extremities more common than upper). Lesions are initially lytic and progressively become sclerotic and hyperostotic. Bilateral symmetrical disease, clavicle involvement, and comorbid inflammatory conditions (dermatologic disorders, inflammatory bowel disease) support the diagnosis.

■ Diagnosis

Metastatic neuroblastoma with left adrenal primary.

✓ Pearls

- Langerhans cell histiocytosis has either no periostitis or lamellated, benign-appearing periosteal reaction.
- Neuroblastoma commonly metastasizes to bone and results in lytic lesions that are most often metaphyseal.

- Secondary osseous non-Hodgkin lymphoma typically results in permeative, lytic lesions.
- Bilateral symmetrical disease and/or clavicle lesions suggest chronic recurrent multifocal osteomyelitis.

Suggested Readings

Bousson V, Rey-Jouvin C, Laredo JD, et al. Fibrous dysplasia and McCune-Albright syndrome: imaging for positive and differential diagnoses, prognosis, and follow-up guidelines. Eur J Radiol. 2014; 83(10):1828–1842

Khanna G, Sato TS, Ferguson P. Imaging of chronic recurrent multifocal osteomyelitis. Radiographics. 2009; 29(4):1159–1177

Papaioannou G, McHugh K. Neuroblastoma in childhood: review and radiological findings. Cancer Imaging. 2005; 5:116–127

Case 120

Karen M. Ayotte

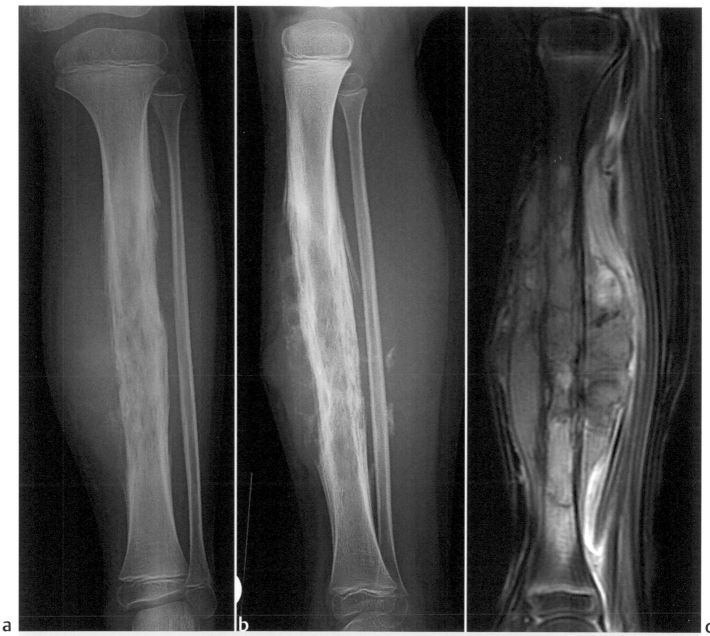

Fig. 120.1 Frontal view of the tibia and fibula demonstrates a permeative diaphyseal lesion with aggressive periosteal reaction and a soft-tissue mass **(a)**. Lateral view shows spiculated soft-tissue calcification **(b)**. T2-W fat-suppressed sagittal image shows extensive heterogeneous marrow signal with surrounding edema and a large, lobulated soft-tissue mass **(c)**.

■ **Clinical Presentation**

A 6-year-old boy with leg pain (▶Fig. 120.1).

■ Key Imaging Finding

Aggressive bone lesion.

■ Top Three Differential Diagnoses

- **Osteomyelitis.** Osteomyelitis has such a wide spectrum of radiographic appearances (including—in the early stage—normal) that it may be difficult if not impossible to conclusively exclude the diagnosis. A clinical history of fever or recent infection is helpful but not specific. Common radiological findings include a lytic lesion with variably aggressive features, bone resorption, periostitis, sclerotic nidus, draining cloaca, and subcutaneous gas. Osteomyelitis is most common in the metaphysis but may extend to the epiphysis or diaphysis. The degree of sclerosis within and around the lesion varies depending upon the organism, duration of infection, and age and overall health of the patient. CT and MRI are most useful if the clinical diagnosis is in doubt or if medical treatment fails.
- **Osteosarcoma.** Osteosarcoma is the most common primary bone malignancy of childhood, with a peak incidence at age 10 to 20 years. The classic description is an aggressive lesion in the metaphysis of a long bone, with abnormal new bone proliferation. Highly aggressive lesions may appear predominantly lytic.

The more unusual telangiectatic osteosarcoma may have fluid-fluid levels, resembling aneurysmal bone cyst. MRI is useful for detecting nearby "skip" lesions. Nuclear medicine bone scan (or PET-CT) is especially useful during initial workup to identify metastatic foci.
- **Ewing sarcoma.** Ewing sarcoma is the second most common primary bone malignancy of childhood, with a peak incidence at age 10 to 15 years. The classic description of this small round blue cell tumor is of a moth-eaten or permeative, medullary-based metadiaphyseal lesion in a long bone, with aggressive periosteal reaction. A large soft-tissue mass is common. However, the appearance ranges from purely lytic to predominantly sclerotic. Long bone lesions are more common in younger patients, and flat bone origin is more common in adolescents and young adults. Patients often present with pain. Constitutional findings such as fever and elevated inflammatory markers are common. MRI is critical for local staging.

■ Additional Differential Diagnoses

- **Langerhans cell histiocytosis (LCH).** LCH may present as solitary or multifocal lytic bone lesions. The radiographic appearance is notoriously variable. Therefore, LCH is a reasonable diagnostic consideration for many bone lesions, benign or aggressive, in patients younger than 30 years.
- **Metastases.** Secondary malignancies commonly affect bones via hematogenous dissemination. Leukemia is the most

common entity to involve long bones in pediatric patients. Other common neoplasms that metastasize to bone include neuroblastoma and lymphoma. Metastases typically present as lytic foci with a permeative or moth-eaten appearance. Lymphoma may also arise in bone as a primary lesion.

■ Diagnosis

Ewing sarcoma.

✓ Pearls

- Osteosarcoma usually presents as an aggressive metaphyseal long bone lesion with bone proliferation.
- Ewing sarcoma typically presents as a lytic medullary lesion with aggressive periosteal reaction.

- Osteomyelitis has a wide variety of imaging appearance; history of fever is helpful but not specific.
- Bone scan is useful to evaluate for metastases, multifocal lesions, or skip lesions as seen in osteosarcoma.

■ Suggested Readings

Jaramillo D, Dormans JP, Delgado J, Laor T, St Geme JW III. Hematogenous osteomyelitis in infants and children: imaging of a changing disease. Radiology. 2017; 283(3):629–643

Kaste SC. Imaging pediatric bone sarcomas. Radiol Clin North Am. 2011; 49(4):749–765, vi–vii

Khanna G, Bennett DL. Pediatric bone lesions: beyond the plain radiographic evaluation. Semin Roentgenol. 2012; 47(1):90–99

Nichols RE, Dixon LB. Radiographic analysis of solitary bone lesions. Radiol Clin North Am. 2011; 49(6):1095–1114, v

Wyers MR. Evaluation of pediatric bone lesions. Pediatr Radiol. 2010; 40(4):468–473

Case 121

James S. Chalfant

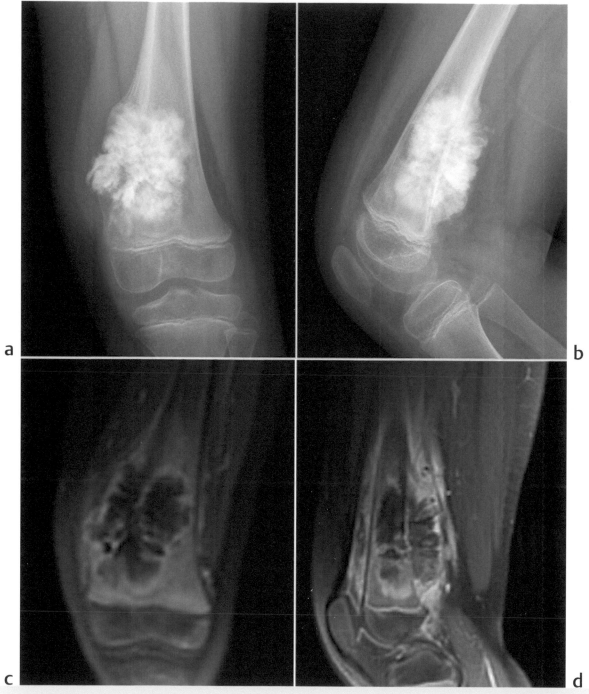

Fig. 121.1 Frontal **(a)** and lateral **(b)** views of the knee show an amorphous, dense metaphyseal lesion with lamellated and sunburst periosteal reaction and cortical destruction. T1-W fat-saturated gadolinium-enhanced coronal **(c)** and sagittal **(d)** MRI images show a heterogeneous, hypointense, calcific metaphyseal lesion with peripheral enhancement and a large soft-tissue component.

■ **Clinical Presentation**

An 8-year-old with a knee mass (►Fig.121.1).

■ Key Imaging Finding

Aggressive dense osseous lesion.

■ Top Three Differential Diagnoses

• **Chronic osteomyelitis.** Chronic osteomyelitis appears as heterogeneous sclerosis with dense, ossified endosteal and periosteal thickening that forms an involucrum. An isolated, dense sequestrum, consisting of necrotic bone, may serve as a nidus for ongoing infection. Chronic osteomyelitis appears hypointense on T1 and hyperintense on T2; the rim and granulation tissue enhance. A bony sequestrum, if present, is hypointense on both T1 and T2 and does not enhance. A draining cloacal tract may also be seen.

• **Osteosarcoma.** Osteosarcoma is the most common primary bone malignancy in children. There are several subtypes, with conventional high-grade intramedullary osteosarcoma representing 75%. Lesions usually originate in the metaphysis of long bones (distal femur, proximal tibia, humerus) during puberty. Radiographs classically reveal an aggressive, ill-defined, fluffy lesion with osteoid matrix, medullary and cortical destruc-

tion, aggressive periosteal reaction, and a soft-tissue mass. However, the extent of matrix ossification/calcification varies, and most lesions are mixed lytic and sclerotic. MRI appearance varies, with lytic regions appearing hypointense on T1 and hyperintense on T2 and mineralized regions hypointense on both sequences. Skip lesions occur in up to 15% of cases, making evaluation of the entire bone essential.

• **Ewing sarcoma.** Ewing sarcoma is the second most common primary bone malignancy in children and occurs in long bones (femur, tibia, humerus) and flat bones (ribs, scapula, pelvis). When in the long bones, most cases are metadiaphyseal or diaphyseal. Radiographs reveal an aggressive, permeative lesion with periosteal reaction (classically laminated, or "onion-skin"), variable sclerosis, and a soft-tissue mass. There may be patchy sclerosis due to reactive new bone formation.

■ Additional Differential Diagnoses

• **Lymphoma.** Primary bone lymphoma is almost always non-Hodgkin lymphoma. It appears permeative/lytic and often involves the metaphysis of long bones without periostitis. Secondary bone lymphoma often involves the spine and can be non-Hodgkin or, rarely, Hodgkin lymphoma. Hodgkin lymphoma is typically at least partly sclerotic.

• **Metastasis.** In the absence of known malignancy, osseous metastases are rare in children. When they do occur, they are often widespread and lytic.

• **Langerhans cell histiocytosis.** This has many different appearances and is difficult to exclude with imaging. Flat and long bones may be affected. Typically, these lesions are intramedullary and lytic with little sclerosis.

■ Diagnosis

Osteosarcoma.

✓ Pearls

• Presence of a bony sequestrum makes chronic osteomyelitis likely.
• Osteosarcoma is the most common primary bone malignancy in children and has an osteoid matrix in 90%.

• Ewing sarcoma is permeative and classically has onion-skin periosteal reaction.
• Lymphoma commonly lacks periosteal reaction.

Suggested Readings

Kim SH, Smith SE, Mulligan ME. Hematopoietic tumors and metastases involving bone. Radiol Clin North Am. 2011; 49(6):1163–1183, vi

Rajiah P, Ilaslan H, Sundaram M. Imaging of primary malignant bone tumors (non-hematological). Radiol Clin North Am. 2011; 49(6):1135–1161, v

Toma P, Granata C, Rossi A, Garaventa A. Multimodality imaging of Hodgkin disease and non-Hodgkin lymphomas in children. Radiographics. 2007; 27(5):1335–1354

Case 122

Jennifer L. Nicholas

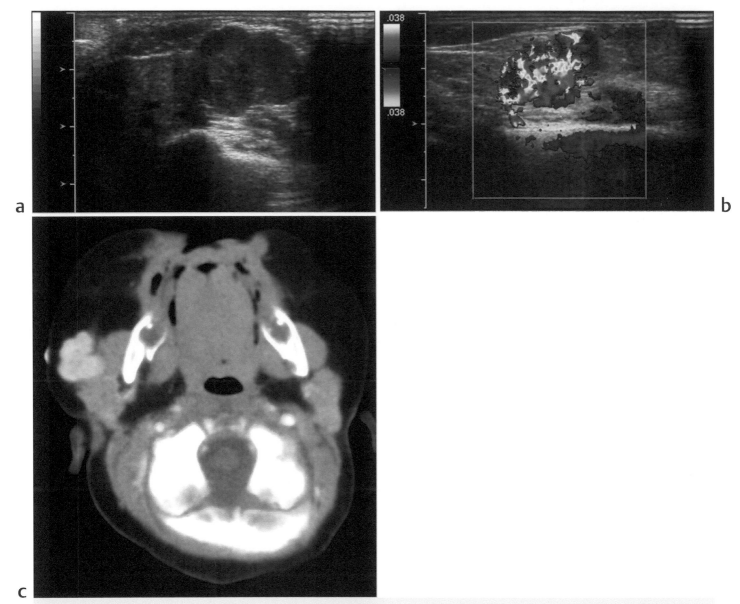

Fig. 122.1 US of the right cheek using a high-frequency linear transducer shows a well-defined, lobulated mass in the subcutaneous soft tissues that abuts but does not clearly involve the adjacent musculature; the mass is heterogeneous and slightly hypoechoic relative to surrounding tissues and was noted to be compressible (**a**). Color Doppler US interrogation shows the lesion is hypervascular with relatively homogeneous flow (**b**). Contrast-enhanced CT shows a lobulated, well-circumscribed, vigorously enhancing mass (**c**).

■ **Clinical Presentation**

A 1-month-old infant with a soft-tissue mass on the right cheek (▶Fig. 122.1).

■ Key Imaging Finding

Soft-tissue mass in an infant.

■ Top Three Differential Diagnoses

- **Infantile hemangioma.** Infantile hemangioma is the most common tumor of infancy, affecting up to 10% of Caucasian children. Many are noted within the first month of life. There may be an associated cutaneous lesion, such as a pale spot, telangiectatic or macular red stain, or bruiselike pseudoecchymotic patch. About 60% occur in the craniofacial region, 25% on the trunk, and 15% on the extremities. About 80% are solitary. At US, these high-flow lesions usually appear solid, well defined, hypoechoic, and hypervascular, with homogeneous flow. MRI appearance varies with lesion phase. Multiple cutaneous hemangiomas may be a harbinger of hemangiomas elsewhere (usually the liver) and should prompt further imaging. Infantile hemangiomas typically proliferate in the first year of life and involute by age 5 years.
- **Infantile myofibroma.** This benign, nodular soft-tissue tumor also occurs in muscle, bones, and viscera. Although rare, it is the most common fibrous tumor of infancy. Most infantile myofibromas present by age 2 years. The tumors may be solitary or multifocal (myofibromatosis). US appearance ranges from homogeneous and slightly hyperechoic to nearly anechoic with a thick rim. Many of these lesions regress without intervention. Treatment if needed is surgical excision.
- **Fibrous hamartoma of infancy.** Most fibrous hamartomas of infancy present as solitary painless nodules. Some have overlying skin changes, including altered pigmentation, eccrine gland hyperplasia, or hair. Most occur within the first year of life, and about one-fourth are present at birth. The lesions are usually located in the subcutaneous soft tissues and lower dermis of the axilla, upper arm, upper trunk, inguinal region, and external genital area. US shows a heterogeneously hyperechoic mass with a "serpentine" pattern and ill-defined or lobulated margins without substantial blood flow. Fibrous hamartomas sometimes regress spontaneously, but the treatment of choice is local excision.

■ Additional Differential Diagnoses

- **Infantile fibrosarcoma.** This large, rapidly growing tumor is the most common malignant soft-tissue mass in infants and is usually encountered in the extremities. US typically shows a heterogeneous, infiltrative, hypervascular lesion. MRI appearance is nonspecific. The prognosis is better in children than in adults.
- **Neuroblastoma metastasis.** Neuroblastoma metastases are usually solid, vascular lesions. They are primarily hyperechoic and may contain calcifications. Calcifications are readily recognized at CT.

■ Diagnosis

Infantile hemangioma.

✓ Pearls

- Infantile hemangiomas should be well defined and compressible and show high-velocity flow.
- US appearance of infantile myofibromas varies from homogeneous and slightly echogenic to almost anechoic with a thick rim.
- Fibrous hamartoma of infancy should be in the subcutaneous soft tissues and lower dermis and is generally heterogeneously hyperechoic with a "serpentine" pattern.
- Infantile fibrosarcomas grow rapidly, are heterogeneous, and are poorly defined.

Suggested Readings

Dickey GE, Sotelo-Avila C. Fibrous hamartoma of infancy: current review. Pediatr Dev Pathol. 1999; 2(3):236–243
Lee S, Choi YH, Cheon JE, Kim MJ, Lee MJ, Koh MJ. Ultrasonographic features of fibrous hamartoma of infancy. Skeletal Radiol. 2014; 43(5):649–653
North PE. Pediatric vascular tumors and malformations. Surg Pathol Clin. 2010; 3(3):455–494
Schurr P, Moulsdale W. Infantile myofibroma: a case report and review of the literature. Adv Neonatal Care. 2008; 8(1):13–20

Case 123

Rebecca Stein-Wexler

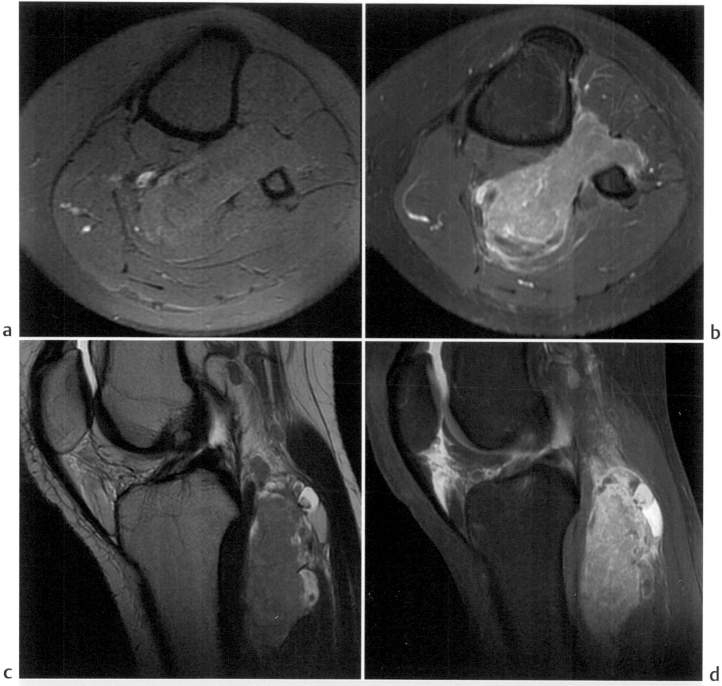

Fig. 123.1 Axial T1-W fat-suppressed image shows an ill-defined, slightly hyperintense mass between and posterior to the tibia and fibula (**a**). Axial T1-W fat-suppressed gadolinium-enhanced image better delineates this mildly heterogeneous, moderately enhancing bilobed lesion (**b**). Sagittal T2-W image shows the mass is predominantly hypointense, with peripheral, hyperintense lobulations (**c**). Sagittal T1-W gadolinium-enhanced image shows cystic and solid areas in this heterogeneously enhancing mass (**d**).

■ Clinical Presentation

A 17-year-old with a slowly growing knee mass (▶Fig. 123.1).

■ Key Imaging Finding

Large soft-tissue mass in an older child.

■ Top Three Differential Diagnoses

- **Rhabdomyosarcoma (RMS).** Most pediatric soft-tissue masses are benign, but large size (>10 cm), deep, nonfascial location, older age, and heterogeneous noncircumscribed appearance increase the likelihood of malignancy. RMS is the most common pediatric soft-tissue sarcoma overall. However, infantile sarcoma (in infants) and synovial cell sarcoma (in older children) are more common in the extremities. Extremity RMS usually affects older children. Despite the name, it occurs in a variety of tissues—not just muscle. Extremity RMS is usually of the alveolar subtype, which has a worse prognosis than botryoid, which affects the head/neck and genitourinary tract. Radiographs and US show a nonspecific soft-tissue mass without calcification, which enhances intensely but heterogeneously at CT and MRI. It is dark on T1 and bright on T2, and there may be areas of necrosis. CT/MRI appearance is nonspecific but useful for evaluating disease extent. Complete surgical resection significantly improves prognosis.
- **Lymphoma.** Lymphoma can involve almost any organ in the body and should be considered in the differential diagnosis of any puzzling lesion. When localized to the soft tissues, it is usually of the non-Hodgkin variety. Soft-tissue lymphoma may represent primary disease or result from contiguous or distant spread. The mass crosses fascial planes, engulfing more often than displacing vessels. Mass effect on vessels may cause distal soft-tissue swelling. Soft-tissue lymphoma is homogeneously hypoechoic on US and homogeneous on CT. Intermediate signal on T1-W MRI, it is intermediate to hyperintense on T2. Both CT and MRI commonly show soft-tissue stranding and enhancement due to infiltration. Adjacent nodal stations may demonstrate confluent lymphadenopathy, which is unusual in other soft-tissue sarcomas. Chemotherapy and radiation therapy are the mainstays of treatment.
- **Synovial sarcoma.** This highly malignant tumor arises from primitive mesenchyme. Often misdiagnosed as a benign lesion, it may appear small and encapsulated at diagnosis. The mass may have been present for months to years. Although it is usually found within 7 cm of a joint, it does not arise from synovial tissue. Synovial sarcoma most often occurs at the hands and feet or knee. About one-third calcify, and another one-third demonstrate "triple signal": hyperintense hemorrhage, isointense necrosis, and hypointense fibrosis. Resectable disease has an excellent prognosis, but metastatic disease (lung, bone, lymph nodes) is often fatal.

■ Additional Differential Diagnosis

- **Desmoid tumor (aggressive fibromatosis).** This infiltrative lesion does not metastasize but may be difficult to completely resect, so recurrence is common. It is most often encountered in adolescents and young adults. Usually located in muscle and adjacent fascia, it may encase nerves and vessels. Superficial soft tissues are rarely involved. MRI signal varies with cellularity, vascularity, and the amount of collagen and water.

■ Diagnosis

Synovial sarcoma.

✓ Pearls

- Although most pediatric soft-tissue masses are benign, risk of malignancy increases in older children and if the mass is greater than 10 cm, deep, heterogeneous, and noncircumscribed.
- Of all soft-tissue sarcomas, synovial sarcoma most often resembles a benign lesion.
- One-third of synovial sarcomas calcify, and another one-third show "triple signal" of hemorrhage, necrosis, and fibrosis.
- Desmoid tumor does not metastasize but is very infiltrative and hence difficult to resect.

Suggested Readings

Brisse HJ, Orbach D, Klijanienko J. Soft tissue tumours: imaging strategy. Pediatr Radiol. 2010; 40(6):1019–1028

McCarville MB, Spunt SL, Skapek SX, Pappo AS. Synovial sarcoma in pediatric patients. AJR Am J Roentgenol. 2002; 179(3):797–801

Roper GE, Stein-Wexler R. Soft tissue masses. In Stein-Wexler R, Wootton-Gorges SL, Ozonoff MB, eds. Pediatric Orthopedic Imaging. Berlin/Heidelberg: Springer; 2015:715–770

Case 124

Rebecca Stein-Wexler

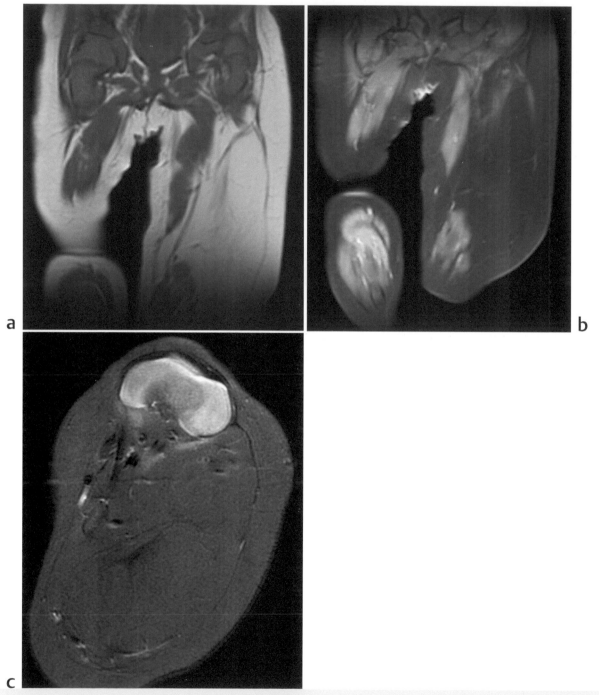

Fig. 124.1 Coronal T1-W image shows a large, infiltrative fatty mass with a few hypointense septations; the left hip is dislocated **(a)**. Gadolinium-enhanced T1-W fat-suppressed image shows strands enhance minimally **(b)**. Axial inversion-recovery fat-suppressed image shows the mass suppresses completely **(c)**.

■ Clinical Presentation

A 7-month-old boy with a soft, slowly growing thigh mass (▶ Fig. 124.1).

■ Key Imaging Finding

Fatty soft-tissue mass.

■ Top Three Differential Diagnoses

- **Lipoblastoma.** This rare tumor of embryonal white fat usually presents before age 4 years. It is considerably more common in boys than in girls. Patients are brought to medical attention because of a bulky, painless mass or its effect on adjacent structures. The mass consists of fat cells in various stages of maturation, along with myxoid stroma and a rich capillary network. Imaging appearance depends on the ratio of adipose cells to stroma. Radiographs may show a relatively lucent mass. Cross-sectional imaging shows a mass that resembles fatty tissue elsewhere, except there may be an increased amount of fibrous tissue (hypointense on all sequences on MRI). Enhancement may exceed that of adjacent fat due to a rich capillary network. Treatment is usually excision, but if untreated lipoblastoma will eventually evolve into lipoma.
- **Lipoblastomatosis.** Lipoblastomatosis resembles lipoblastoma but infiltrates muscle and other adjacent tissues. Because of this, resection is difficult and therefore recurrence is relatively common.
- **Lipoma.** In patients older than 10 years of age, fatty tumors are more likely to represent lipoma than lipoblastoma or lipoblastomatosis. As in adults, lipomas in children appear homogeneous and well circumscribed. Imaging characteristics are identical to those of subcutaneous fat.

■ Additional Differential Diagnoses

- **Teratoma.** Mature teratomas are generally considered benign, with very low risk of malignant transformation. They present as a large, heterogenous mass of fat and soft tissue that displaces and does not invade structures. Most are partly cystic, and one-fourth are partly calcified. Immature teratomas are typically predominantly soft-tissue density with smaller calcific and fatty foci. These tumors usually occur in the chest, abdomen, pelvis, and head/neck region.
- **Liposarcoma.** Liposarcoma is extremely rare in pediatric patients and usually presents in teens. In children, liposarcoma is almost always the myxoid subtype. Imaging and histology are nondiagnostic, and delineation of a t(12;16) translocation is needed for diagnosis. At imaging, liposarcoma may resemble lipoblastoma, with more admixed soft tissue than would be seen with lipoma. Sometimes myxoid elements appear cystic, and occasionally the mass shows no fatty characteristics at all.

■ Diagnosis

Lipoblastomatosis, with altered mechanics leading to hip dislocation.

✓ Pearls

- Lipoblastoma usually occurs in young children and—unlike lipoma—has myxoid stroma admixed with immature white fat.
- Lipoblastomatosis is more infiltrative than lipoblastoma and often recurs.
- Lipomas are common in children older than 10 years; they appear and behave similar to lipomas in adults.
- Liposarcoma is rare in children, is usually of the myxoid cell type, may contain no demonstrable fat, and must be diagnosed by molecular imaging.

Suggested Readings

Chen CW, Chang WC, Lee HS, Ko KH, Chang CC, Huang GS. MRI features of lipoblastoma: differentiating from other palpable lipomatous tumor in pediatric patients. Clin Imaging. 2010; 34(6):453–457

Murphey MD, Carroll JF, Flemming DJ, Pope TL, Gannon FH, Kransdorf MJ. From the archives of the AFIP: benign musculoskeletal lipomatous lesions. Radiographics. 2004; 24(5).1433–1466

Roper GE, Stein-Wexler R. Soft tissue masses. In Stein-Wexler R, Wootton-Gorges SL, Ozonoff MB eds. Pediatric Orthopedic Imaging. Berlin/Heidelberg: Springer; 2015:715–770

Case 125

Shruthi Ram

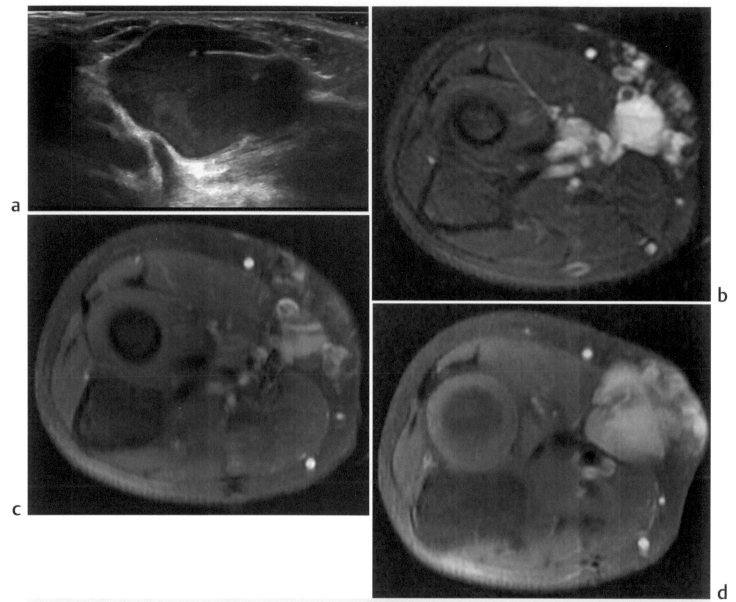

Fig. 125.1 US of the upper arm shows a well-circumscribed, septated mass containing hypoechoic material that was noted to swirl at real-time evaluation **(a)**. Axial T2-W fat-suppressed MRI shows a lobulated, hyperintense mass with at least one fluid–fluid level and a phlebolith (superficial round hypointensity); there is also signal void within a more anterior vessel **(b)**. T1-W gadolinium-enhanced fat-suppressed images show diffuse enhancement within the mass; the phlebolith remains hypointense **(c,d)**. (These images are provided courtesy of Gerald Behr.)

■ Clinical Presentation

A 7-year-old boy with a soft, compressible, bluish upper arm mass present since birth, growing proportionally to his somatic growth (▶Fig. 125.1).

■ Key Imaging Finding

Multiseptated cystic soft-tissue mass.

■ Top Three Differential Diagnoses

• **Venous malformation.** Venous malformations are low-flow lesions composed of endothelial-lined vascular sinusoids. They present in childhood or early adulthood as a blue, soft, compressible, nonpulsatile mass that grows proportionally with the body. At US, the mass typically appears multiseptated and cystic, with multiple sinusoidal spaces. Real-time US may demonstrate "to-and-fro" motion of echoes within the spaces due to slow-moving debris, and spectral Doppler may show venous flow. MRI shows a septated, lobulated fluid signal mass that crosses tissue planes. The absence of flow voids distinguishes it from a high-flow vascular malformation. The presence of phleboliths and gradual enhancement differentiates venous from lymphatic malformation, but venous and lymphatic elements may occur in a single lesion.

• **Lymphatic malformation.** Lymphatic malformations are another type of low-flow lesion, consisting of embryonic lymphatic sacs. Clinical and imaging features overlap with venous malformations, and the hybrid venolymphatic malformations contain elements of both. Enhancement pattern differs from that of venous malformations. Macrocystic lymphatic malformations show rim and septal enhancement. Microcystic lesions show no to minimal diffuse enhancement. Both venous and lymphatic malformations are treated with percutaneous sclerotherapy.

• **Infantile fibrosarcoma.** Infantile fibrosarcoma is a rare, malignant neoplasm of infancy, with better prognosis than the adult form. It is in the differential of any rapidly growing painless soft-tissue mass in an infant. Imaging shows a heterogeneous, hypervascular soft-tissue mass. Treatment is complete excision.

■ Additional Differential Diagnoses

• **Infantile hemangioma.** This high-flow vascular lesion is a true neoplasm formed of proliferating endothelial cells. A characteristic feature is rapid early proliferation and subsequent involution. Hemangiomas appear solid and often hypoechoic at US; MRI appearance varies with lesion phase.

• **Arteriovenous malformation.** This high-flow vascular malformation consists of enlarged arterial feeding vessels, along with the distinguishing feature of early draining veins. Dynamic MR angiography is useful for diagnosis. Arteriovenous malformations are treated with transarterial embolization.

■ Diagnosis

Venous malformation.

✓ Pearls

• Vascular malformations are categorized into low- and high-flow lesions, based on the presence of flow voids, enhancement pattern, and spectral Doppler characteristics.

• Venous malformations are multiseptated lesions that contain slow-moving fluid and demonstrate enhancement; there may also be phleboliths.

• Lymphatic malformations may be macrocystic, in which case the rims and septa enhance, or microcystic, in which case there is usually no or occasionally minimal diffuse enhancement.

Suggested Readings

Ahuja AT, Richards P, Wong KT, Yuen EH, King AD. Accuracy of high-resolution sonography compared with magnetic resonance imaging in the diagnosis of head and neck venous vascular malformations. Clin Radiol. 2003; 58(11):869–875

Ainsworth KE, Chavhan GB, Gupta AA, Hopyan S, Taylor G. Congenital infantile fibrosarcoma: review of imaging features. Pediatr Radiol. 2014; 44(9):1124–1129

Flors L, Leiva-Salinas C, Maged IM, et al. MR imaging of soft-tissue vascular malformations: diagnosis, classification, and therapy follow-up. Radiographics. 2011; 31(5):1321–1340, discussion 1340–1341

Case 126

Stephen Henrichon

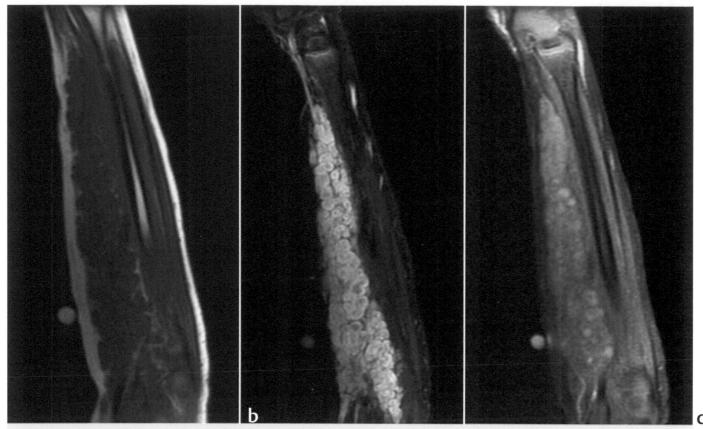

Fig. 126.1 Sagittal T1-W MRI of the forearm shows a lobulated, elongated soft-tissue mass that is isointense to muscle **(a)**. The mass is markedly hyperintense on inversion recovery (IR), with multiple areas of central hypointensity **(b)**. Gadolinium-enhanced fat-suppressed T1-W image shows mild enhancement **(c)**.

■ Clinical Presentation

A 7-year-old boy with overgrowth of the right forearm (▶Fig. 126.1).

■ Key Imaging Finding

Overgrowth of an extremity.

■ Top Three Differential Diagnoses

- **Posttraumatic.** Fractures may lead to limb length discrepancy by two mechanisms. Fracture-related hyperemia may cause an extremity to enlarge. Alternatively, physeal injury may limit growth, leading to relative enlargement of the other side. Residual bony deformity may suggest the etiology.
- **Plexiform neurofibroma.** Thirty percent of patients with neurofibromatosis type 1 (NF1) have plexiform neurofibromas, but only 10% of neurofibromas occur in patients with NF1. Plexiform neurofibromas are infiltrative, nodular, ropey masses that follow along deep and superficial branches of nerves and may lead to enlargement of an extremity. If superficial, they appear as a "bag of worms" on clinical exam. MRI shows a multilobulated, serpiginous mass (or masses) of intermediate T1 signal intensity. Enhancement is heterogeneous. Fluid-sensitive sequences show central hypointensity and peripheral hyperintensity, resulting in the classic "target" sign. Malignant degeneration occurs in a small percentage of cases and may manifest as new-onset pain, increasing size, and loss of the target appearance. Plaquelike neurofibromas, which are also a feature of NF1, infiltrate the superficial subcutaneous soft tissues and result in thickened skin. Localized neurofibromas are more common than plexiform or plaquelike neurofibromas both in patients with NF1 and in the general population; they appear as focal, fusiform enlargement of a usually superficial nerve.
- **Beckwith–Wiedemann syndrome (BWS).** BWS is usually sporadic and causes hemihypertrophy along with macroglossia, macrosomia, and abdominal wall defects. Extremity radiographs and cross-sectional imaging simply show asymmetrical osseous and soft-tissue enlargement. During their first decade, patients are at increased risk for embryonal tumors, usually Wilms tumor and hepatoblastoma. If an extremity is enlarged but other findings of BWS are absent, tumor risk is lower.

■ Additional Differential Diagnoses

- **Klippel–Trénaunay–Weber syndrome.** The classic triad of this disorder is limb hypertrophy, port wine stain, and congenital varicosities/venous malformations. Vascular malformations are venous and/or lymphatic and usually affect one leg, extending into the pelvis. X-rays show limb hypertrophy with bony and soft-tissue overgrowth, cortical thickening, fat hypertrophy, phleboliths, and serpiginous opacities in the soft tissues. MRI shows the infiltrative venolymphatic malformation along with fatty hyperplasia and muscle atrophy.
- **Macrodystrophia lipomatosa.** This spontaneous condition usually leads to enlargement of the second and third digits, rarely affecting an entire extremity. It presents at birth. Although there is hamartomatous overgrowth of all mesenchymal elements, adipose tissue and nerves are most severely affected.

■ Diagnosis

Plexiform neurofibroma.

✓ Pearls

- The MRI "target" appearance of plexiform neurofibroma helps exclude malignant degeneration.
- Most neurofibromas occur in patients who do not have NF1.
- Patient with Beckwith–Wiedemann syndrome have increased risk of embryonal tumors, such as Wilms tumor and hepatoblastoma.
- Lymphaticovenous malformations are an important feature of Klippel–Trénaunay–Weber syndrome.

Suggested Readings

Monsalve J, Kapur J, Malkin D, Babyn PS. Imaging of cancer predisposition syndromes in children. Radiographics. 2011; 31(1):263–280

Prada CE, Rangwala FA, Martin LJ, et al. Pediatric plexiform neurofibromas: impact on morbidity and mortality in neurofibromatosis type 1. J Pediatr. 2012; 160(3):461–467

Uller W, Fishman SJ, Alomari AI. Overgrowth syndromes with complex vascular anomalies. Semin Pediatr Surg. 2014; 23(4):208–215

Case 127

Aleksandar Kitich

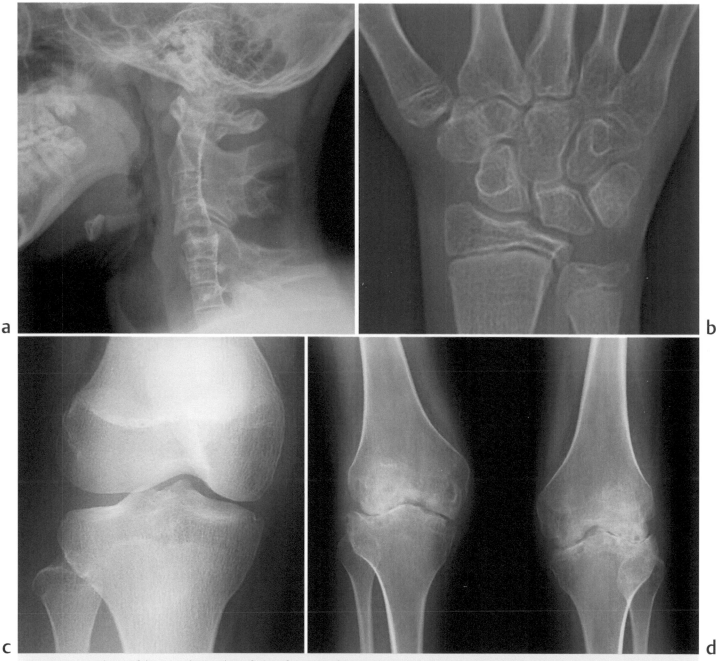

Fig. 127.1 Lateral view of the cervical spine shows fusion of posterior elements at C2–C4 and C5–T1 with partial fusion of the vertebral bodies; the intervertebral disk at C4–C5 is wide, and there is subluxation at this level **(a)**. (This image is provided courtesy of Tal Laor.) A frontal view of the wrist shows erosive changes in the carpus with areas of joint space narrowing, especially at the capitate and trapezoid **(b)**. Frontal view of the knee demonstrates subtle early erosions at the medial aspect of the right tibial plateau **(c)**. Frontal view of both knees in a patient with more advanced disease show cortical erosions, ballooning of the distal femurs with deformity of the articular surfaces, and reactive sclerosis **(d)**.

■ **Clinical Presentation**

Radiographs from several teens with joint pain (▶Fig. 127.1).

■ Key Imaging Finding

Cervical spine fusion, joint space narrowing with juxta-articular erosions, and ballooning of the femoral condyles.

■ Diagnosis

Juvenile idiopathic arthritis (JIA). JIA is a heterogeneous group of chronic arthropathies that develop before the age of 16 years and last at least 6 weeks. Diagnosis is based on clinical and laboratory findings. The disease is stratified based on the number of joints affected, along with the presence or absence of other clinical findings. If fewer than five joints are involved at diagnosis, the disease is considered oligoarticular, whereas with polyarticular disease five or more joints are involved. Fevers, rash, and hepatosplenomegaly suggest Still disease, a severe form of JIA.

Imaging is widely used in diagnosis and follow-up. Initial radiographs are often unremarkable, but as disease progresses osteopenia, bony erosions, and joint deformities develop. Due to their higher sensitivity for early signs of arthritis, MRI and US are employed more and more for initial diagnosis, evaluating disease severity, and assessing response to therapy.

Joints of the hand, cervical spine, and knee are most often involved. Radiographs are usually normal early on, or they may show soft-tissue swelling, joint effusion, and possibly osteopenia. They are important for excluding other osseous pathology and providing a baseline for follow-up. With disease progression, hyperemia leads to epiphyseal overgrowth. Thick cartilage in children initially protects bone from erosions, but eventually joint space narrowing and erosions may develop. With advanced disease, there may be ankylosis, growth disturbance, angular deformity, and contractures. Ankylosis is most common in the carpal bones, tarsal bones, and cervical spine. Soft-tissue periarticular calcifications may develop.

Contrast-enhanced MRI is most sensitive for detecting synovitis and early bone erosions. Erosions are best visualized using spin echo or fast spin echo MRI. Fluid-sensitive fat-suppressed techniques are best for evaluating joint fluid, marrow edema, and cartilage integrity. However, MRI is expensive, often requires contrast administration or patient sedation, and may not be readily available. Alternatively, US allows for evaluation of joint effusions, synovial proliferation, and cartilage thickness within smaller joints. Together, radiography, MRI, and US play an important role in diagnosis and management of JIA.

✓ Pearls

• On radiographs, early juvenile idiopathic arthritis appears as soft-tissue swelling, joint effusions, and periarticular osteopenia.
• Late radiographic findings include joint space narrowing, erosions, and subluxation.
• US is particularly useful for evaluating for joint effusions, synovial thickening, and tenosynovitis in the small joints.

• A severe form of juvenile idiopathic arthritis complicated by systemic manifestations such as fevers, rash, hepatosplenomegaly, lymphadenopathy, and anemia is known as Still disease.

Suggested Readings

Jordan A, McDonagh JE. Juvenile idiopathic arthritis: the paediatric perspective. Pediatr Radiol. 2006; 36(8):734–742

Kan JH. Juvenile idiopathic arthritis and enthesitis-related arthropathies. Pediatr Radiol. 2013; 43 Suppl 1:S172–S180

Ording Muller LS, Humphries P, Rosendahl K. The joints in juvenile idiopathic arthritis. Insights Imaging. 2015; 6(3):275–284

Sheybani EF, Khanna G, White AJ, Demertzis JL. Imaging of juvenile idiopathic arthritis: a multimodality approach. Radiographics. 2013; 33(5):1253–1273

Case 128

Leslie E. Grissom

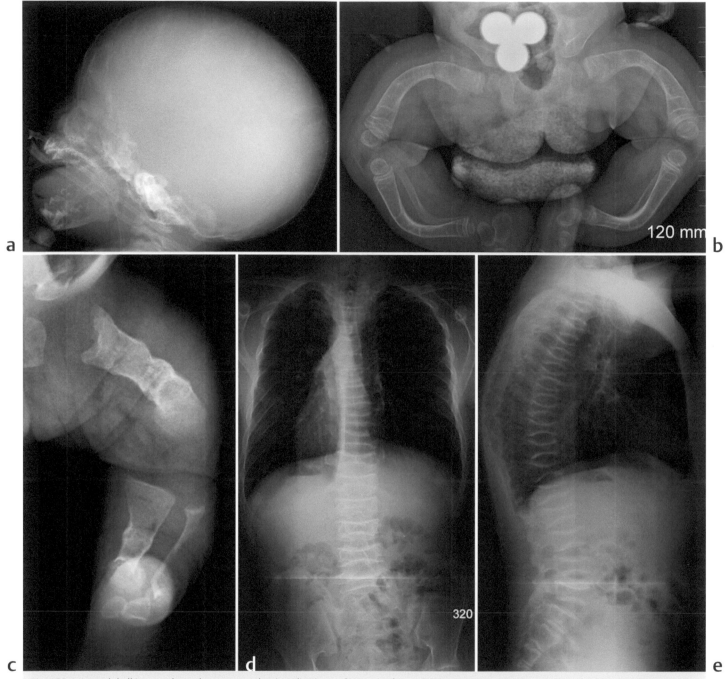

Fig. 128.1 Lateral skull in a newborn shows severe demineralization and Wormian bones (a). Lower extremities in an 11-month-old girl are bowed and very osteoporotic (b). Lower extremity in a newborn is crumpled, short, and thick (c). Spine radiographs in a 12-year-old boy show biconcave vertebrae and mild kyphoscoliosis (d,e).

■ Clinical Presentation

Several patients of different ages with the same disorder (▶Fig. 128.1).

■ Key Imaging Finding

Osteopenia, Wormian bones, bowing deformities, and multilevel spine fractures.

■ Diagnosis

Osteogenesis imperfecta (OI; also known as "brittle bone disease"). First described in 1788, osteogenesis imperfecta is a heterogeneous group of disorders characterized by some or all of the following: osteopenia, multiple fractures, blue sclerae, hypoplastic teeth/caries, easy bruising, joint hypermobility, and premature deafness. The incidence is about 6 per 100,000 births. Various genetic defects lead to at least 16 different subtypes. Abnormal type 1 collagen is seen in most of these disorders. Most cases are autosomal dominant, but some are autosomal recessive or result from new mutations. Types I through IV are the most common.

Patients with type I OI, which is the mildest, may present as children or adults with fractures from insignificant trauma. Type II is lethal in the perinatal period, and these patients are frequently diagnosed in utero with multiple rib and long bone fractures, leading to severe deformities. The skull bones are very poorly ossified. Patients with type III OI often have fractures at birth, but fractures may be delayed until age 2 years; they develop moderately short stature, scoliosis, and progressive deformity. Type IV is moderate in severity. Clinical features of these (and other) subtypes overlap, and therefore the disease may be described best as mild, moderate, marked, and lethal.

In general, bones are osteoporotic, and trabeculae are relatively thin. Patients with the lethal form of OI are born with beaded ribs, crumpled, short, thick long bones, and biconcave vertebrae. Patients with *severe* OI usually have fractures at birth. Bones are gracile and somewhat short, and biconcave deformity of the vertebrae leads to severe kyphoscoliosis. Patients with moderate OI have moderately fragile bones, and some have short stature; one-fourth have fractures at birth. Finally, those with mild OI have gracile bones that may be bowed; fractures are especially common in the lower extremities. Striking features of OI include excessive callus formation, popcorn calcifications about the epiphyses, large skull with frontal bossing, thin calvarium, Wormian bones, and basilar impression/invagination.

Treatment with bisphosphonates leads to thin metaphyseal bands, which resemble growth arrest lines. Intramedullary rods are commonly placed across fractures or across particularly gracile bones. Joint replacement and spine surgery may be required to preserve function.

Steroid-induced osteoporosis, idiopathic juvenile osteoporosis, metabolic bone disease, and neuromuscular disease may also lead to osteoporosis and multiple fractures, but clinical findings usually differentiate these entities from OI. Similarly, patients with dysplasias such as neurofibromatosis 1 and camptomelic dysplasia may have bowing of the extremities, but they also have features typical of their disease. Finally, multiple fractures are seen in patients with nonaccidental trauma, but they should not have Wormian bones and, in the absence of malnutrition, bone density is normal.

✓ Pearls

- Lethal osteogenesis imperfecta presents perinatally with beaded ribs, crumpled long bones, and biconcave vertebrae.
- Severe kyphoscoliosis develops in patients with severe osteogenesis imperfecta, and fractures are commonly present at birth.

- Patients with mild osteogenesis imperfecta may have gracile, bowed bones, but presentation may be delayed until childhood or early adulthood.

Suggested Readings

Burnei G, Vlad C, Georgescu I, Gavriliu TS, Dan D. Osteogenesis imperfecta: diagnosis and treatment. J Am Acad Orthop Surg. 2008; 16(6):356–366

Renaud A, Aucourt J, Weill J, et al. Radiographic features of osteogenesis imperfecta. Insights Imaging. 2013; 4(4):417–429

Sillence D. Osteogenesis imperfecta: an expanding panorama of variants. Clin Orthop Relat Res. 1981(159):11–25

Van Dijk FS, Pals G, Van Rijn RR, Nikkels PG, Cobben JM. Classification of osteogenesis imperfecta revisited. Eur J Med Genet. 2010; 53(1):1–5

Case 129

Rebecca Stein-Wexler

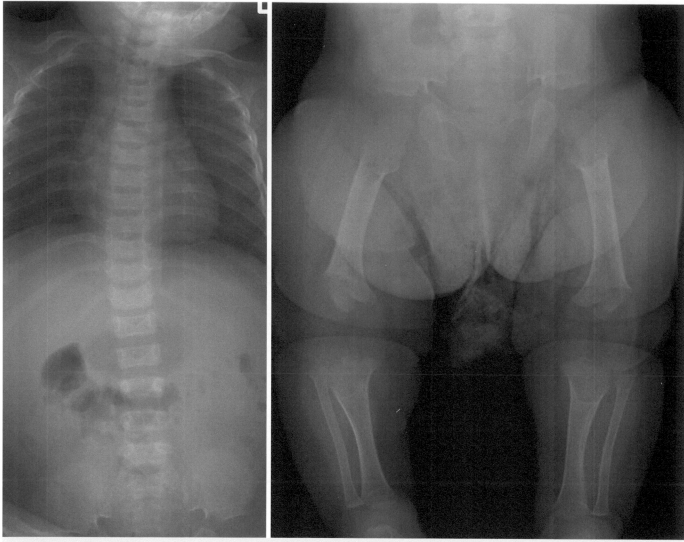

Fig. 129.1 Frontal radiograph of the chest and abdomen shows decreased interpediculate distances at the lower lumbar spine **(a)**. Frontal view of the pelvis and lower extremities shows the pelvis has "tombstone" iliac bones secondary to decreased acetabular angles and a "champagne glass" pelvic inlet. There is rhizomelic (proximal) limb shortening and an inverted "V" configuration of the distal femurs **(b)**.

a

b

■ Clinical Presentation

Infant with short stature and limb deformities (▶Fig. 129.1).

■ Key Imaging Finding

Decreased lower lumbar interpediculate distances, "tombstone" iliac bones, "champagne glass" pelvic inlet, and rhizomelic limb shortening.

■ Diagnosis

Achondroplasia. The most common nonlethal skeletal dysplasia, achondroplasia is a genetic disorder that results from autosomal-dominant inheritance or from spontaneous mutation. It is characterized by skeletal abnormalities attributable to decreased cartilage matrix production and endochondral ossification. Rhizomelic (proximal) limb shortening, metaphyseal flaring, and decreased interpediculate distance within the lower lumbar spine are characteristic.

Neurological problems are common. The foramen magnum and the skull base are small, which may result in brainstem compression. Restricted flow of CSF in this area sometimes causes hydrocephalus. The skull vault is large. The typical spine findings of narrow interpediculate distance and short pedicles may cause spinal cord compression. This may lead to weakness and numbness of the lower extremities.

The pelvis has a typical "tombstone" appearance due to squared iliac bones with decreased acetabular angles. The inner pelvic contour, with small sacrosciatic notches, has a "champagne glass" configuration.

The upper femurs and humeri of infants appear oval, and they are relatively lucent. Long bones are short and tubular, and the metaphyses slope more than usual. As the child matures, the tubular bones appear to become abnormally thick, although this just reflects normal width increase but lack of lengthening. Metaphyses develop irregular contour at sites of muscle insertion. Bullet-shaped phalanges of the hand taper above broad metastases. The hand has a "trident" shape.

Achondroplasia may be diagnosed by prenatal US at 25 weeks, with femur length often below the third percentile, a large head, a small chest, and polyhydramnios.

A less severe form of achondroplasia is termed "hypochondroplasia." In this condition, findings are mild, sometimes limited to the spine. Patients usually present with short stature and short limbs after age 2 to 4 years. Vertebral abnormalities are limited to decreased lumbar interpediculate distance. Limb shortening is usually rhizomelic but may be mesomelic (middle). The skull, pelvis, and hands appear normal, unlike with achondroplasia.

It is important not to confuse achondroplasia with "pseudo-achondroplasia," which is a completely unrelated syndrome that resembles multiple epiphyseal dysplasia.

✓ Pearls

- Achondroplasia shows decreased interpediculate distance, "champagne glass" pelvis, and "tombstone" iliac bones.
- The findings of hypochondroplasia are milder than with achondroplasia and may be limited to decreased lumbar interpediculate distance, although some patients have limb shortening as well.

Suggested Readings

Glass RB, Norton KI, Mitre SA, Kang E. Pediatric ribs: a spectrum of abnormalities. Radiographics. 2002; 22(1):87–104

Lemyre E, Azouz EM, Teebi AS, Glanc P, Chen MF. Bone dysplasia series. Achondroplasia, hypochondroplasia and thanatophoric dysplasia: review and update. Can Assoc Radiol J. 1999; 50(3):185–197

Parnell SE, Phillips GS. Neonatal skeletal dysplasias. Pediatr Radiol. 2012; 42 Suppl 1:S150–S157

Case 130

James S. Chalfant

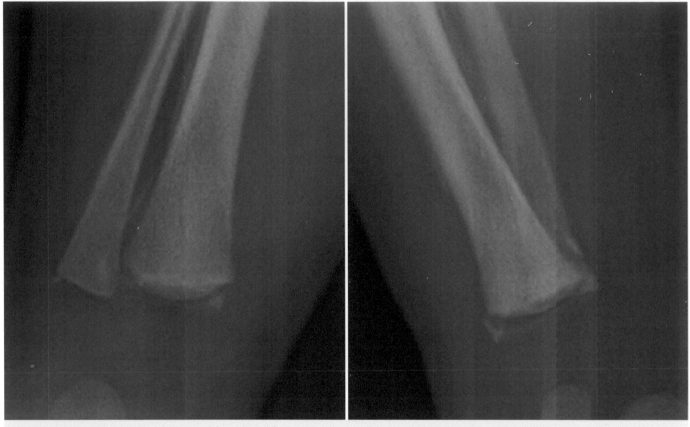

Fig. 130.1 Frontal **(a)** and lateral **(b)** views of the tibia and fibula show subacute metaphyseal fractures with periosteal reaction.

a

b

■ Clinical Presentation

A 2-month-old infant who is irritable (▶Fig. 130.1).

■ Key Imaging Finding

Classic metaphyseal lesions.

■ Diagnosis

Nonaccidental trauma (NAT). Fractures are the second most common finding in NAT, after cutaneous injuries. While metabolic disorders, skeletal dysplasias, and birth trauma may result in fractures that mimic abuse, the presence of suspicious fractures must prompt further evaluation, at which point other etiologies may also be explored. Radiography is usually sufficient to identify osseous injuries, and multiple professional societies including the American College of Radiology have published recommended skeletal survey protocols. The value of the skeletal survey decreases with age. A more focused examination should be performed for children older than 2 years based on clinical history, symptoms, and physical exam. A total body radiograph (babygram) is not appropriate in the evaluation of NAT, as it offers poor bone detail. Bone scintigraphy may augment the NAT workup if radiographs are negative.

In children younger than 3 years without significant known trauma, the positive predictive value of rib fractures for abuse is 95%. Commonly, fractures occur in the rib head or neck due to anteroposterior compression from squeezing. However, fractures due to abuse may be seen anywhere along the rib. Acute, nondisplaced fractures may be very difficult to see. Repeat imaging after 2 weeks may reveal sclerosis, periosteal reaction, and callus formation and thus help identify occult fractures.

Classic metaphyseal lesions (corner and bucket handle fractures) are highly specific for abuse in children younger than 1 year. Transmetaphyseal disruption of trabeculae from shearing forces during shaking causes these fractures. The classically described corner and bucket handle fractures represent the same pattern of metaphyseal injury viewed in different projections. A corner fracture (triangular-shaped bone fragment) is apparent when imaged tangentially, while a bucket handle fracture (crescent-shaped bone fragment) is seen when imaged at an angle.

Long bone fractures raise concern for abuse if the patient is nonambulatory. Other fractures that are associated with abuse include scapular, spinous process, and sternal fractures. Multiple bilateral fractures, injuries incompatible with the provided history, or findings indicating delay in seeking medical attention should also raise suspicion. Fractures of different ages are worrisome, with the caveat that fracture dating may be difficult and should be done cautiously given its role in legal proceedings. Repeat imaging may assist in dating and reveal fractures that were occult on the initial skeletal survey.

Intra-abdominal injuries such as hepatic/splenic lacerations and duodenal hematomas may accompany skeletal injuries. NAT may also result in hypoxic–ischemic brain injury, along with subdural and parenchymal hemorrhage. If there is high suspicion or evidence of abuse, cross-sectional imaging may be appropriate. While the need for cross-sectional imaging is case based, the American College of Radiology's Appropriateness Criteria deems a CT head without contrast as "usually appropriate" for children 24 months of age or younger with high-risk features (rib fractures, multiple fractures, facial injury, younger than 6 months), even in the absence of focal neurologic signs or symptoms.

✓ Pearls

- Rib fractures and classic metaphyseal lesions are highly specific for nonaccidental trauma.
- A complete skeletal survey is indicated for nonaccidental trauma workup in children younger than 2 years.
- A more focused examination can be performed for children older than 2 years based on areas of suspected injury.
- Fractures in unusual locations, of different ages, or incompatible with history should raise suspicion.

Suggested Readings

Kraft JK. Imaging of non-accidental injury. Orthop Trauma. 2011; 25:109–118

Offiah A, van Rijn RR, Perez-Rossello JM, Kleinman PK. Skeletal imaging of child abuse (non-accidental injury). Pediatr Radiol. 2009; 39(5):461–470

Stoodley N. Neuroimaging in non-accidental head injury: if, when, why and how. Clin Radiol. 2005; 60(1):22–30

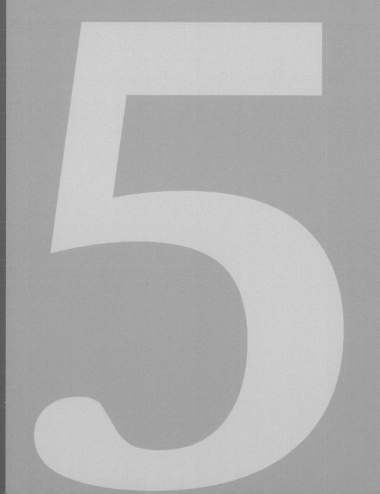

Part 5

Head and Neck Imaging

Case 131

Rebecca Stein-Wexler and Duy Quang Bui

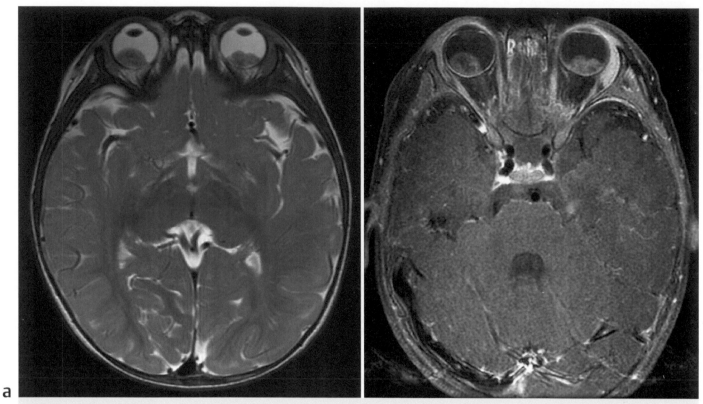

a   b

Fig. 131.1 Axial T2-W MRI shows bilateral intraocular masses that are slightly hypointense to gray matter **(a)**. T1-W fat-suppressed gadolinium-enhanced axial image shows the masses enhance **(b)**.

■ Clinical Presentation

An 8-year-old with leukocoria (▶Fig. 131.1).

■ **Key Imaging Finding**

Intraocular mass.

■ **Top Three Differential Diagnoses**

• **Retinoblastoma.** This is the most common intraocular malignancy in children. Most cases are diagnosed by age 5 years. The tumor is often sporadic. Inherited disease is more likely to be bilateral and to have additional suprasellar and pineal tumors. Patients usually present with leukocoria (white reflex), strabismus, or occasionally vision loss. Calcification is a near-constant feature, important to diagnosis. On MRI, the tumor is slightly hyperintense on T1 and hypointense on T2; it enhances avidly. It is important to evaluate the intra- and extraocular extent, as well as additional CNS disease. Metastases may involve regional lymph nodes, lung, liver, and bones.

• **Persistent fetal vasculature (PFV; formerly persistent hyperplastic primary vitreous).** PFV is a congenital condition that occurs when the primary vitreous (mesenchymal tissue that occupies the posterior chamber of the orbit) fails to regress and instead proliferates, forming fibrofatty tissue. Typically unilateral, PFV presents with leukocoria and microphthalmia and is usually diagnosed soon after birth. On CT, the orbit is small, with hyperdense vitreous that is typically hyperintense on T1 and T2. The hyperdense material assumes a V shape due to retinal detachment, a central remnant hyaloid stalk, and a retrolental mass.

• **Coats disease.** This retinal telangiectasia leads to breakdown of the blood–retina barrier and accumulation of fat and fluid in the retina and subretinal space. Patients present with leukocoria, progressive vision loss, and eventual retinal detachment, usually around age 6 to 8 years. CT and MRI show a noncalcified intraocular lesion that does not enhance. The lesion is denser than vitreous on CT and hyperintense on T1 and T2.

■ **Additional Differential Diagnosis**

• **Retinopathy of prematurity.** Also known as retrolental fibroplasia, this vascular disorder of the retina is usually seen in premature infants weighing less than 1.5 kg who received oxygen therapy. Vascular scarring and retinal detachment develop. Imaging shows an abnormal retrolental density, retinal detachment—sometimes with a fluid–fluid level, and microphthalmia. Calcification is rare except in advanced disease.

■ **Diagnosis**

Retinoblastoma.

✓ **Pearls**

• Retinoblastoma usually calcifies and shows avid enhancement on MRI.
• Persistent fetal vasculature is characterized by micropthalmos with V-shaped vitreous that is hyperdense on CT and hyperintense on both T1- and T2-W MRI.

• Coat disease also has hyperdense vitreous that like persistent fetal vasculature is T1/T2 hyperintense, but without a central stalk.

Suggested Readings

Burns NS, Iyer RS, Robinson AJ, Chapman T. Diagnostic imaging of fetal and pediatric orbital abnormalities. AJR Am J Roentgenol. 2013; 201(6):W797–W808

Chung EM, Specht CS, Schroeder JW. From the archives of the AFIP: pediatric orbit tumors and tumorlike lesions: neuroepithelial lesions of the ocular globe and optic nerve. Radiographics. 2007; 27(4):1159–1186

Rauschecker AM, Patel CV, Yeom KW, et al. High-resolution MR imaging of the orbit in patients with retinoblastoma. Radiographics. 2012; 32(5):1307–1326

Case 132

Patrick J. Sanchez

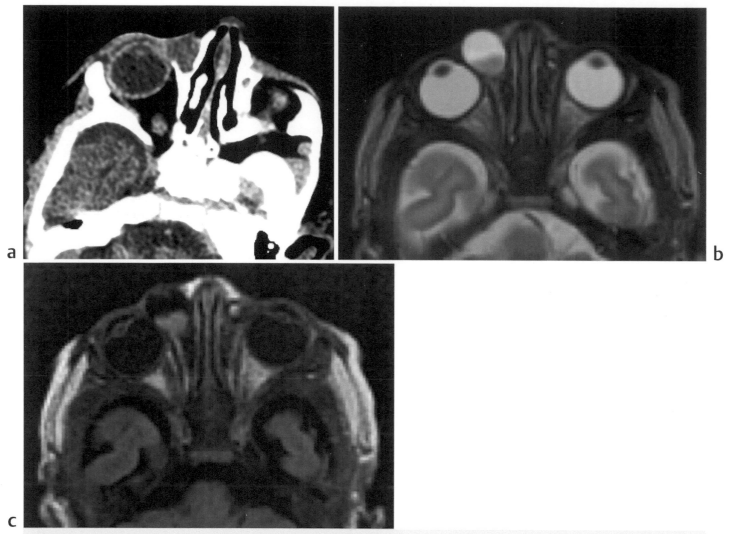

Fig. 132.1 Axial CT demonstrates a homogeneous, well-defined, thin-walled cystic lesion in the medial right canthus near the nasolacrimal duct **(a)**. Axial T2-W MRI shows a fluid-debris level, with hyperintense T2 fluid layered above hypointense material **(b)**. Axial T2 fluid-attenuated inversion recovery (FLAIR) MRI demonstrates suppression of fluid signal within the lesion **(c)**.

■ Clinical Presentation

A 3-year-old with intermittent swelling of the right eye (▶Fig. 132.1).

■ Key Imaging Finding

Cystic lesion in the anteromedial orbit.

■ Top Three Differential Diagnoses

- **Dacryocystocele.** A dacryocystocele is a benign, usually congenital cystic mass that forms at the inferomedial canthus due to obstruction of the proximal and distal ends of the nasolacrimal duct. Patients typically present with a triad of imaging findings, including a medial canthal mass, an enlarged nasolacrimal duct, and an intranasal mass. CT shows a cystic mass at the medial canthus and nasal cavity with mostly homogeneous fluid attenuation. On MRI, a dacryocystocele appears as a high-T2 cystic lesion in the medial canthal region extending into the nasal cavity, where it displaces the inferior turbinate and nasal septum. Internal debris may result in heterogeneous signal characteristics. There may be thin peripheral enhancement.
- **Dacryocystitis.** Dacryocystitis is inflammation of the nasolacrimal duct sac along the medial canthus and is typically a clinical diagnosis. It sometimes complicates dacryocystocele.

Imaging, if performed, demonstrates a round mass in the medial canthus with peripheral rim enhancement. If untreated, dacryocystitis may progress to abscess or orbital cellulitis.
- **Dermoid/epidermoid.** Dermoid and epidermoid cysts of the orbit are common congenital orbital lesions in children. Both are developmental, resulting from either incomplete separation of ectoderm from the neural tube or complex ectodermal in-folding during facial development. Both appear as well-circumscribed, cystic masses with smooth remodeling of adjacent bone. MRI characteristics vary, since epidermoids contain fluid, whereas dermoids contain lipid. Epidermoids demonstrate low T1 and high T2 signal intensity (similar to CSF but without suppression of signal on FLAIR). They have increased signal on DWI. Dermoid cysts in contrast are hypodense on CT and hyperintense on T1-W MRI.

■ Additional Differential Diagnoses

- **Encephalocele.** A naso-orbital encephalocele is a congenital neural tube defect with herniation of cranial contents through a defect in the midline anterior skull base. On MRI, it appears as a heterogeneous mass contiguous with intracranial structures. Signal characteristics are similar to those of brain and CSF.

- **Abscess.** An orbital abscess may result from untreated or progressive periorbital cellulitis. CT and MRI show heterogeneous attenuation and signal characteristics within the orbit, with peripheral enhancement and restricted diffusion. A distinct fluid collection may be observed.

■ Diagnosis

Dacryocystocele.

✓ Pearls

- Dacryocystocele results from obstruction of the nasolacrimal duct and appears as a cystic medial canthal mass.
- Dacryocystitis is inflammation of the nasolacrimal duct sac and may complicate a dacryocystocele.

- Since dermoids are lipid, they resemble fat on MRI, whereas epidermoids resemble simple fluid.

Suggested Readings

LeBedis CA, Sakai O. Nontraumatic orbital conditions: diagnosis with CT and MR imaging in the emergent setting. Radiographics. 2008; 28(6):1741–1753

Lowe LH, Booth TN, Joglar JM, Rollins NK. Midface anomalies in children. Radiographics. 2000; 20(4):907–922, quiz 1106–1107, 1112

Case 133

Rebecca Stein-Wexler

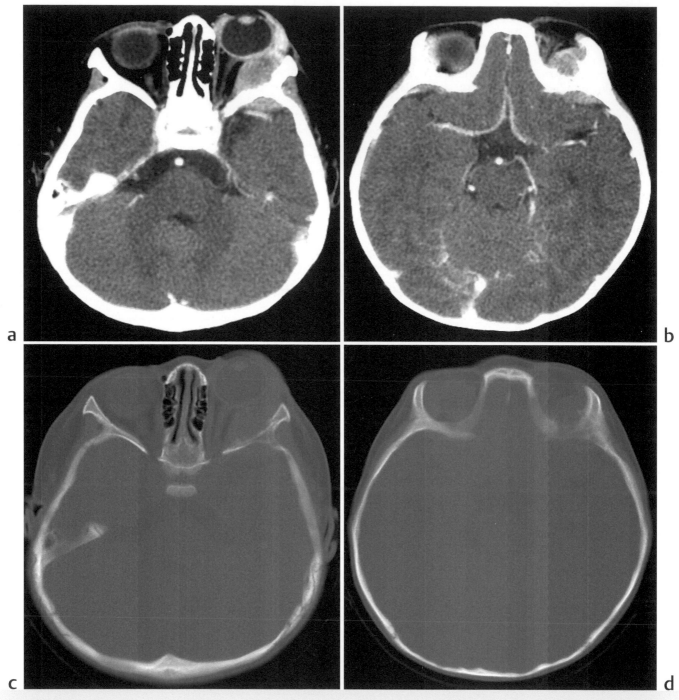

Fig. 133.1 Axial contrast-enhanced CT images show a left orbital mass centered at the posterolateral orbital roof, with a large soft-tissue component that causes proptosis and also extends intracranially to exert mass effect on the left frontal lobe (**a,b**). Bone windows show bone destruction along with subtle aggressive periosteal reaction (**c,d**).

■ Clinical Presentation

A 3-year-old with proptosis (▶Fig. 133.1).

■ Key Imaging Finding

Solid extraconal orbital mass.

■ Top Three Differential Diagnoses

- **Rhabdomyosarcoma (RMS).** RMS is the most common extra-ocular orbital malignancy in children. About 10% of RMS occurs in the orbit (superomedial or inferior). This soft-tissue tumor is aggressive, growing rapidly and usually presenting with proptosis. Most RMS is extraconal, though there may be intraconal extension. Bony erosion and invasion of the paranasal sinuses are fairly common. Homogeneous on CT, the tumor enhances diffusely. It appears more heterogeneous on MRI, especially if it has bled. RMS encases or displaces—but does not enlarge—the ocular muscles. The eyelid may be thickened without being infiltrated by tumor. Metastases (lung and bone) are less common than with RMS elsewhere.

- **Neuroblastoma (NB) metastasis.** Most pediatric orbital metastatic disease is NB, bilateral in about half of patients. Orbital NB is usually associated with an abdominal primary and is most common in patients younger than 2 years. Lytic lesions are often present elsewhere. Proptosis and periorbital ecchymosis result in the "raccoon eye" appearance. The tumor usually arises from the bony roof or lateral orbital wall and is extraconal. Preseptal extension is uncommon. There is permeative bone destruction, aggressive periosteal reaction, and often scattered intratumoral calcification. NB is hyperdense on unenhanced CT. Hemorrhage and/or necrosis lead to a heterogeneous appearance on T2-W MRI, along with heterogeneous enhancement. Dural metastases may cause dural widening. Urine vanillylmandelic acid (VMA) is often elevated.

- **Langerhans cell histiocytosis (LCH).** The superior or superolateral orbit is a relatively common site of eosinophilic granuloma (another name for the individual lesion in LCH). LCH usually develops before age 4 years. Identification of disease in the orbit should prompt a search for skeletal involvement elsewhere (technetium-99m bone scan, radiographs, and/or whole-body MRI). LCH is usually osteolytic, and beveled margins are typical of skull lesions. CT and MRI show a mass that destroys bone and may extend into the orbit, temporal fossa, face, and epidural region. Enhancement is moderate to marked. The mass is intermediate on T1 and usually hyperintense or occasionally hypointense on T2. It may be bilateral. Patients may present with diabetes insipidus (DI), which indicates pituitary involvement.

■ Additional Differential Diagnosis

- **Granulocytic sarcoma (GS, chloroma).** This soft-tissue tumor may precede systemic disease in patients with acute myelogenous leukemia (AML), develop during the course of disease, or be the first sign of relapse. Most GS occurs in children younger than 10 years. GS is usually unilateral. Orbital GS typically originates in the subperiosteal lateral orbital wall and does not erode bone. It encases rather than invades adjacent structures, such as the lacrimal gland and extraocular muscles. GS is homogeneous and does not calcify. It enhances uniformly. Iso- or hypointense compared with muscle on T1, it is heterogeneously iso- to hyperintense on T2.

■ Diagnosis

Neuroblastoma metastasis.

✓ Pearls

- Orbital rhabdomyosarcoma is most common in the superomedial or inferior orbit and invades bone and sinuses.
- Neuroblastoma metastasis is most common in the superior or lateral orbit wall and shows bone destruction.
- Granulocytic sarcoma may precede development of AML, is lateral within the orbit, and does not erode bone.
- Bilateral extraocular intraorbital masses are most likely neuroblastoma, granulocytic sarcoma, or Langerhans cell histiocytosis.

Suggested Readings

Chung EM, Smirniotopoulos JG, Specht CS, Schroeder JW, Cube R. From the archives of the AFIP: pediatric orbit tumors and tumorlike lesions: nonosseous lesions of the extraocular orbit. Radiographics. 2007; 27(6):1777–1799

Chung EM, Murphey MD, Specht CS, Cube R, Smirniotopoulos JG. From the archives of the AFIP. Pediatric orbit tumors and tumorlike lesions: osseous lesions of the orbit. Radiographics. 2008; 28(4):1193–1214

Case 134

Patrick J. Sanchez

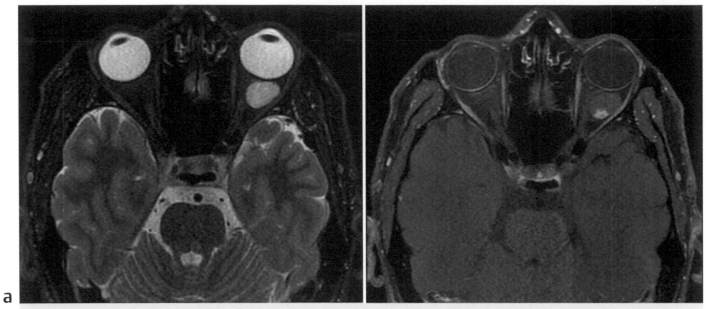

Fig. 134.1 Axial T2-W MRI shows a well-circumscribed T2-bright lesion in the intraconal space of the left orbit, displacing the adjacent optic nerve medially and lateral rectus muscle laterally **(a)**. Axial T1-W fat-suppressed gadolinium-enhanced MRI shows a small focus of avid enhancement **(b)**.

■ **Clinical Presentation**

A 4-month-old with proptosis (▶Fig. 134.1).

■ Key Imaging Finding

Hypervascular intraconal mass.

■ Top Three Differential Diagnoses

- **Hemangioma.** Capillary hemangiomas are one of the most common vascular lesions of the orbit in children. They develop shortly after birth and undergo a proliferative phase that lasts up to 1 year, followed by an involutional phase. CT shows a lobulated soft-tissue mass that enhances intensely, most often found in the extraconal space. On MRI, the lesion appears well circumscribed, isointense to hyperintense on T1, and moderately hyperintense on T2 (relative to muscle). Enhancement is intense. Flow voids and thin internal septa may be seen. Orbital capillary hemangiomas may occur in the setting of PHACES (posterior fossa malformations, hemangiomas, arterial anomalies, cardiac defects, eye abnormalities, sternal cleft, and supraumbilical raphe) syndrome. Maffucci syndrome is characterized by multiple enchondromas and soft-tissue hemangiomas that may involve the orbit.
- **Venolymphatic malformation (VLM).** VLM is composed of variable amounts of lymphatic and venous vessels. Although a

fairly common vascular lesion of the orbit, it is relatively rare in children. VLM appears as a poorly circumscribed, irregular, lobulated intraorbital mass that often involves both the intra- and extraconal spaces. Lesions may have small, cystic areas. CT may show bony remodeling and calcified phleboliths. MRI is preferred, typically demonstrating fluid–fluid levels that are isointense to slightly hyperintense on T1 and hyperintense on T2 (relative to brain). Enhancement on CT and MRI varies but is typically less intense than with orbital hemangiomas.

- **Dermoid/epidermoid.** These lesions may occur in the deep as well as anterior orbit and should be considered in the setting of a pediatric orbital mass. Epidermoids demonstrate low T1 and high T2 signal intensity (similar to CSF, but without suppression of signal on FLAIR). They have increased signal on diffusion. Dermoid cysts in contrast are hypodense on CT and hyperintense on T1-W MRI.

■ Additional Differential Diagnosis

- **Optic nerve glioma.** Optic nerve gliomas are uncommon tumors of the orbit, typically seen in the setting of neurofibromatosis type 1. CT and MRI show fusiform enlargement of the

optic nerve. The lesion may be T1 isointense to hypointense and T2 hyperintense (compared to the contralateral optic nerve). Enhancement is common.

■ Diagnosis

Hemangioma.

✓ Pearls

- Hemangiomas of the orbit are vascular lesions that demonstrate intense contrast enhancement.
- Optic nerve gliomas demonstrate fusiform enlargement of the optic nerve and usually occur in patients with neurofibromatosis type 1.

- Venolymphatic malformations of the orbit are less common in children than in adults and appear as a variably enhancing lobulated mass that may have phleboliths or fluid–fluid levels.

Suggested Readings

Chung EM, Smirniotopoulos JG, Specht CS, Schroeder JW, Cube R. From the archives of the AFIP: pediatric orbit tumors and tumorlike lesions: nonosseous lesions of the extraocular orbit. Radiographics. 2007; 27(6):1777–1799

Smoker WR, Gentry LR, Yee NK, Reede DL, Nerad JA. Vascular lesions of the orbit: more than meets the eye. Radiographics. 2008; 28(1):185–204, quiz 325

Case 135

Patrick J. Sanchez

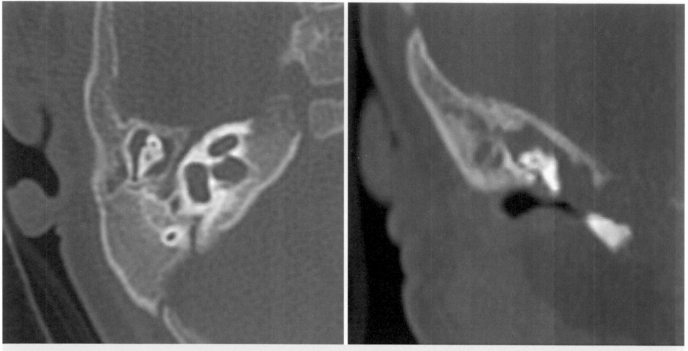

Fig. 135.1 Axial (a) and coronal (b) CT images of the temporal bone demonstrate a homogeneous, expansile soft-tissue density mass filling nearly the entire middle ear, with fluid in the mastoid air cells. The middle ear ossicles are preserved without erosion.

■ **Clinical Presentation**

A child presenting with hearing loss (▶Fig. 135.1).

■ Key Imaging Finding

Soft-tissue mass in the middle ear.

■ Top Three Differential Diagnoses

- **Otitis media.** Acute otitis media is typically a disease of infancy and early childhood. It does not require imaging if uncomplicated. CT/MRI show fluid and debris within the middle ear and mastoid air cells, sometimes with air fluid levels. Bony structures are preserved, including the middle ear ossicular chain, mastoid trabeculae, and overlying cortex. Chronic otitis media due to underlying eustachian tube dysfunction may be complicated by granulation tissue formation and development of an acquired cholesteatoma.
- **Congenital cholesteatoma.** Cholesteatomas are classified as congenital or acquired, with the congenital form typically presenting in children. Congenital cholesteatomas arise from the embryonic inclusion of epithelial rest cells within the temporal bone and are therefore composed primarily of tissue derived from epithelium, such as keratin and cholesterol. They may occur anywhere within the temporal bone, including the middle ear. CT demonstrates an expansile soft-tissue mass. MRI shows a well-marginated lesion that may erode the ossicles and scutum. It is dark on T1 and usually brighter than CSF on T2. Lesions do not typically attenuate on FLAIR. There is no central enhancement, although some lesions may demonstrate thin peripheral enhancement.
- **Aberrant internal carotid artery (ICA).** An aberrant ICA is a collateral pathway of the normal ICA, resulting from involution of the first embryonic portion of the ICA. The reduced caliber ICA consequently passes through the tympanic canal into the middle ear, returning to its normal course in the petrous carotid canal. The normal bone that should cover the carotid canal is absent. CT and MRI show a soft-tissue mass continuous with the ICA. MRI shows signal flow void, and postcontrast images demonstrate avid arterial enhancement. Middle ear surgery performed on an unrecognized aberrant ICA can be catastrophic.

■ Diagnosis

Congenital cholesteatoma.

✓ Pearls

- Acute otitis media demonstrates soft-tissue opacification of the middle ear and mastoids, without bony erosion.
- A congenital cholesteatoma appears as a soft-tissue mass that causes bony erosion, typically in the setting of conductive hearing loss.
- It is important to evaluate for continuity with the ICA in order to exclude aberrant ICA.

Suggested Readings

Baráth K, Huber AM, Stämpfli P, Varga Z, Kollias S. Neuroradiology of cholesteatomas. AJNR Am J Neuroradiol. 2011; 32(2):221–229

Juliano AF, Ginat DT, Moonis G. Imaging review of the temporal bone: part I. Anatomy and inflammatory and neoplastic processes. Radiology. 2013; 269(1):17–33

Case 136

Rebecca Stein-Wexler

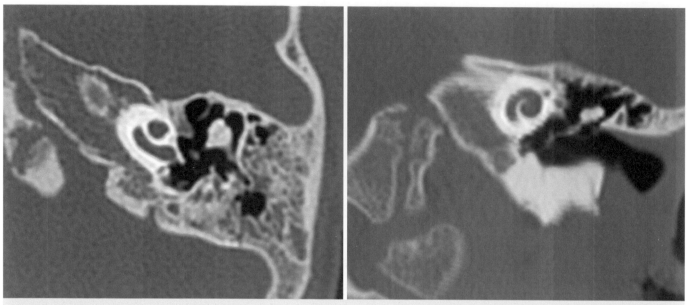

a   b

Fig. 136.1 Axial temporal bone CT shows the basal turn of the cochlea and an apical cyst instead of the middle and apical turns **(a)**. Coronal reformatted image shows only two turns of the cochlea **(b)**.

■ Clinical Presentation

A 4-year-old girl with sensorineural hearing loss (▶ Fig. 136.1).

■ Key Imaging Finding

Inner ear congenital malformation.

■ Top Three Differential Diagnoses

- **Enlarged vestibular aqueduct (VA).** Enlarged VA is by far the most common cause of sensorineural hearing loss (SNHL). Hearing loss is often progressive and may be exacerbated by trauma. In addition, enlarged VA accompanies inner ear anomalies in almost 85% of patients. The condition is often bilateral. On CT, the upper normal for the midpoint of the VA is 1.5 mm. MRI demonstrates enlargement of the endolymphatic duct and sac.
- **Incomplete partition type 2 (IP2; Mondini malformation).** SNHL due to this and the following malformations is usually diagnosed in infancy. Temporal bone MRI and CT play complementary roles. Brain MRI is useful for diagnosing frequently coexistent brain abnormalities. With IP2, the modiolus is incomplete, and there is no interscalar septum or osseous spiral lamina. The cochlea makes only 1.5 turns. The basal turn is normal, but the middle and apical turns fuse to form an apical cyst. In addition, the VA is often enlarged, whereas the semicircular canals tend to be normal.
- **Common cavity.** With common cavity, there is no differentiation between the cochlea and vestibule, so they form a confluent cystic cavity that completely lacks internal architecture. The cavity is usually wider than it is tall. The semicircular canals are usually also deformed.

■ Additional Differential Diagnoses

- **Cochlear hypoplasia.** In this condition, a small cochlear bud (1–3 mm) protrudes from a usually normal vestibule. It completes at most one turn. The internal auditory canal (IAC) is usually small, and the vestibule and semicircular canals are usually abnormal.
- **Incomplete partition type 1 (IP1; cystic cochleovestibular malformation).** With IP1, there is no modiolus, so the cochlea appears cystic. Unlike with common cavity, the dilated vestibule is separate from the cochlea. Axial imaging shows a circle-of-8 or snowman appearance. The VA is normal and the IAC dilated, increasing risk of meningitis.

■ Diagnosis

Incomplete partition type 2 (Mondini malformation).

✓ Pearls

- Enlarged vestibular aqueduct is the most common cause of sensorineural hearing loss, and in addition this condition accompanies many inner ear anomalies.
- With incomplete partition type 2, the modiolus is incomplete; the middle and apical turns of the cochlea fuse to form an apical cyst.
- With incomplete partition type 1, the dilated vestibule is separate from the cochlea, but with common cavity they form a confluent cystic cavity.
- A tiny cochlear bud protrudes from the vestibule in cochlear hypoplasia.

Suggested Readings

DeMarcantonio M, Choo DI. Radiographic evaluation of children with hearing loss. Otolaryngol Clin North Am. 2015; 48(6):913–932

Joshi VM, Navlekar SK, Kishore GR, Reddy KJ, Kumar EC. CT and MR imaging of the inner ear and brain in children with congenital sensorineural hearing loss. Radiographics. 2012; 32(3):683–698

Sennaroglu L, Saatci I. A new classification for cochleovestibular malformations. Laryngoscope. 2002; 112(12):2230–2241

Case 137

Anna E. Nidecker

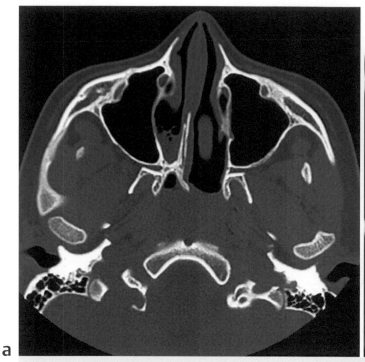
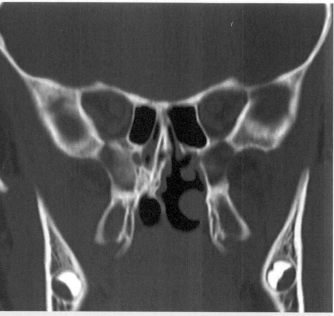

a   b

Fig. 137.1 Axial CT shows bone bridging the nasal aperture on the right (a). Coronal reformat shows the nasal septum is deviated to the right, and bone extends from the lateral aspect of the nasal septum to the medial aspect of the nasal cavity (b).

■ Clinical Presentation

A 10-year-old boy with nasal stuffiness (▶Fig. 137.1).

■ Key Imaging Finding

Narrowed choanae (posterior nasal passage).

■ Top Three Differential Diagnoses

- **Choanal atresia/stenosis.** Bilateral choanal atresia is the most common cause of neonatal nasal obstruction, but if unilateral this may present in older children. It occurs when the posterior part of the nasal passage is congenitally stenotic or occluded, blocking air passage to the posterior nasopharynx and oropharynx. The choana is normally about 3 mm wide in children younger than 2 years. Atresia is osseous (90%) or membranous (10%) and is unilateral in about half of cases. Since infants are obligate nasal breathers, affected neonates typically show signs of respiratory distress or even cyanosis at birth. Crying relieves respiratory distress by opening the oral airway. Rhinorrhea and the inability to pass a nasal cannula are other important clinical signs that should initiate investigation. Bilateral choanal atresia is a life-threatening condition, and an oral airway must be established immediately. The condition is best diagnosed on CT, where soft tissue or bone bridges the posterior nasal passage on one or both sides.
- **Nasal aperture stenosis.** The nasal (pyriform) aperture is the bony inlet of the nose, formed by the nasal and maxillary bones. The maxillary spine marks its inferior border. Stenosis of the aperture is a very rare cause of nasal obstruction in infants. It is typically associated with other severe congenital midline anomalies, such as holoprosencephaly. There is no standardized size for the aperture, so diagnosis can be difficult. Findings on CT include inward bowing of the maxillary spine and bone or soft tissue extending across the nostrils just inside the nares.
- **Stenosis of entire nasal airway.** This is usually osseous and may be associated with prematurity. It is also seen in Apert syndrome (maxillary hypoplasia). This extremely rare condition may be asymptomatic in the newborn period, as stenosis may be incomplete.

■ Additional Differential Diagnosis

- **Congenital nasal mass.** Congenital masses in the midline nasal region resulting from defective neural tube closure include anterior encephaloceles, nasal gliomas, and dermoids/ epidermoids. These can result in nasal obstruction. MRI and CT demonstrate a cystic or soft-tissue mass in the nasal passageway.

■ Diagnosis

Unilateral choanal atresia.

✓ Pearls

- Choanal atresia can be bony or soft tissue.
- Bilateral choanal atresia presents in neonates with respiratory distress as well as constant nasal drainage (rhinorrhea) and inability to pass a nasal cannula.
- The diagnosis of unilateral choanal atresia may be delayed because the infant is able to use one nostril to breathe.
- Choanal atresia is much more common than nasal aperture stenosis or stenosis of the entire airway.

Suggested Readings

Lowe LH, Booth TN, Joglar JM, Rollins NK. Midface anomalies in children. Radiographics. 2000; 20(4):907–922, quiz 1106–1107, 1112

Vanzieleghem BD, Lemmerling MM, Vermeersch HF, et al. Imaging studies in the diagnostic workup of neonatal nasal obstruction. J Comput Assist Tomogr. 2001; 25(4):540–549

Case 138

Anna E. Nidecker

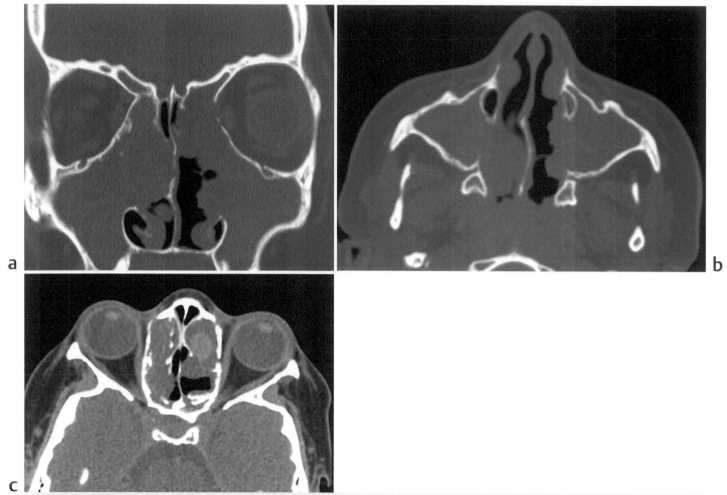

Fig. 138.1 Coronal reformatted CT in bone windows shows pan sinus opacification with demineralization of the bony portions of the ostiomeatal complex and ethmoid sinuses **(a)**. Axial CT in bone windows shows polypoid soft-tissue fills the maxillary sinuses and extends into the nasal cavity; the nasal septum is intact **(b)**. Axial CT in soft-tissue windows shows focal hyperdensity within soft tissue that almost fills the ethmoid air cells **(c)**.

■ Clinical Presentation

Child complaining of chronic nasal stuffiness (▶Fig. 138.1).

■ **Key Imaging Finding**

Opacified paranasal sinuses.

■ **Top Three Differential Diagnoses**

- **Underpneumatization.** Pneumatization of the paranasal sinuses is a gradual process, so the paranasal sinuses of infants and small children are often dense and may be mistaken for inflammatory sinus disease. Furthermore, crying may lead to transient opacification of the paranasal sinuses.
- **Sinusitis.** As in adults, both acute and chronic sinusitis commonly causes opacification of the paranasal sinuses. The bony margins of the paranasal sinuses may be unusually thick in cases of chronic infection. Bone erosion and inflammation in adjacent structures, such as orbits and facial fat, should raise suspicion for malignancy or an aggressive—possibly fungal—infection. Increased density also suggests fungal etiology.
- **Cystic fibrosis.** Cystic fibrosis is an autosomal-recessive hereditary disease caused by a defect in the cystic fibrosis trans-

membrane conductance regulator (CFTR) gene. This gene is involved in the production of sweat, digestive enzymes, and mucus, which become abnormally thick in patients with cystic fibrosis. The diagnosis can be made with a "sweat test" (testing for abnormally high chloride levels) or by genetic testing. Mucus is unusually thick and accumulates, impairing the ability of cilia to clear it from the lungs. A similar process in the sinuses causes mucus buildup, obstruction of drainage pathways, and subsequent infection. The appearance resembles sinus inflammation from other causes. Difficult-to-treat sinus infections with concomitant lung infection and failure to thrive can be signs of cystic fibrosis.

■ **Additional Differential Diagnoses**

- **Granulomatosis with polyarteritis (GPA).** Previously known as Wegener granulomatosis, GPA is a systemic, probably autoimmune vasculitis affecting small- and medium-sized vessels in many organ systems. Necrotizing granulomas form, and lung and kidney damage can be fatal. Chronic paranasal sinus inflammation that does not respond to routine therapy is a common presentation. Inflammation in the mucosal vessels leads to destruction of the mucosa and surrounding structures, including cartilage and bone. Hallmarks include "saddle

nose" deformity (from collapsed nasal cartilage) and obliterated nasal septum.
- **Kartagener syndrome.** Also known as primary ciliary dyskinesia, this autosomal-recessive disorder causes abnormal motility of the cilia lining the respiratory tract, including the trachea, lungs, paranasal sinuses, eustachian tubes, and middle ears. Poor mucociliary clearance and increased incidence of infections in the sinuses and lungs result. The triad of bronchiectasis, abnormal situs, and sinusitis characterize this syndrome.

■ **Diagnosis**

Cystic fibrosis with focus of fungal super infection.

✓ **Pearls**

- With cystic fibrosis, thick mucus impairs the ability of cilia to function properly.
- Granulomatosis with polyarteritis commonly presents with chronic paranasal sinus inflammation that does not respond to therapy.

- Kartagener syndrome is characterized by bronchiectasis, abnormal situs, and sinusitis.

Suggested Readings

Gysin C, Alothman GA, Papsin BC. Sinonasal disease in cystic fibrosis: clinical characteristics, diagnosis, and management. Pediatr Pulmonol. 2000; 30(6):481–489

Momeni AK, Roberts CC, Chew FS. Imaging of chronic and exotic sinonasal disease: review. AJR Am J Roentgenol. 2007; 189(6) Suppl:S35–S45

Case 139

Rebecca Stein-Wexler and Duy Quang Bui

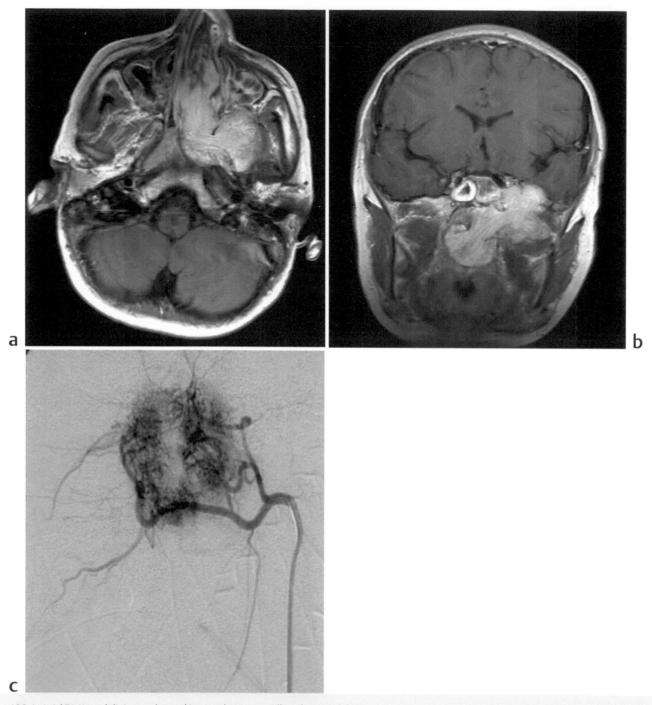

Fig. 139.1 Axial T1-W gadolinium-enhanced image shows an avidly enhancing lobulated mass that is centered in the sphenopalatine fossa but extends into the nasal cavity and pterygopalatine fossa **(a)**. Coronal T1-W gadolinium-enhanced image shows extension into the middle cranial fossa **(b)**. Digital subtraction angiography (DSA) demonstrates hypervascular tumor blush **(c)**.

■ **Clinical Presentation**

A 12-year-old boy with epistaxis (▶Fig. 139.1).

■ Key Imaging Finding

Aggressive nasal cavity/nasopharyngeal mass.

■ Top Three Differential Diagnoses

- **Lymphoma.** Lymphoma is the most common malignancy of the head and neck in children. Most cases manifest as cervical lymphadenopathy due to Hodgkin disease. The nasopharynx is more likely to be affected by non-Hodgkin lymphoma. Lymphomatous lymph nodes are less T2 intense than reactive nodes, and enhancement is both less intense and more variable.
- **Rhabdomyosarcoma (RMS).** This is a common pediatric soft-tissue malignancy, and about one-third of cases occur in the head and neck. It is most often encountered in young children (mean age 5–6 years) but has a second peak in adolescence. RMS typically occurs in the orbits (proptosis), nasal sinuses (obstruction, epistaxis), and neck (mass). This aggressive tumor shows bone remodeling and destruction on CT. MRI is best for evaluating intracranial extension as well as both

local and perineural spreads. RMS is homogeneous, with variable but usually homogeneous contrast enhancement.
- **Juvenile nasopharyngeal angiofibroma.** Benign but aggressive, this highly vascular tumor presents in adolescent males (median age 15 years) with unilateral nasal obstruction and epistaxis. CT and MRI show an avidly enhancing nasal mass that involves the sphenopalatine fossa, nasopharynx, nasal cavity, and/or sphenoid sinus. It causes bone remodeling and destruction. Fibrous tissue may cause the tumor to appear hypointense on T2. Flow voids are prominent, and there is intense enhancement. Intracranial extension into the middle cranial fossa occurs infrequently. Due to the degree of hypervascularity, preoperative embolization is commonly performed to assist with hemostasis during resection.

■ Additional Differential Diagnosis

- **Nasopharyngeal squamous cell carcinoma.** This rare, aggressive tumor occurs in adolescents, often with a history of Epstein–Barr virus infection. Patients present with cervical lymphadenopathy, nasal obstruction, otitis media, and/or

rhinorrhea, and are often initially treated for infection. Imaging shows a soft-tissue mass that usually destroys the skull base and may also destroy the bone of the paranasal sinuses.

■ Diagnosis

Juvenile nasopharyngeal angiofibroma.

✓ Pearls

- Although head/neck lymphoma usually presents with cervical adenopathy, it may manifest as a nasopharyngeal mass.
- Both rhabdomyosarcoma and the far less common nasopharyngeal squamous cell carcinoma are aggressive, homogeneous soft-tissue masses that tend to destroy bone.

- Juvenile nasopharyngeal angiofibroma is a benign, very vascular, aggressive tumor that presents in adolescent boys as an avidly enhancing nasal sinus mass.

Suggested Readings

Boghani Z, Husain Q, Kanumuri VV, et al. Juvenile nasopharyngeal angiofibroma: a systematic review and comparison of endoscopic, endoscopic-assisted, and open resection in 1047 cases. Laryngoscope. 2013; 123(4):859–869

Freling NJ, Merks JH, Saeed P, et al. Imaging findings in craniofacial childhood rhabdomyosarcoma. Pediatr Radiol. 2010; 40(11):1723–1738, quiz 1855

Stambuk HE, Patel SG, Mosier KM, Wolden SL, Holodny AI. Nasopharyngeal carcinoma: recognizing the radiographic features in children. AJNR Am J Neuroradiol. 2005; 26(6):1575–1579

Case 140

Anna E. Nidecker

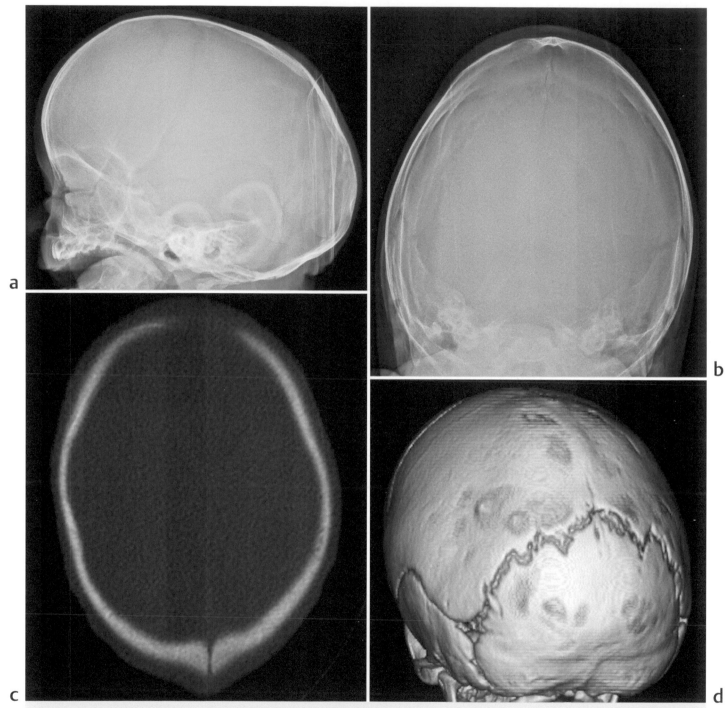

Fig. 140.1 Lateral skull radiograph shows an elongated skull shape (**a**). Townes view shows bone bridging the sagittal suture (**b**). Axial CT in bone windows shows bone heaped up at the knife-sharp sagittal suture (**c**). Surface volume–rendered reconstruction shows bone bulging at the expected position of the sagittal suture (**d**).

■ **Clinical Presentation**

An infant with a funny-looking head (▶Fig. 140.1).

■ Key Imaging Finding

Premature sutural synostosis.

■ Top Three Differential Diagnoses

- **Sagittal synostosis.** Cranial synostosis occurs when the fibrous sutures of the skull close prematurely. Open sutures allow the skull to expand as the brain grows. When a suture fuses prematurely, the skull grows parallel to the closed suture, leading to abnormal head shape. Clinical examination is usually diagnostic. A low-dose head CT with three-dimensional (3D) surface-rendered reconstructions confirms sutural synostosis. In cases of sagittal synostosis, compensatory growth occurs forward at the coronal suture and backward at the lambdoid suture. The skull becomes elongated in the anteroposterior plane, leading to frontal bossing and scaphocephaly (*scapho*, meaning boat), also called dolichocephaly (*dolicho*, meaning elongated). During early stages, the suture margin loses its normal serrated contour and appears knife sharp and dense. With progressive closure, bone bridges the suture and eventually obliterates it. Isolated sagittal synostosis is usually idiopathic.
- **Metopic synostosis.** Premature fusion of this anterior suture leads to a triangular-shaped frontal bone, or trigonocephaly. (*trigon*, meaning triangle). The orbits may appear quizzical, due to upward slanting of their medial portion. About one-third of cases are syndromic.
- **Coronal synostosis.** Premature fusion of one coronal suture leads to anterior flattening, or plagiocephaly, whereas fusion of both leads to an abnormally wide, brachycephalic skull (*brachi*, meaning arms). The condition may also be recognized by the appearance of the "harlequin eye," due to upward slanting of the lateral orbital roof as a result of hypoplasia of the supraorbital ridge. Bilateral coronal synostosis is often syndromic, whereas unilateral synostosis is typically idiopathic.

■ Additional Differential Diagnoses

- **Lambdoid synostosis.** Lambdoid synostosis leads to posterior plagiocephaly, or flattening of the posterior skull. If both sutures fuse, the skull shape is tall. Both unilateral and bilateral lambdoid synostoses are rare.
- **Kleeblattschädel skull.** This clover-leaf-shaped skull results from fusion of the sagittal, coronal, and lambdoid sutures. It may be seen with thanatophoric dysplasia and both Apert and Crouzon syndromes.
- **Positional plagiocephaly.** Children with positional plagiocephaly present with posterior skull flattening, mimicking lambdoid synostosis. However, this skull contour is due to unchanged positioning of the head slightly to the side while lying supine. Persistent pressure on one side of the posterior skull causes bony remodeling. Positional plagiocephaly may be distinguished from synostotic posterior plagiocephaly by the position of the ipsilateral ear relative to the contralateral ear. In synostotic plagiocephaly, the ipsilateral ear is displaced anteriorly. The forehead may also jut out anteriorly in patients with posterior synostotic plagiocephaly. If they cannot be distinguished clinically, a head CT allows evaluation of the lambdoid suture.

■ Diagnosis

Premature synostosis of the sagittal suture.

✓ Pearls

- With early fusion, the suture loses its serrated contour; its edges become dense and sharp before fusing completely.
- Sagittal and unilateral coronal synostoses are usually idiopathic, whereas others are often syndromic.

- Abnormal anterior position of the ipsilateral ear relative to the contralateral ear distinguishes lambdoid synostosis from positional plagiocephaly.

Suggested Readings

Badve CA, Mallikarjunappa MK, Iyer RS, Ishak GE, Khanna PC. Craniosynostosis: imaging review and primer on computed tomography. Pediatr Radiol. 2013; 43(6):728–742, quiz 725–727

Nagaraja S, Anslow P, Winter B. Craniosynostosis. Clin Radiol. 2013; 68(3):284–292

Case 141

Anna E. Nidecker

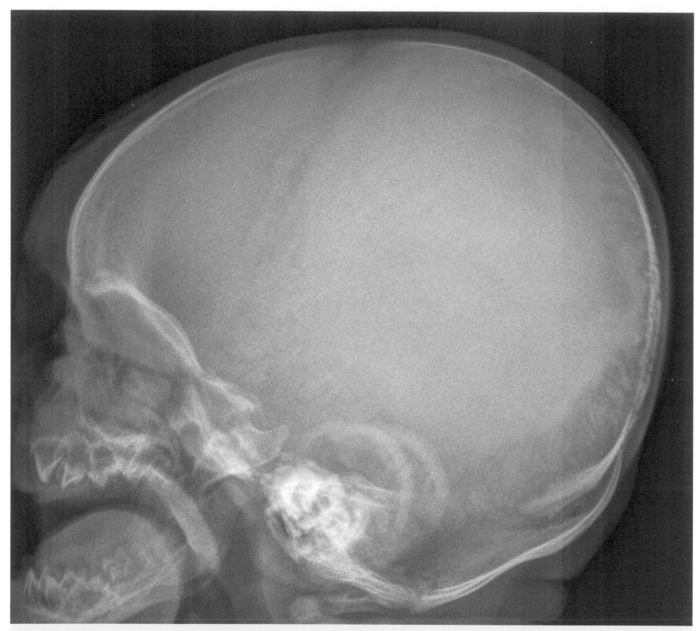

Fig. 141.1 There are many small islands of bone within the lambdoid suture.

■ Clinical Presentation

A 3-month-old infant who fell from the changing table (▶Fig. 141.1).

■ Key Imaging Finding

Wormian bones.

■ Top Three Differential Diagnoses

- **Idiopathic.** Wormian bones, which are small areas of ossification within the sutures of the cranium, are also known as intrasutural bones. They typically have irregular, well-corticated margins. Wormian bones are most common in the lambdoid suture, which is more tortuous than other sutures. The presence of a few wormian bones is typically idiopathic. However, if there are more than 10, or if they are very large, the likelihood of an associated disorder is increased.
- **Osteogenesis imperfecta (OI).** OI is a group of genetic disorders resulting in a defect in type I collagen that leads to excessive bone fragility and multiple fractures. Other tissues are also affected, with blue sclera, short stature, hearing loss, and breathing problems also occurring in some of these patients.

There are eight subtypes (I–VIII). Type I is the mildest, and type II is the most severe. Patients with OI have an increased incidence of wormian bones. The most severely affected are likely to have more numerous wormian bones.

- **Cleidocranial dysostosis.** This rare genetic disorder results in abnormal ossification of midline structures, particularly the skull and clavicles (hence the name). These patients have an increased incidence of wormian bones in the skull, in addition to an abnormally thin and poorly ossified calvarium. Patients also have nonunion of the mandibular symphysis and hypoplastic or absent clavicles. Other findings include hypoplastic paranasal sinuses, cleft palate, and wide symphysis pubis.

■ Additional Differential Diagnosis

- **Other associated disorders.** Wormian bones are associated with many other syndromes, including trisomy 21 and pycno- dysostosis. Patients with rickets and hypothyroidism may also demonstrate wormian bones.

■ Diagnosis

Wormian bones.

✓ Pearls

- Wormian bones are focal islands of ossification within sutures, with irregular but well-corticated margins.
- Wormian bones are usually idiopathic.
- The larger the number and size of wormian bones, the more likely there is an underlying abnormality; if there are more than 10, osteogenesis imperfecta is the most likely diagnosis.

- Additional findings of multiple fractures (fragile bones) or absent midline bones (clavicles, mandible), respectively, suggest osteogenesis imperfecta or cleidocranial dysostosis.

Suggested Readings

Offiah AC, Hall CM. Radiological diagnosis of the constitutional disorders of bone. As easy as A, B, C? Pediatr Radiol. 2003; 33(3):153–161

Panda A, Gamanagatti S, Jana M, Gupta AK. Skeletal dysplasias: A radiographic approach and review of common non-lethal skeletal dysplasias. World J Radiol. 2014; 6(10):808–825

Warman ML, Cormier-Daire V, Hall C, et al. Nosology and classification of genetic skeletal disorders: 2010 revision. Am J Med Genet A. 2011; 155A(5):943–968

Case 142

Anna E. Nidecker

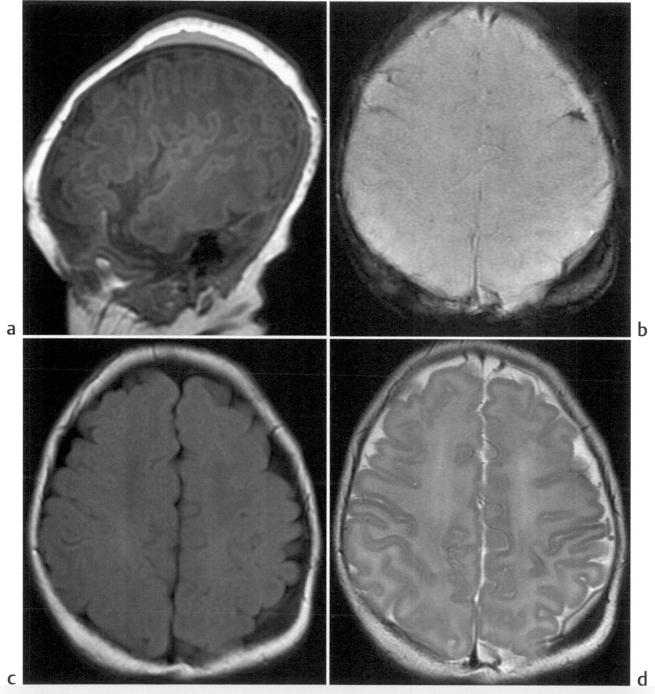

Fig. 142.1 Sagittal 3D spoiled gradient (SPGR) image shows a mildly hyperintense lentiform lesion, superficial to the calvarium, that does not cross the coronal or lambdoid sutures (**a**). Axial gradient echo (GRE) image shows the fluid is hypointense, and there is blooming artifact (**b**). Axial T2 FLAIR image shows the collection is hypointense (**c**). It is also hypointense on axial T2-W image (**d**).

■ Clinical Presentation

An 8-day-old with head swelling (▶ Fig. 142.1).

■ Key Imaging Finding

Scalp fluid collection in the neonate.

■ Top Three Differential Diagnoses

- **Cephalohematoma.** Fluid collections and hematomas external to the skull are distinguished by their location relative to the periosteum and also relative to the galeal aponeurosis. The galeal aponeurosis is a fibrous band that covers the skull. It merges anteriorly with the frontalis muscle and posteriorly with the occipitalis muscle. In the case of a true cephalohematoma, hemorrhage is confined to the area beneath both the galeal aponeurosis and the periosteum of the outer table of the skull. This means that the collection cannot cross suture lines and therefore has limited potential for causing catastrophic blood loss.
- **Subgaleal hematoma.** A true subgaleal hematoma is also located beneath the galeal aponeurosis. However, it is superficial to the periosteum of the outer table of the calvarium, and therefore hemorrhage is not limited by suture lines. Subgaleal hematomas can be large, and they hold greater potential for catastrophic blood loss in infants. Most (90%) of these hematomas result from applying a vacuum to the head at delivery, which ruptures emissary veins superficial to the periosteum. Swelling may occur immediately after delivery or begin 12 to 72 hours later. Hemorrhage may be extensive and spread across the entire head. Distinguishing a true subgaleal hematoma from a cephalohematoma is not always possible on imaging.
- **Caput succedaneum.** This is the most superficial of the scalp hematomas in infants. It forms where vacuum forceps were applied. This collection of serosanguineous fluid is located beneath the skin, superficial to the galeal aponeurosis. It is not fluctuant, does not grow, and is infrequently imaged.

■ Additional Differential Diagnosis

- **Nonaccidental trauma (NAT).** NAT should always be considered when encountering an infant with evidence of head trauma. The fluid collections mentioned earlier are more common in the perinatal period, however. If superficial blood and/or fluid is identified, it is important to correlate findings with birth history. The entities discussed earlier are correlated with vaginal birth, are located at the top (crown) of the head, and typically become clinically apparent within 72 hours of birth. Signs that may suggest NAT include presence of subdural hematomas, retinal hemorrhages, and fractures, which are very rare in delivery.

■ Diagnosis

Cephalohematoma.

✓ Pearls

- Scalp hematomas are very common following vaginal delivery, especially if there has been birth trauma or vacuum-assisted devices have been used.
- While it may be difficult to distinguish subgaleal hematomas from cephalohematomas on imaging, an important distinction is that subgaleal hematomas can cross suture lines and therefore hold greater potential for blood loss.
- The presence of other findings, such as retinal hemorrhages, subdural hematomas of varying ages, and fractures, should raise suspicion for nonaccidental trauma.

Suggested Readings

Firlik KS, Adelson PD. Large chronic cephalohematoma without calcification. Pediatr Neurosurg. 1999; 30(1):39–42

Foerster BR, Petrou M, Lin D, et al. Neuroimaging evaluation of non-accidental head trauma with correlation to clinical outcomes: a review of 57 cases. J Pediatr. 2009; 154(4):573–577

Glass RB, Fernbach SK, Norton KI, Choi PS, Naidich TP. The infant skull: a vault of information. Radiographics. 2004; 24(2):507–522

Case 143

Karen M. Ayotte

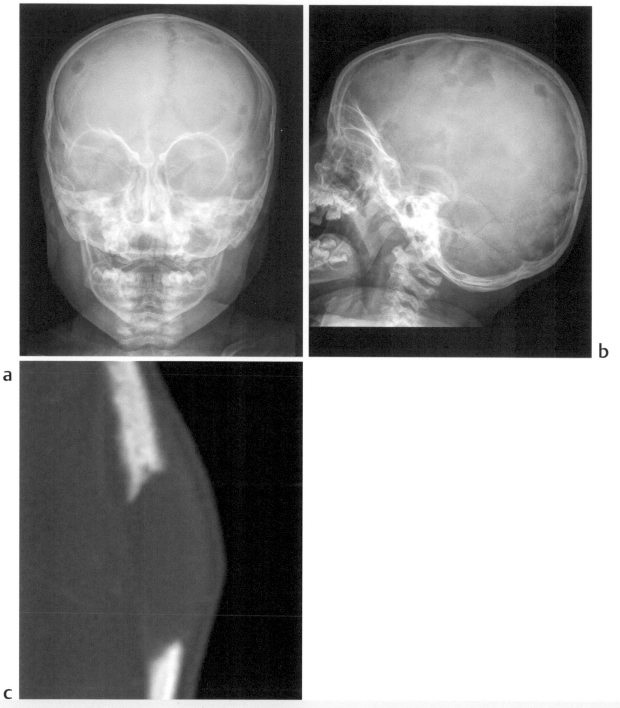

Fig. 143.1 Frontal **(a)** and lateral **(b)** skull radiographs show multiple well-circumscribed, lytic calvarial lesions. Left temporal bone CT at bone windows shows well-defined beveled margins and a small soft-tissue mass **(c)**.

■ **Clinical Presentation**

A 20-month-old boy with headache (▶Fig. 143.1).

■ Key Imaging Finding

Lytic skull lesions.

■ Top Three Differential Diagnoses

- **Langerhans cell histiocytosis (LCH).** The skull is the most common site of osseous involvement in LCH. The classic lesion is well defined and lytic, without sclerotic borders. A "beveled edge" appearance, or "hole within hole," results from greater involvement of the inner than outer table of the skull. LCH may also present as a round, radiolucent skull defect with a central dense nidus or sequestrum of intact bone, referred to as a "button sequestrum." The most common clinical presentation includes pain, palpable mass, and/or systemic symptoms.
- **Epidermoid cyst.** Epidermoid cysts result from abnormal deposition of epithelial rests within the diploic space during development. They are the second most common etiology for

solitary skull lesions that lead to biopsy in the pediatric population. When an epidermoid cyst involves the diploic space, the radiographic appearance overlaps that of LCH. Epidermoid cysts are typically well-defined, expansile lesions without a central matrix. The rim may or may not be sclerotic.
- **Neoplasm.** Leukemia, Ewing sarcoma, and metastatic neuroblastoma may produce poorly defined osteolytic lucencies in all bones, including the skull. Metastatic deposits in the skull cause lytic destruction and expansion. Localized areas of bone destruction in leukemia are frequently surrounded by normal bone and likely represent tumor metastases. These lesions tend to have an aggressive appearance.

■ Additional Differential Diagnoses

- **Infection.** Osteomyelitis has a wide range of imaging manifestations, and it may even appear normal or mimic an aggressive neoplasm. In the skull, bone destruction may lead to a lytic lesion, typically with poorly defined margins. There may be overlying soft-tissue edema. Subacute and chronic infection may present radiographically as a round, radiolucent, more well-defined skull defect with a central dense nidus or sequestrum of necrotic bone. This "button sequestrum" serves as a nidus for infection.
- **Leptomeningeal cyst.** The term leptomeningeal cyst (growing skull fracture) signifies a well-defined bone defect that arises when traumatic laceration of the dura exposes the skull to the pulsations of CSF within the subarachnoid space. Pulsatile pressure gradually widens the fracture line. Leptomeningeal cysts are an uncommon complication of skull fractures (0.6%) and are usually seen in children younger than 3 years.

■ Diagnosis

Langerhans cell histiocytosis.

✓ Pearls

- Langerhans cell histiocytosis classically presents as a lytic skull lesion with nonsclerotic, beveled margins.
- Langerhans cell histiocytosis and osteomyelitis may have "button sequestra" and systemic symptoms.

- Common metastatic skull lesions in children include neuroblastoma and leukemia.
- A leptomeningeal cyst (growing skull fracture) is caused by CSF pulsations after disruption of the dura.

Suggested Readings

D'Ambrosio N, Soohoo S, Warshall C, Johnson A, Karimi S. Craniofacial and intracranial manifestations of langerhans cell histiocytosis: report of findings in 100 patients. AJR Am J Roentgenol. 2008; 191(2):589–597

Gibson SE, Prayson RA. Primary skull lesions in the pediatric population: a 25-year experience. Arch Pathol Lab Med. 2007; 131(5):761–766

Glass RB, Fernbach SK, Norton KI, Choi PS, Naidich TP. The infant skull: a vault of information. Radiographics. 2004; 24(2):507–522

Krasnokutsky MV. The button sequestrum sign. Radiology. 2005; 236(3):1026–1027

Case 144

Rebecca Stein-Wexler

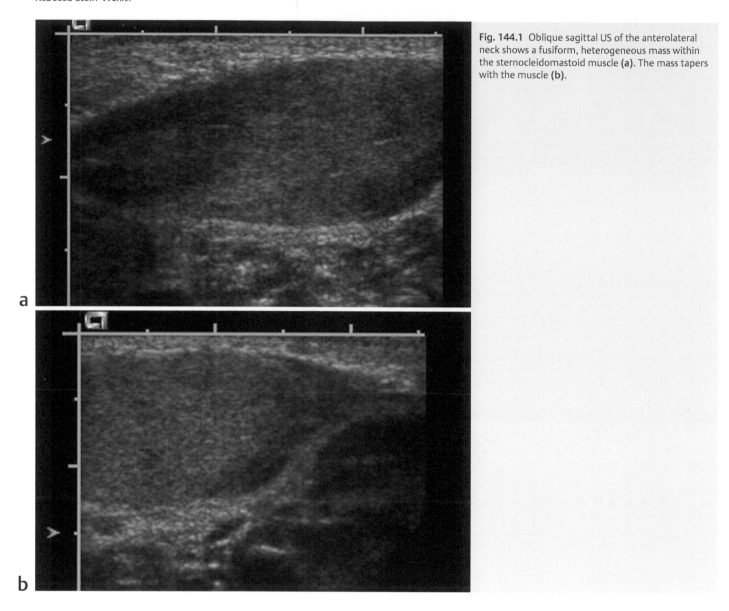

Fig. 144.1 Oblique sagittal US of the anterolateral neck shows a fusiform, heterogeneous mass within the sternocleidomastoid muscle (**a**). The mass tapers with the muscle (**b**).

■ Clinical Presentation

A 2-week-old with torticollis and a neck mass (▶Fig. 144.1).

■ Key Imaging Finding

Solid neck mass in an infant.

■ Top Three Differential Diagnoses

• **Fibromatosis colli.** Infants with this pseudotumor present in the first few weeks of life with a palpable mass in the sterno-cleidomastoid muscle. It causes the chin to turn slightly away from and the head to tilt toward the affected side. The mass may be due to compression of venous outflow from the ster-nocleidomastoid during difficult delivery, leading to muscle fibrosis. US shows fusiform expansion of the muscle, with a focal hyperechoic mass or a diffusely heterogeneous muscle. The mass does not extend beyond the sternocleidomastoid, and tissue planes are preserved. MRI is rarely necessary. The mass enlarges over the first few weeks of life and then stabi-lizes in size, resolving between age 4 and 8 months.

• **Lymphadenopathy.** Infectious or neoplastic lymphadenopa-thy may cause a unilateral neck mass. A variety of organisms may cause reactive adenopathy or lymphadenitis. Malignant adenopathy may be secondary (often neuroblastoma or rhab-domyosarcoma) or primary. Non-Hodgkin lymphoma (NHL) presents in the head/neck in about one-third of cases, often as unilateral cervical lymphadenopathy. However, this would be unusual in an infant. US helps distinguish reactive from lymphomatous adenopathy. Neoplastic lymph nodes often lose their oval structure and lack an echogenic hilum. They may have subcapsular instead of hilar vessels. Lymphoma-tous lymph nodes enhance less at CT and show little or no fat stranding. Signal intensity is decreased on T2-W MRI. Nodes infiltrated by metastatic neuroblastoma may show stippled calcification.

• **Neuroblastoma.** Most neuroblastoma encountered in the neck represents metastatic disease. Primary cervical neuro-blastoma represents about 5% of all cases of neuroblastoma and has a relatively good prognosis. It typically presents in girls younger than 3 years, as an indolent mass in the lateral neck. Patients may also present with Horner syndrome or cra-nial nerve IX–XII palsy, or with respiratory distress and feed-ing difficulties depending on the location of the mass. MRI is essential to evaluate the relationship of the mass to neurovas-cular structures, including the brachial plexus and extension into neural foramina. Imaging appearance is similar to neuro-blastoma elsewhere.

■ Additional Differential Diagnoses

• **Rhabdomyosarcoma.** This soft-tissue tumor is more common in children than in infants. However, it should be considered if a mass resembles fibromatosis colli but extends beyond the sternocleidomastoid muscle.

• **Fibrosarcoma.** This large, vascular mass is the most com-mon malignant soft-tissue mass in infants but is usually encountered in the extremities. The prognosis is better than for fibrosarcoma in adults. Imaging appearance is nonspecific, with the tumor showing marked, heterogeneous enhance-ment on T1-W contrast-enhanced MRI and also appearing heterogeneous on T2-W sequences.

■ Diagnosis

Fibromatosis colli.

✓ Pearls

• Fibromatosis colli appears as expansion of the sternoclei-domastoid muscle in the first few weeks of life, with the US appearance of a focal mass or diffuse heterogeneity.

• Lymphadenopathy is usually infectious, but imaging features may suggest neoplastic disease.

• Primary cervical neuroblastoma is less common than meta-static involvement of cervical lymph nodes.

Suggested Readings

Fefferman NR, Milla SS. Ultrasound imaging of the neck in children. Ultrasound Clin. 2009; 4:553–569

Robson CD. Imaging of head and neck neoplasms in children. Pediatr Radiol. 2010; 40(4):499–509

Tranvinh E, Yeom KW, Iv M. Imaging neck masses in the neonate and young infant. Semin Ultrasound CT MR. 2015; 36(2):120–137

Case 145

Patrick J. Sanchez

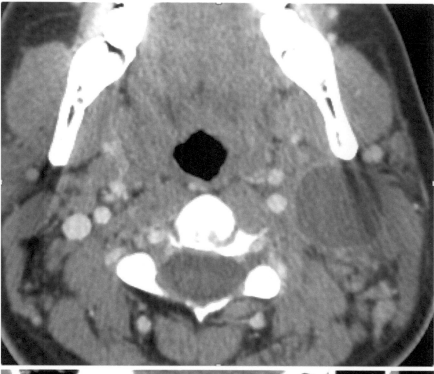

a

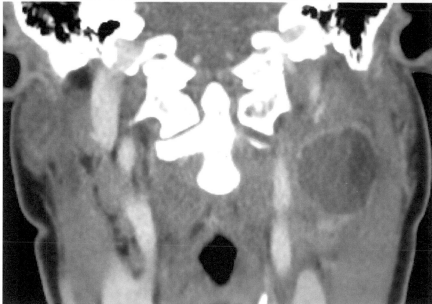

b

Fig. 145.1 Axial contrast-enhanced CT shows a well-circumscribed, hypodense cystic lesion in the left lateral neck that displaces the carotid arteries medially and demonstrates thin peripheral enhancement **(a)**. Coronal reformat also shows the circumscribed cystic lesion **(b)**.

■ Clinical Presentation

A 14-year-old boy with fever and facial fullness (▶ Fig. 145.1).

■ Key Imaging Finding

Cystic superficial lateral neck mass.

■ Top Three Differential Diagnoses

- **Suppurative lymphadenopathy.** Liquefaction of lymph nodes in cases of severe infectious adenitis may lead to intranodal abscess formation, usually due to bacterial infection. US shows hypoechoic to anechoic lymphadenopathy, with increased vascularity and internal septations. Nodes are hypointense on CT, showing peripheral enhancement and perinodal inflammation. A similar appearance is seen with tuberculosis, but in that case multiple conglomerate nodes are usually affected. Necrotic lymphadenopathy due to malignancy typically shows less surrounding inflammation.
- **Branchial cleft cyst.** Most branchial cleft cysts are type 2. These congenital cystic remnants of the second branchial cleft apparatus typically present as a fluctuant neck mass in adolescence or early adulthood. The cysts are usually located along the anterior border of the sternocleidomastoid muscle, although they may present anywhere along the course of the second branchial cleft, from the palatine tonsil to the skin. The cyst is hypodense on CT, bright on T2, and variable on T1, depending on its protein content. Extension of the cyst between the internal and external carotid arteries results in the "notch" or "beak" sign. Type 1 cysts, which are less common, are located near the base of the ear, in the parotid or submandibular gland, or at the angle of the mandible.
- **Venolymphatic malformation (VLM).** Venous and lymphatic malformations are often grouped together, since behavior and treatment are similar and a single lesion often has elements of both. Although other vascular anomalies also occur in the neck (high-flow infantile hemangiomas and arteriovenous malformations), VLMs are more common and most likely to appear as a cystic mass. These low-flow lesions are usually lobulated and septated. Venous elements may demonstrate flow voids and phleboliths. Lymphatic elements have cystic spaces that may contain complex hemorrhagic or proteinaceous fluid; septa enhance, and there may be fluid–fluid levels. VLMs infiltrate tissue planes and depending on location may extend into the mediastinum or face. Like arteriovenous malformations, their growth is proportional to that of the child, whereas hemangiomas initially show marked proliferation.

■ Additional Differential Diagnoses

- **Thyroglossal duct cyst.** The characteristic midline location of this congenital cystic remnant of the thyroglossal duct helps distinguish it from a branchial cleft cyst.
- **Laryngocele.** A laryngocele is an acquired dilatation of the laryngeal ventricle within the larynx.

■ Diagnosis

Branchial cleft cyst type 2.

✓ Pearls

- Suppurative lymphadenopathy appears as multiple enlarged lymph nodes with central hypoattenuation in the setting of an upper respiratory infection (usually bacterial).
- Type 2 branchial cleft cyst should be the leading diagnosis for a cyst along the anterior margin of the sternocleidomastoid muscle, especially in the adolescent age group.
- Venous and lymphatic elements often coexist within a venolymphatic malformation and thus lesions may demonstrate both venous (phleboliths, flow voids) and lymphatic (septal enhancement) characteristics.

Suggested Readings

Flors L, Leiva-Salinas C, Maged IM, et al. MR imaging of soft-tissue vascular malformations: diagnosis, classification, and therapy follow-up. Radiographics. 2011; 31(5):1321–1340, discussion 1340–1341

Koeller KK, Alamo L, Adair CF, Smirniotopoulos JG. Congenital cystic masses of the neck: radiologic-pathologic correlation. Radiographics. 1999; 19(1):121–146, quiz 152–153

Ludwig BJ, Wang J, Nadgir RN, Saito N, Castro-Aragon I, Sakai O. Imaging of cervical lymphadenopathy in children and young adults. AJR Am J Roentgenol. 2012; 199(5):1105–1113

Case 146

Anna E. Nidecker

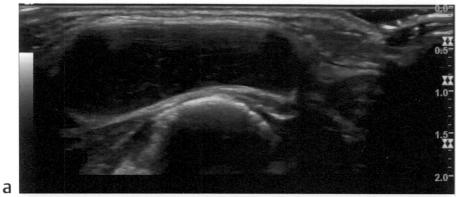

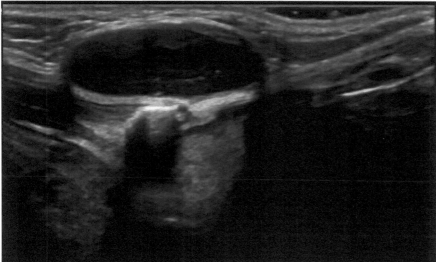

Fig. 146.1 Transverse US just above the thyroid gland demonstrates a well-circumscribed oval cystic mass with mildly complex fluid (a). Longitudinal midline US above the thyroid gland shows a similar appearance (b).

■ **Clinical Presentation**

An infant with stridor (▶ Fig. 146.1).

■ Key Imaging Finding

Anterior midline cystic neck mass.

■ Top Three Differential Diagnoses

- **Thyroglossal duct cyst.** The thyroglossal duct follows the embryonic path of the thyroid gland from the foramen cecum at the base of the tongue to the anterior lower neck. Thyroglossal duct cysts arise in remnants of this duct. Most are infrahyoid in location. They account for 70% of congenital neck masses in children. The lesions are soft, mobile, and unattached to the skin. They are attached to the hyoid and move with swallowing. On US, they appear well defined, with variable echogenicity due to occasional internal hemorrhage and proteinaceous debris. CT shows a thin-walled cystic structure. Sagittal MRI is best for demonstrating lesions at the tongue base, whereas cysts elsewhere along the thyroglossal duct are better seen in the axial plane. Superimposed infection may alter the imaging appearance and cause the cysts to become symptomatic.
- **Dermoid cyst.** Only about 7% of dermoid cysts occur in the head and neck, most often in the midline anterior suprahyoid neck (sublingual or submandibular spaces). However, they can occur anywhere. Dermoid cysts typically present in the second or third decade. They are lined by epithelium and differ from epidermoid cysts in that they contain skin appendages, such as sebaceous glands and hair follicles. Clinical manifestations are similar to thyroglossal duct cysts, but they do not move with swallowing. On CT, dermoid cysts appear as unilocular cystic structures with variable attenuation due to the presence of fat or calcification. Occasionally, small lobules of fat are seen within the fluid, giving the pathognomonic "sack-of-marbles" appearance.
- **Vallecular cyst.** Vallecular cysts are essentially mucoceles caused by obstruction of a mucous gland duct in the larynx. They are typically very small (1–5 mm) and asymptomatic. If infected, they may lead to epiglottitis, which can obstruct the airway and be life-threatening.

■ Additional Differential Diagnosis

- **Venolymphatic malformation.** These congenital lesions contain venous and lymphatic components. Some lesions are predominantly venous, while others contain mostly lymphatic tissue. Both present as multicystic masses that cross tissue planes, and both may have fluid–fluid levels. Those with a predominantly venous component may show slow flow within the cystic areas and may contain phleboliths. Those that are mostly lymphatic may show blood flow and enhancement in the intervening septa. They are usually located in the lateral or posterior neck and are not typically in the anterior midline.

■ Diagnosis

Thyroglossal duct cyst.

✓ Pearls

- Thyroglossal duct cysts may be located anywhere from the tongue base to the thyroid gland.
- Thyroglossal duct cysts are the most common congenital neck mass in children.
- Dermoid cysts are uncommon in the head/neck and usually located above the hyoid bone.

Suggested Readings

Koeller KK, Alamo L, Adair CF, Smirniotopoulos JG. Congenital cystic masses of the neck: radiologic-pathologic correlation. Radiographics. 1999; 19(1):121–146, quiz 152–153

Puttgen KB, Pearl M, Tekes A, Mitchell SE. Update on pediatric extracranial vascular anomalies of the head and neck. Childs Nerv Syst. 2010; 26(10):1417–1433

Case 147

Rebecca Stein-Wexler and Duy Quang Bui

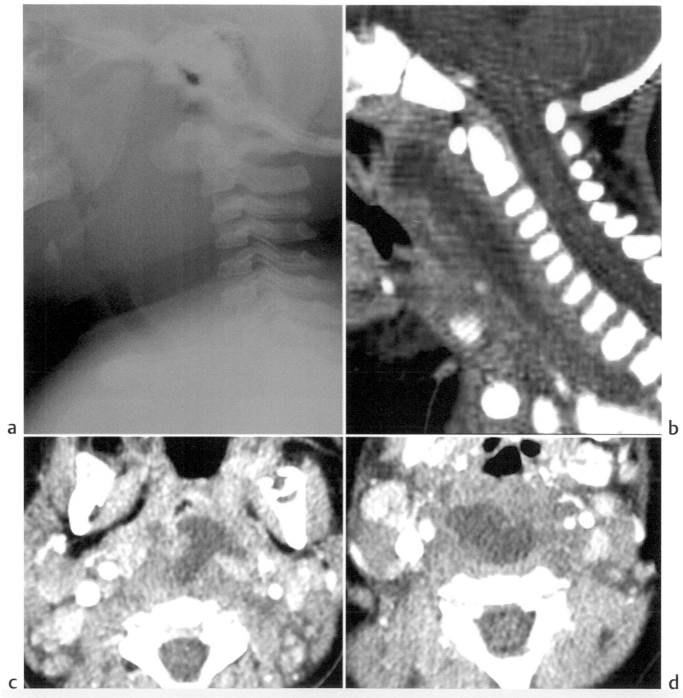

Fig. 147.1 Lateral neck radiograph shows marked prevertebral soft-tissue swelling with narrowed hypopharynx **(a)**. Sagittal reformatted contrast-enhanced neck CT shows retropharyngeal hypodensity tracking toward the mediastinum **(b)**. Axial contrast-enhanced CT shows an irregularly shaped hypodensity at the level of the oropharynx **(c)** and hypopharynx **(d)**.

■ Clinical Presentation

A 5-month-old infant with fever and stridor (▶ Fig. 147.1).

■ Key Imaging Finding

Prevertebral soft-tissue swelling.

■ Top Three Differential Diagnoses

- **Redundant soft tissue.** On a lateral neck X-ray, the prevertebral soft tissues from C1 through C3/C4 normally measure up to half of the anteroposterior (AP) diameter of a vertebral body. Below this, prevertebral thickness should not exceed the AP diameter of one vertebral body (the esophagus contributes the increased thickness). However, normal prevertebral soft tissues may appear abnormally thick if a radiograph is performed in flexion and/or exhalation. The hypopharynx should be well distended on a proper study obtained in inhalation. A repeat view with optimum technique should be obtained if findings are questionable.
- **Suppurative retropharyngeal lymph node.** This consists of infection of a retropharyngeal lymph node, with the inflammation confined to the nodal capsule. Patients may present with dysphagia or odynophagia. CT shows a hypodense lesion with a smooth, thin, enhancing rim. The shape is typically ovoid or rounded. The suppurative lymph node is more likely than retropharyngeal abscess to be unilateral within the retropharyngeal space. It is important to make the distinction between retropharyngeal abscess and suppurative lymph node as the latter is treated medically if the patient is stable.
- **Retropharyngeal abscess.** This usually results from rupture of a suppurative lymph node and is most often encountered in children younger than 6 years old. The inflammation is contained by adjacent anterior visceral fascia and lateral carotid fascia. Patients typically present with acute to subacute dysphagia or odynophagia. CT with contrast shows a round or ovoid fluid collection with peripheral enhancement that is thicker and more irregular than with a suppurative retropharyngeal lymph node. Important complications include airway compromise and extension of abscess into the mediastinum via the danger space. Treatment is surgical.

■ Additional Differential Diagnosis

- **Hematoma.** This is usually encountered in the setting of trauma, typically a whiplash-type injury. It may be accompanied with cervical vertebral fractures. Unenhanced CT shows hyperdense retropharyngeal soft tissue. On MRI, the signal corresponds to hemorrhage, with the appearance depending on its stage of evolution. In the acute setting, hemorrhage will be T1 hyperintense.

■ Diagnosis

Retropharyngeal abscess.

✓ Pearls

- If prevertebral soft tissues appear abnormally thick on a lateral neck radiograph, consider whether the appearance could be due to exhalation and flexion, in which case a repeat study may be performed.
- The marginal enhancement of a suppurative lymph node is thinner and smoother than with retropharyngeal abscess.

- Retropharyngeal suppurative lymphadenitis is limited to the nodal capsule and often unilateral, whereas retropharyngeal abscess is typically central in location and more extensive.
- It is important to evaluate for mediastinal spread of retropharyngeal abscess via the danger space.

Suggested Readings

Grisaru-Soen G, Komisar O, Aizenstein O, Soudack M, Schwartz D, Paret G. Retropharyngeal and parapharyngeal abscess in children: epidemiology, clinical features and treatment. Int J Pediatr Otorhinolaryngol. 2010; 74(9):1016–1020

Hoang JK, Branstetter BF, IV, Eastwood JD, Glastonbury CM. Multiplanar CT and MRI of collections in the retropharyngeal space: is it an abscess? AJR Am J Roentgenol. 2011; 196(4):W426–W432

Meuwly JY, Lepori D, Theumann N, et al. Multimodality imaging evaluation of the pediatric neck: techniques and spectrum of findings. Radiographics. 2005; 25(4):931–948

Case 148

Rebecca Stein-Wexler and Duy Quang Bui

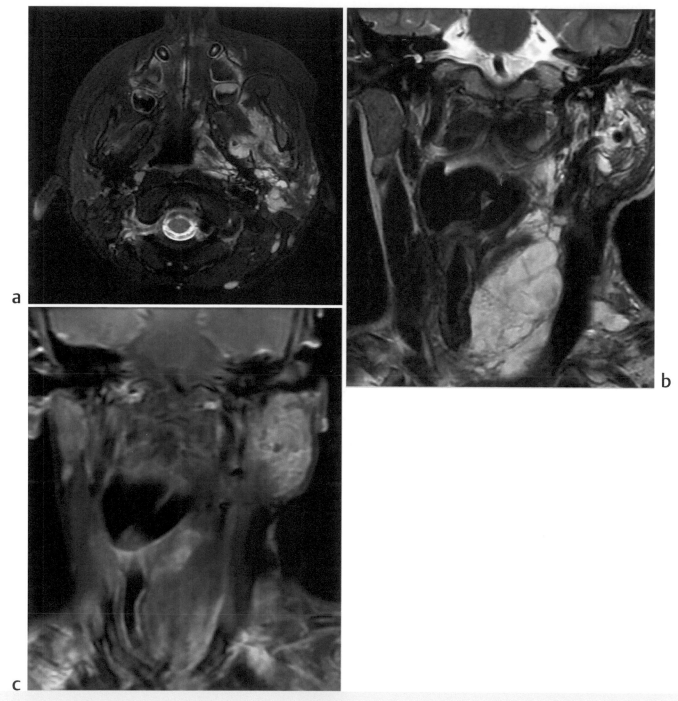

Fig. 148.1 Axial STIR image shows an infiltrative multicystic lesion in the left parapharyngeal space **(a)**. Coronal T2-W image shows it exerts mass effect, displacing the trachea to the right, and also extends laterally toward the superficial soft tissues **(b)**. Coronal fat-saturated gadolinium-enhanced T1-W image shows mild enhancement in the septa of the lesion **(c)**.

■ Clinical Presentation

A 9-year-old girl with left neck swelling (▶Fig. 148.1).

■ Key Imaging Finding

Vascular anomaly.

■ Top Three Differential Diagnoses

- **Lymphatic malformation.** Vascular anomalies are categorized as vascular neoplasms, which undergo mitosis and cell proliferation, and vascular malformations, which do not. Hemangiomas are considered neoplasms. Lymphatic malformations, venous malformations, and arteriovenous malformations are vascular malformations, which are further categorized according to having fast or slow blood flow depending on whether or not there is arterial flow. Lymphatic malformations may be pure, or they may also have venous elements, making them venolymphatic malformations. Both appear as multicystic masses that cross tissue planes, and both may have fluid–fluid levels. Lymphatic components show no blood flow and may show enhancement within septa but not within the intervening cystic spaces. Macrocystic lymphatic malformations have definable cysts, whereas the less common microcystic lesions appear solid. Although lymphatic malformations may occur anywhere, they are common in the head and neck region, especially the posterior cervical triangle. They often extend deep into the mediastinum or face. Hemorrhage and infection may cause the lesions to increase in size. The intralesional fluid is often simple, appearing hypoechoic on US, hypodense on CT, and T1 dark/T2 bright. However, hemorrhage or infection may cause the fluid to appear more complex. They are associated with Noonan, Turner, Down, and other syndromes.
- **Venous malformation.** Like lymphatic malformations, venous malformations appear as multicystic masses that may cross tissue planes. They may be solitary or multiple, and sometimes they are well circumscribed. They too may have fluid–fluid levels. Portions of the lesion will demonstrate slow, venous flow. The presence of phleboliths is pathognomonic. Adjacent bone may be remodeled but should not be destroyed. The enhancement pattern is typically heterogeneous, due to variable, slow intralesional flow.
- **Hemangioma.** Hemangiomas are benign vascular neoplasms. Congenital lesions are present on day 1 of life, whereas infantile lesions appear during the first 2 months. Hemangiomas grow rapidly during their proliferative phase, generally until about age 1 year. Growth then plateaus. Involution occurs over the next few years, and lesions should resolve by about age 5 years. They usually appear as a cutaneous or subcutaneous ovoid soft-tissue mass. They are solid and hypoechoic at US. MRI appearance varies with lesion phase. When proliferating, they show early enhancement and are T2 hyperintense. Hemangioendotheliomas and angiosarcomas are much less common vascular neoplasms.

■ Additional Differential Diagnosis

- **Arteriovenous malformation.** These fast-flow vascular malformations are rare in children. They consist of enlarged arterial feeding vessels, along with the distinguishing feature of early draining veins. Dynamic MR angiography is useful for diagnosis. This lesion is treated with transarterial embolization.

■ Diagnosis

Macrocystic lymphatic malformation.

✓ Pearls

- Lymphatic malformations and venous malformations may coexist together; both may have fluid–fluid levels.
- With venous malformations, the cystic spaces may enhance, whereas with lymphatic malformation, the intervening septa may enhance.
- The presence of phleboliths in a trans-spatial multicystic mass suggests venous malformation.

Suggested Readings

Dubois J, Alison M. Vascular anomalies: what a radiologist needs to know. Pediatr Radiol. 2010; 40(6):895–905

Gaddikeri S, Vattoth S, Gaddikeri RS, et al. Congenital cystic neck masses: embryology and imaging appearances, with clinicopathological correlation. Curr Probl Diagn Radiol. 2014; 43(2):55–67

Case 149

Rebecca Stein-Wexler

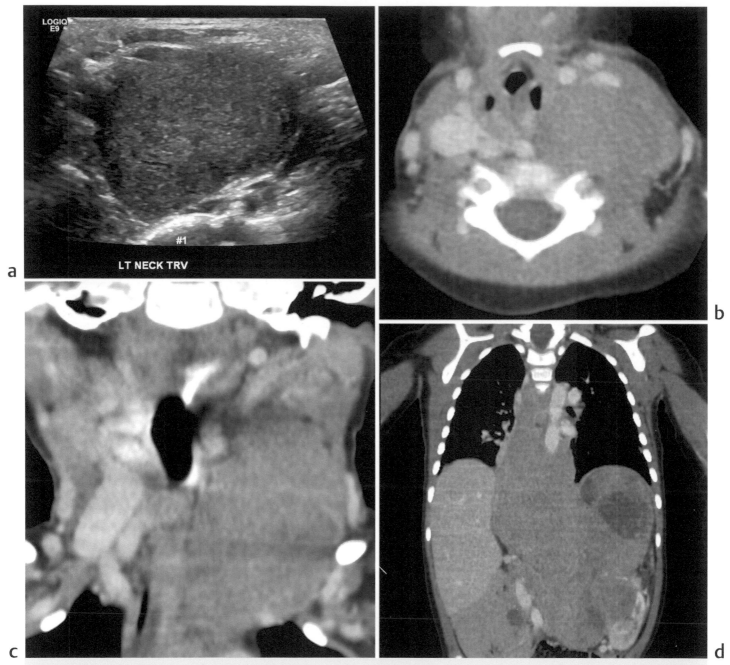

Fig. 149.1 Transverse US of the neck shows a mildly heterogeneous mass **(a)**. Axial contrast-enhanced CT shows a homogeneous mass displaces airway and vessels **(b)**. Coronal reformatted image shows the mass extends into the mediastinum **(c)**. Coronal reformatted image of the chest and abdomen shows there is a mixed cystic and solid left upper quadrant mass that extends into the posterior mediastinum **(d)**.

■ Clinical Presentation

A 3-year-old girl with a firm neck mass (▶Fig. 149.1).

■ Key Imaging Finding

Solid neck mass after infancy.

■ Top Three Differential Diagnoses

- **Infectious lymphadenopathy.** Infection with a variety of organisms may cause reactive lymphadenopathy or lymphadenitis, resulting in a unilateral or bilateral neck mass. Inflamed lymph nodes classically retain their ovoid shape, hilar vessels, and echogenic hilum. Lymphadenopathy secondary to tuberculosis typically has a more matted, conglomerate appearance, whereas with bacterial or viral lymphadenopathy the individual nodes appear more distinct.
- **Neoplastic lymphadenopathy.** Neoplastic lymphadenopathy in the neck in children is usually due to lymphoma, with neuroblastoma and rhabdomyosarcoma metastases accounting for most other cases. Lymphoma causes most malignancy of the head and neck in children, usually Hodgkin disease. However, non-Hodgkin lymphoma presents in the head/neck in about one-third of cases, often as unilateral cervical lymphadenopathy. US helps distinguish reactive from lymphomatous lymphadenopathy. Lymphomatous lymph nodes often lose their oval structure and lack an echogenic hilum. They may have subcapsular instead of hilar vessels. They enhance less at CT and show little or no fat stranding. Lymphomatous nodes are more homogeneous on MRI and show lower signal intensity on T2-W sequences. They enhance less intensely and more variably. Metastases secondary to neuroblastoma may demonstrate calcifications.
- **Rhabdomyosarcoma (RMS).** This is a common pediatric soft-tissue malignancy, and about one-third of cases occur in the head and neck. Most RMSs are seen in young children (mean age 5–6 years), but there is a second peak in adolescence. RMS typically develops in the orbits (proptosis), nasal sinuses (obstruction, epistaxis), and neck (mass). This aggressive tumor shows bone remodeling and destruction on CT. MRI is best for evaluating intracranial extension of this aggressive-appearing mass, as well as both local and perineural spread. RMS is homogeneous, with variable but usually homogeneous contrast enhancement.

■ Additional Differential Diagnosis

- **Neuroblastoma.** Although primary neuroblastoma may occur in the neck, most cases in this area are metastatic. Primary cervical neuroblastoma has a relatively good prognosis but is uncommon, representing about 5% of all cases of neuroblastoma. It typically presents in girls younger than 3 years, as an indolent mass in the lateral neck. Patients may also present with Horner syndrome or cranial nerve IX–XII palsy, or with respiratory distress and feeding difficulties, depending on the location of the mass. MRI is essential to evaluate the relationship of the mass to neurovascular structures, including the brachial plexus and extension into neural foramina. Imaging appearance is similar to neuroblastoma elsewhere.

■ Diagnosis

Metastatic neuroblastoma.

✓ Pearls

- Neoplastic lymphadenopathy in the neck is usually due to lymphoma; the lymph nodes tend to be round and lack both hilar vessels and an echogenic hilum.
- Rhabdomyosarcoma appears aggressive, destroying bone and showing perineural spread.
- Neuroblastoma in the neck is usually metastatic.

Suggested Readings

Freling NJ, Merks JH, Saeed P, et al. Imaging findings in craniofacial childhood rhabdomyosarcoma. Pediatr Radiol. 2010; 40(11):1723–1738, quiz 1855

Turkington JR, Paterson A, Sweeney LE, Thornbury GD. Neck masses in children. Br J Radiol. 2005; 78(925):75–85

Case 150

Patrick J. Sanchez

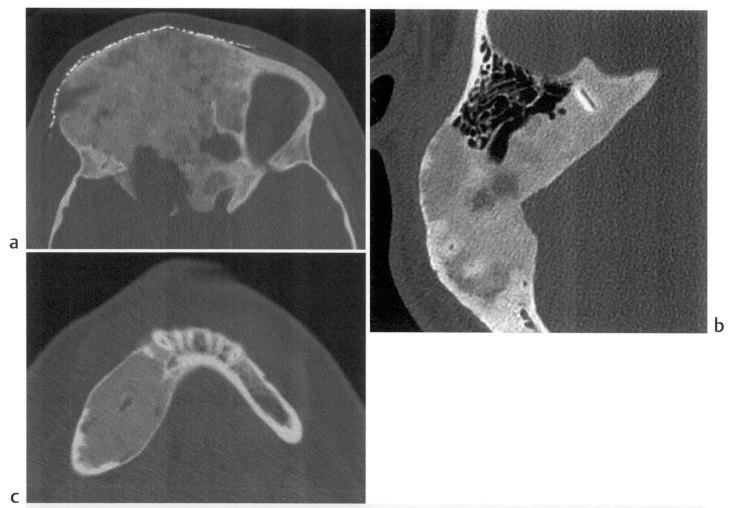

Fig. 150.1 Axial CT image in bone window demonstrates an expansile lesion involving the supraorbital bone, with ground glass attenuation; metallic mesh along the anterior aspect of the lesion is from a debulking procedure (**a**). Axial CT through the temporal bone shows a similar ground glass appearance, with cortex intact (**b**). The mandible has a similar appearance (**c**).

■ Clinical Presentation

A child with facial deformity and history of reconstructive surgery (►Fig. 150.1).

■ Key Imaging Finding

Ground glass, expansile lesions involving the facial bones.

■ Diagnosis

Fibrous dysplasia. Fibrous dysplasia is a non-neoplastic skeletal developmental abnormality secondary to defects in osteoblastic differentiation and maturation. In this condition, normal bone matrix is replaced with fibrous stroma. Almost any bone in the body can be affected. Of the facial bones, the mandible and maxilla are most often involved. Fibrous dysplasia may be monostotic or polyostotic, with 50% of polyostotic cases involving the facial bones. On both radiographs and CT, lesions have a characteristic "ground glass" matrix. The affected bones are expanded, and the outer cortex preserved. Mixed regions of heterogeneous lucency and sclerosis may also be observed. MRI is not usually required in the evaluation of fibrous dysplasia. The MRI appearance of heterogeneous T1 and T2 signal intensity and heterogeneous contrast enhancement is less specific than the appearance on CT. On MRI, fibrous dysplasia can be mistaken for malignancy.

If fibrous dysplasia is polyostotic, McCune–Albright syndrome should be considered. These patients also have café au lait spots and precocious puberty. The café au lait spots are often more numerous on one side of the body. Patients with McCune–Albright syndrome may have other endocrine abnormalities as well, including hyperthyroidism and Cushing syndrome.

Cherubism is a fibrous dysplasialike syndrome involving only the maxilla and mandible. Originally thought to be a variant of fibrous dysplasia, it is now considered a separate clinical entity. Cherubism is a rare autosomal-dominant disorder with variable penetrance. It typical presents in early childhood with bilateral jaw fullness and expansile, multiloculated cystic masses involving the mandible and maxilla. Histological features are similar to a giant cell granuloma. Imaging shows relatively symmetrical lucent, expansile lesions of the mandible and maxilla with a characteristic "soap bubble" appearance.

✓ Pearls

- Fibrous dysplasia involving the facial bones presents with characteristic bone lesions, which are expansile and demonstrate a "ground glass" matrix.
- The diagnosis of fibrous dysplasia is most reliably made with CT, since MRI may be misleading and on pathology fibrous dysplasia may be confused with other fibro-osseous lesions.

- Cherubism is a distinct clinical entity characterized by symmetrical, expansile lesions involving the maxilla and mandible with a characteristic "soap bubble" appearance.

Suggested Readings

Beaman FD, Bancroft LW, Peterson JJ, Kransdorf MJ, Murphey MD, Menke DM. Imaging characteristics of cherubism. AJR Am J Roentgenol. 2004; 182(4):1051–1054

Chung EM, Murphey MD, Specht CS, Cube R, Smirniotopoulos JG. From the Archives of the AFIP. Pediatric orbit tumors and tumorlike lesions: osseous lesions of the orbit. Radiographics. 2008; 28(4):1193–1214

Fitzpatrick KA, Taljanovic MS, Speer DP, et al. Imaging findings of fibrous dysplasia with histopathologic and intraoperative correlation. AJR Am J Roentgenol. 2004; 182(6):1389–1398

Part 6

Brain and Spine Imaging

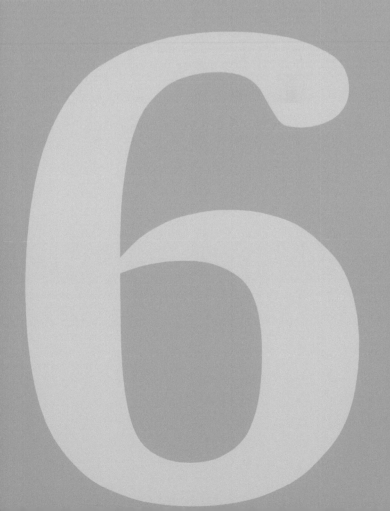

Case 151

Michael Doherty

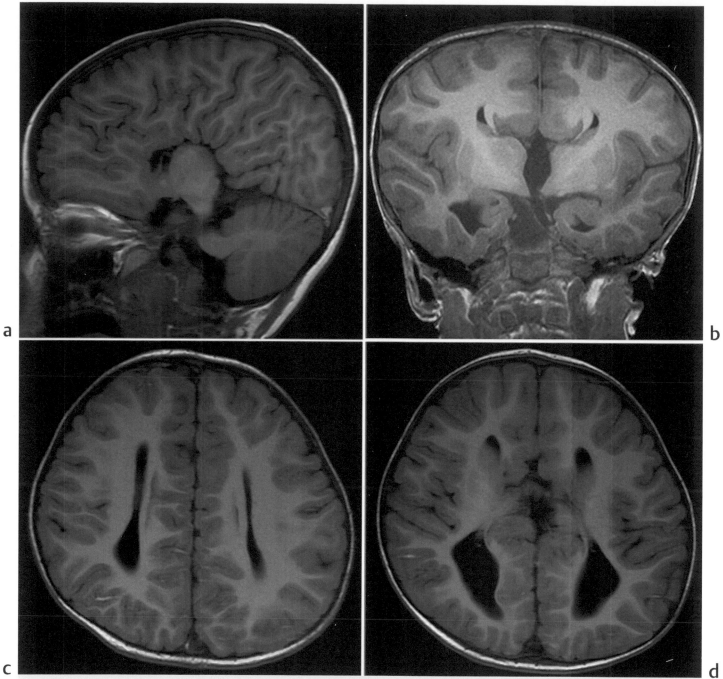

Fig. 151.1 Sagittal T1 FLAIR image shows outward radiation of medial hemispheric sulci from the third ventricle and an abnormal cingulate gyrus (**a**). Coronal 3D fast spoiled gradient (FSPGR) inversion recovery (IR) image shows elevation of the roof of the third ventricle and Probst bundles indenting the lateral ventricles, creating a "bull's horn" configuration (**b**). Axial T1 FLAIR images show dysmorphic gyri (**c,d**), parallel lateral ventricles (**c**), and dilated occipital horns (**d**).

■ **Clinical Presentation**

A 3-year-old girl with developmental delay (▶Fig. 151.1).

■ Key Imaging Finding

Absence of the corpus callosum.

■ Top Three Differential Diagnoses

- **Agenesis of the corpus callosum (ACC).** ACC is caused by failure of axons to form or migrate across the midline. Most patients with isolated ACC are initially clinically normal, but subtle cognitive defects, visual problems, and seizures may develop later. US and MRI performed either prenatally or after birth show similar findings. There is colpocephaly, with parallel configuration of lateral ventricles and dilated occipital horns. Midline images show a high riding third ventricle. The corpus callosum and cingulate sulcus are absent, and the gyri radiate out from the third ventricle. On coronal imaging, Probst bundles run parallel to interhemispheric fissure and indent the lateral ventricles, creating a "bull's horn" configuration. About 15% of cases initially thought to be isolated turn out to be associated with other abnormalities, conferring a worse prognosis. Postnatal MRI and karyotype evaluation help assess for associated anomalies.
- **Chiari 2 malformation with colpocephaly.** This complex hindbrain malformation is closely associated with neural tube defects. Most patients are diagnosed at prenatal screening with elevated alpha-fetoprotein and abnormal US. Most others present at birth with hydrocephalus and myelomeningocele, but milder cases may present later with varying degrees of lower extremity paresis/spasticity, clubfoot, bowel/bladder dysfunction, and epilepsy. On MRI, the characteristic findings include a crowded posterior fossa, callosal agenesis/dysgenesis, tectal beaking, inferior tonsillar and vermian displacement, and medullary kinking. Prenatal US classically shows cerebellar compression (banana sign), frontal bone concavity (lemon sign), and ventriculomegaly. Prenatal folate reduces the incidence of Chiari 2 malformation. Myelomeningocele is surgically repaired within 48 hours of birth, and hydrocephalus may be treated with CSF shunt.
- **Secondary damage to the corpus callosum.** The corpus callosum may be injured due to head trauma or in the course of neurosurgery. In addition, patients with extensive periventricular leukomalacia of prematurity—and other periventricular white matter injury—may develop severe thinning of the corpus callosum. The corpus callosum may also be so stretched by hydrocephalus that it appears extremely thin. Even after hydrocephalus has resolved, the corpus callosum may remain abnormal.

■ Additional Differential Diagnosis

- **Holoprosencephaly.** This condition consists of incomplete separation of the cerebral hemispheres. In addition, there is agenesis of part or all of the corpus callosum, corresponding to the degree of anatomical severity (alobar, semilobar, and lobar).

■ Diagnosis

Agenesis of the corpus callosum.

✓ Pearls

- Agenesis of the corpus callosum demonstrates interhemispheric fissures radiating from the third ventricle.
- Chiari 2 malformations are complex hindbrain malformations that usually occur in association with myelomeningocele.
- The corpus callosum may appear defective as a result of trauma, surgery, hydrocephalus, or injury to the periventricular white matter.

Suggested Readings

Cesmebasi A, Loukas M, Hogan E, Kralovic S, Tubbs RS, Cohen-Gadol AA. The Chiari malformations: a review with emphasis on anatomical traits. Clin Anat. 2015; 28(2):184–194

Craven I, Bradburn MJ, Griffiths PD. Antenatal diagnosis of agenesis of the corpus callosum. Clin Radiol. 2015; 70(3):248–253

Case 152

Anna E. Nidecker

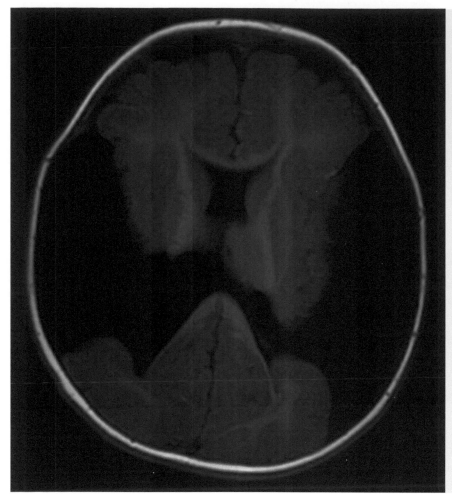

Fig. 152.1 Axial T1-W MRI shows bilateral clefts in the posteroparietal regions connecting lateral ventricles and subarachnoid space. The clefts are lined with gray matter. In addition, there is no septum pellucidum.

■ Clinical Presentation

A 7-month-old boy with developmental delay, hypotonia, and seizures (►Fig. 152.1).

■ **Key Imaging Finding**

CSF-filled cleft/space in a young infant.

■ **Top Three Differential Diagnoses**

- **Schizencephaly.** Schizencephaly results from early destruction of a portion of the germinal matrix and adjacent brain before the hemispheres are fully formed. This results in a gray-matter-lined cleft extending from the body of the lateral ventricle(s) to the outer cortical surface. The cleft is lined with polymicrogyric gray matter. With "closed lip" clefts, the edges of the cleft are fused in a pial-ependymal seam, with no intervening CSF (type I). CSF separates "open lip" clefts (type II); these clefts are usually large and sometimes bilateral. Septo-optic dysplasia is often associated, along with heterotopia and cortical dysplasia. Clinical manifestations include intellectual disability, seizures, and motor dysfunction. More severe malformations (open lip, bilateral, involving motor cortex) result in more severe neurodevelopmental disabilities. Patients with bilateral clefts are severely disabled. MRI and CT show gray matter lining the cleft. A dimple in the ventricle wall indicates the site of closed lip schizencephaly.
- **Porencephaly.** This entity has many definitions, but pathologically it is defined as a cavity within the brain with minimal surrounding gliosis, or astrocyte proliferation. The cyst is lined with dysplastic white matter. Porencephaly is often congenital, due to a fetal cerebrovascular accident or infection. It may develop in early infancy, after head trauma, vascular insult, or infection. It does not usually develop in older children whose brains respond to insult with gliosis rather than necrosis. On cross-sectional imaging, porencephaly appears as one or more unilateral or bilateral cavity(ies) lined with gliotic white matter, usually communicating with the ventricular system or the subarachnoid space. There is ex vacuo dilatation of the adjacent ventricle. Cyst walls are smooth, and adjacent white matter appears bright on inversion recovery (IR) sequences.
- **Arachnoid cyst.** During the development of the brain, the meninges in a limited area may fail to merge, forming a duplicated arachnoid layer that allows interlayer accumulation of CSF. Most occur at the sylvian fissure and are asymptomatic. Arachnoid cysts are well demarcated and hypodense on CT, and they usually follow simple CSF signal on all MR pulse sequences. Occasionally, the contents are slightly complex due to internal hemorrhage. These lesions do not enhance.

■ **Additional Differential Diagnosis**

- **Postinfarct encephalomalacia.** A variety of parenchymal insults in older children may lead to parenchymal volume loss, usually with accompanying ventricular enlargement. The pathological process differs from that preceding porencephaly. The defect often appears wedge-shaped and does not typically communicate with the ventricle or cortex.

■ **Diagnosis**

Bilateral open lip schizencephaly.

✓ **Pearls**

- Schizencephaly consists of a polymicrogyric gray-matter-lined cleft extending from the lateral ventricle to the cortical mantle.
- Closed lip clefts are fused in a pial-ependymal seam, whereas open lip clefts have a gap filled with CSF.
- Porencephalic cysts are lined by white matter, not gray matter.

Suggested Readings

Epelman M, Daneman A, Blaser SI, et al. Differential diagnosis of intracranial cystic lesions at head US: correlation with CT and MR imaging. Radiographics. 2006; 26(1):173–196

Hayashi N, Tsutsumi Y, Barkovich AJ. Morphological features and associated anomalies of schizencephaly in the clinical population: detailed analysis of MR images. Neuroradiology. 2002; 44(5):418–427

Oh KY, Kennedy AM, Frias AE Jr, Byrne JL. Fetal schizencephaly: pre- and postnatal imaging with a review of the clinical manifestations. Radiographics. 2005; 25(3):647–657

Case 153

Geoffrey D. McWilliams

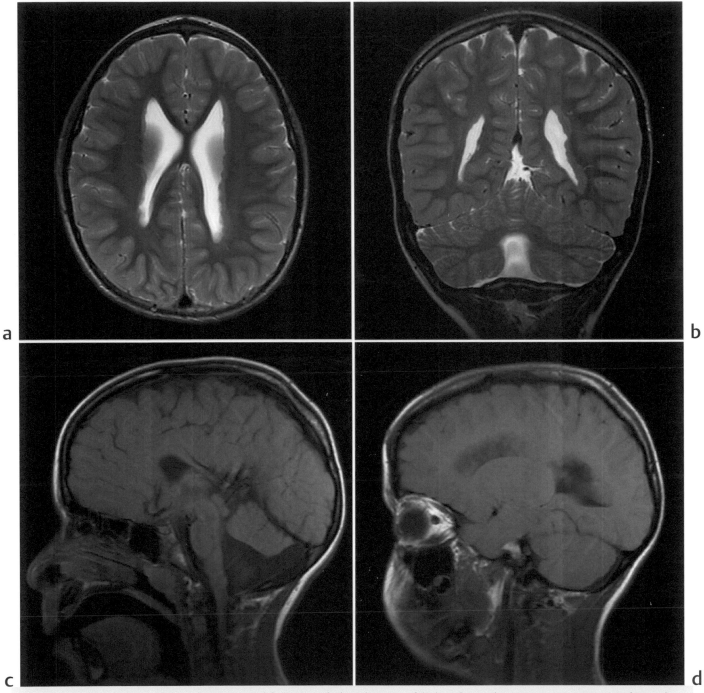

Fig. 153.1 Axial **(a)** and coronal **(b)** T2-W MRI show nodularity along the lateral margins of the lateral ventricles, isointense to gray matter, along with colpocephaly. Sagittal T1-W FLAIR image shows partial agenesis of the corpus callosum and hypoplastic inferior cerebellar vermis **(c)**. Sagittal off-midline T1-W FLAIR image shows innumerable nodules protruding into the lateral ventricle **(d)**.

■ **Clinical Presentation**

A 6-month-old boy with refractory seizures (▶Fig. 153.1).

■ Key Imaging Finding

Nodularity of the ventricular wall.

■ Top Three Differential Diagnoses

- **Gray matter heterotopia.** Gray matter heterotopia refers to anomalous gray matter deposition due to abnormal neuronal migration during fetal development. Patients may present with seizures and/or developmental delay. Heterotopic gray matter may be seen anywhere along the course of neuronal migration but occurs most often in a periventricular nodular pattern. Single or multiple nodules may also be seen in a cortical/subcortical location or on the pial surface. Diffuse patterns of heterotopia include band heterotopia and lissencephaly. Nodules are isointense to cortical gray matter on all sequences and do not enhance.
- **Tuberous sclerosis complex (TSC).** Subependymal hamartomas are a common feature of TSC, which is an acquired or hereditary genetic phakomatosis caused by mutations in TSC1 or TSC2 genes. These genes encode harmartin and tuberin, respectively. TSC is characterized by hamartomatous growths involving multiple organ systems. These include multiple subependymal nodules and cortical/subcortical as well as cerebellar tubers, which progressively calcify in early childhood. Tubers may be T2/FLAIR hyperintense and initially hypodense on CT; if they do not calcify, they may appear cystic. Patients with TSC may develop subependymal giant cell astrocytoma (SEGA), a World Health Organization (WHO) grade 1 tumor that typically forms near the foramen of Monro and demonstrates heterogeneous T1/T2 signal, calcification, strong contrast enhancement, and progressive growth. TSC patients also commonly develop renal angiomyolipomas and cardiac rhabdomyomas. Patients often present with seizures and adenoma sebaceum.
- **Closed lip schizencephaly.** Schizencephaly results from early destruction of a portion of the germinal matrix and adjacent brain before the hemispheres are fully formed. This results in a gray-matter-lined cleft extending from the body of the lateral ventricles to the outer cortical surface. The cleft is lined with polymicrogyric gray matter. With "closed lip" clefts, the edges of the cleft are fused in a pial-ependymal seam, with no intervening CSF (type I). CSF separates "open lip" clefts (type II); these clefts are usually large and sometimes bilateral. Closed lip schizencephaly may be quite subtle on MRI. The presence of slight irregularity in the lateral wall of the lateral ventricle may be the only manifestation on axial MRI. There may be a tiny dimple in the wall where the cleft meets the lateral ventricle, or mild nodularity adjacent to this area. Gray matter may be identified along the cleft at both CT and MRI. Septo-optic dysplasia is often associated, along with heterotopia and cortical dysplasia. Clinical manifestations include intellectual disability, seizures, and motor dysfunction.

■ Diagnosis

Gray matter heterotopia in a patient with Dandy–Walker variant.

✓ Pearls

- Gray matter heterotopia describes a disorder of neuronal migration resulting in nodular or diffuse heterotopic gray matter, most often appearing in a periventricular nodular pattern.
- Tuberous sclerosis complex is a multisystem phakomatosis, which presents with seizures, subependymal nodules, and cerebral and/or cerebellar tubers that progressively calcify; patients are at increased risk for subependymal giant cell astrocytoma.
- Closed lip schizencephaly may be quite subtle, manifesting as a small dimple at the site of the cleft or slight nodularity on either side.

Suggested Readings

Abdel Razek AA, Kandell AY, Elsorogy LG, Elmongy A, Basett AA. Disorders of cortical formation: MR imaging features. AJNR Am J Neuroradiol. 2009; 30(1):4–11

Daghistani R, Rutka J, Widjaja E. MRI characteristics of cerebellar tubers and their longitudinal changes in children with tuberous sclerosis complex. Childs Nerv Syst. 2015; 31(1):109–113

Case 154

Rebecca Stein-Wexler

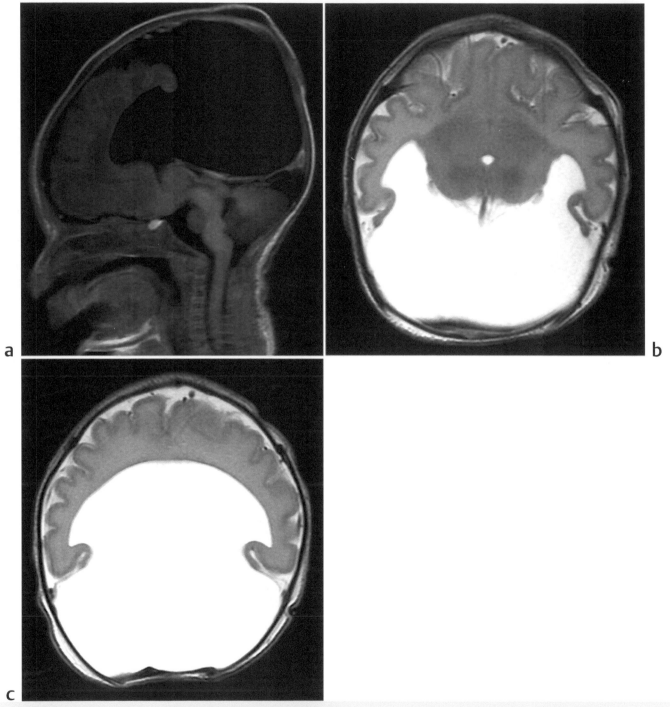

Fig. 154.1 Sagittal two-dimensional (2D) T1-W FLAIR image shows a large dorsal cyst and pancakelike frontal parenchyma (a). Axial 2D FSE T2-W images show fused thalami and basal ganglia (b) and a crescentic monoventricle around the dorsal cyst (c).

■ Clinical Presentation

Newborn with macrocephaly and hypotonia (▶ Fig. 154.1).

■ Key Imaging Finding

Large amount of supratentorial CSF.

■ Top Three Differential Diagnoses

- **Massive hydrocephalus.** Obstruction, overproduction, and/or decreased absorption of CSF may cause ventricular dilatation. If hydrocephalus is severe, the brain appears as an almost imperceptible rim of cortex compressed along the contour of the skull. The presence of a midline falx and absence of thalamic fusion help differentiate this condition from holoprosencephaly, and the presence of a cortical mantle differentiates it from hydranencephaly. This distinction is important, since early shunting of hydrocephalus can allow normal intellect and motor function to develop. In newborns, aqueductal stenosis is a common cause of hydrocephalus affecting the third and lateral ventricles, but neoplasms and posthemorrhagic/infectious obstruction should also be considered. Hemorrhage and infection may also cause communicating hydrocephalus.
- **Hydranencephaly.** A variety of insults between gestational weeks 20 to 27 can lead to massive liquefaction of the supratentorial parenchyma. The inferomedial frontal and temporal lobes as well as the thalami may be normal, the brainstem is atrophic, and the cerebellum is usually normal. The falx is present and the thalami are separate, but there is no cortical mantle, which helps differentiate this entity from massive hydrocephalus and alobar holoprosencephaly. Head circumference varies depending on whether there is also hydrocephalus. Patients are severely neurologically impaired.
- **Alobar holoprosencephaly.** This most severe form of holoprosencephaly develops when the prosencephalon does not divide into separate hemispheres. The cerebral parenchyma is pancakelike or ball-shaped on prenatal US. It is fused anteriorly and surrounds a large dorsal interhemispheric cyst. The corpus callosum, falx, and interhemispheric and sylvian fissures are absent; the basal ganglia, hypothalami, and thalami are fused at the midline. Facial abnormalities are common, including hypotelorism, fused metopic suture (causing trigonocephaly), and cleft palate. About half of cases are associated with a syndrome, often trisomy 13. Lobar holoprosencephaly is the mildest form, characterized by separate thalami but no septum pellucidum and a variable amount of falx. Semilobar holoprosencephaly is intermediate, having fused thalami and intermediate appearance of other structures.

■ Additional Differential Diagnosis

- **Bilateral open lip schizencephaly.** Large bilateral clefts may severely distort anatomy, and a large amount of CSF may accumulate in the defects. Polymicrogyric gray matter should be evident lining the clefts. A falx is present. There may be associated septo-optic dysplasia.

■ Diagnosis

Alobar holoprosencephaly.

✓ Pearls

- Massive hydrocephalus has a thin, sometimes imperceptible, cortical mantle, along with a falx and unfused thalami.
- Patients with hydranencephaly have a falx and separate thalami, but there is no cortical mantle; furthermore, the brainstem is atrophic.
- Alobar holoprosencephaly lacks a falx, and the thalamus is fused in the midline.

Suggested Readings

Barkovich AJ, Raybaud C. Congenital malformations of the brain and skull. In Barkovich AJ, Raybaud C, eds. Pediatric Neuroimaging, 5th ed. Philadelphia, PA: Lippincott Williams & Wilkins; 2012:367–568

Medina LS, Frawley K, Zurakowski D, Buttros D, DeGrauw AJ, Crone KR. Children with macrocrania: clinical and imaging predictors of disorders requiring surgery. AJNR Am J Neuroradiol. 2001; 22(3):564–570

Case 155

Kriti Gwal

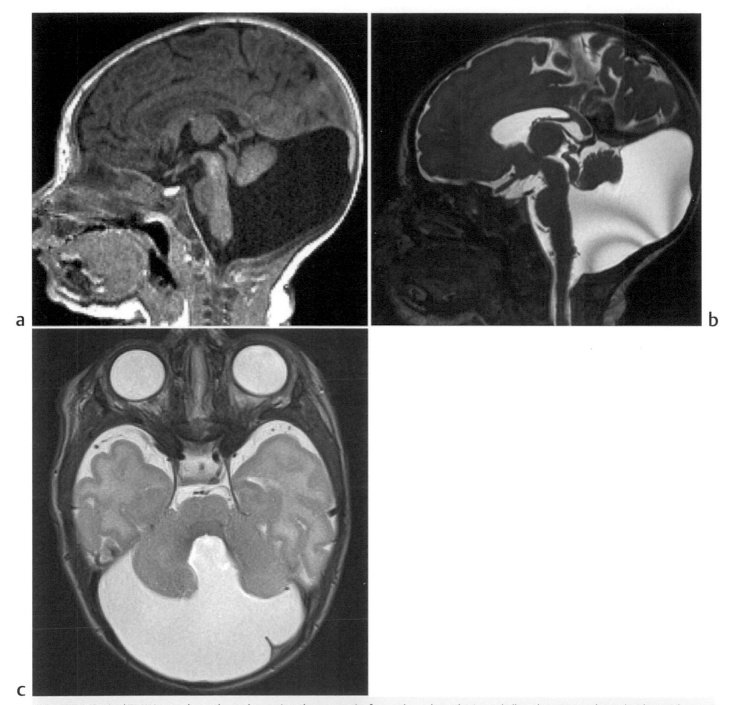

Fig. 155.1 Sagittal T1-W image shows elevated tentorium, large posterior fossa volume, hypoplastic cerebellum that appears elevated and rotated, and large cisterna magna (**a**). Sagittal constructive interference in steady-state (CISS) sequence shows similar findings with an elevated torcula (**b**). Axial T2-W MRI shows the vermian hypoplasia and the large cisterna magna (**c**). (These images are provided courtesy of the Children's Hospital of Philadelphia.)

■ Clinical Presentation

Neonate with abnormal prenatal US (▶ Fig. 155.1).

■ Key Imaging Finding

Posterior fossa cyst in a newborn.

■ Top Three Differential Diagnoses

• **Mega cisterna magna.** Patients with mega cisterna magna have an enlarged cisterna magna but a normal cerebellar vermis and no hydrocephalus. The cisterna magna is considered "mega" when it measures ≥10 mm on sagittal midline images. The fourth ventricle generally appears normal, but the posterior fossa may be enlarged. Isolated mega cisterna magna is considered a normal variant.

• **Dandy–Walker malformation (DWM).** This relatively common posterior fossa malformation is caused by an absent or very small cerebellar vermis, with other portions of the cerebellum also possibly affected. It is often diagnosed prenatally but may present later with developmental delay, hypotonia/spasticity, and ataxia. Classic DWM shows an enlarged posterior fossa with a hypoplastic or occasionally absent cerebellar vermis. A cystlike, dilated fourth ventricle fills the posterior fossa, and there is hypoplasia and rotation of the inferior cerebellar vermis. The severity of hypoplasia of the cerebellar vermis and hemispheres varies. DWM includes elevation of the torcula and transverse dural venous sinuses, as well as the tentorium. Associated malformations include callosal anomalies, polymicrogyria, gray matter heterotopias, and occipital encephaloceles. Hydrocephalus may precipitate diagnosis. The presence of a cerebellar vermis that has normal size and rotation excludes DWM.

• **Blake pouch cyst (BPC).** This results from failure of Blake pouch, a membrane at the floor of the fourth ventricle, to fenestrate normally during development. The BPC is thus a fetal remnant. It herniates from the fourth ventricle through the foramen of Magendie, restricting CSF flow into the subarachnoid space. MRI may show the choroid plexus extending into the cyst, important for diagnosis. Although some patients are asymptomatic, obstructive hydrocephalus is common. Treatment is third ventriculostomy.

■ Additional Differential Diagnoses

• **Arachnoid cyst.** A retrocerebellar or superior vermian posterior fossa arachnoid cyst may cause mass effect, compressing or displacing a normal fourth ventricle. There are usually no associated anomalies.

• **Cerebellar hypoplasia.** Cerebellar hypoplasia is characterized by a small cerebellum with normal size of the fissures and cerebellar folia. Any component of the cerebellum (cerebellar hemispheres or vermis)—or indeed the entire cerebellum— may be hypoplastic. Additional features of Dandy–Walker malformation are absent.

• **Joubert syndrome.** This is defined by the characteristic "molar tooth" appearance on MRI: hypoplastic cerebellar vermis, enlarged and elongated superior cerebellar peduncles that do not decussate and have a horizontal orientation, and a deep interpeduncular fossa. Inheritance is predominantly autosomal recessive.

■ Diagnosis

Dandy–Walker malformation.

✓ Pearls

• The normal cisterna magna measures less than 10 mm at the midline on a sagittal image.
• Dandy–Walker malformation is defined by an enlarged posterior fossa with a hypoplastic cerebellar vermis and is commonly associated with hydrocephalus and additional congenital anomalies.

• Blake pouch cyst may be recognized by the presence of choroid plexus within the cystic space.
• Joubert syndrome features a "molar tooth" appearance of the cerebellum.

Suggested Readings

Barkovich AJ, Raybaud C. Congenital malformations of the brain and skull. In Barkovich AJ, Raybaud C, eds. Pediatric Neuroimaging, 5th ed. Philadelphia, PA: Lippincott Williams & Wilkins; 2012:367–568

Bosemani T, Orman G, Boltshauser E, Tekes A, Huisman TA, Poretti A. Congenital abnormalities of the posterior fossa. Radiographics. 2015; 35(1):200–220

Cornips EM, Overvliet GM, Weber JW, et al. The clinical spectrum of Blake's pouch cyst: report of six illustrative cases. Childs Nerv Syst. 2010; 26(8):1057–1064

Case 156

Kriti Gwal

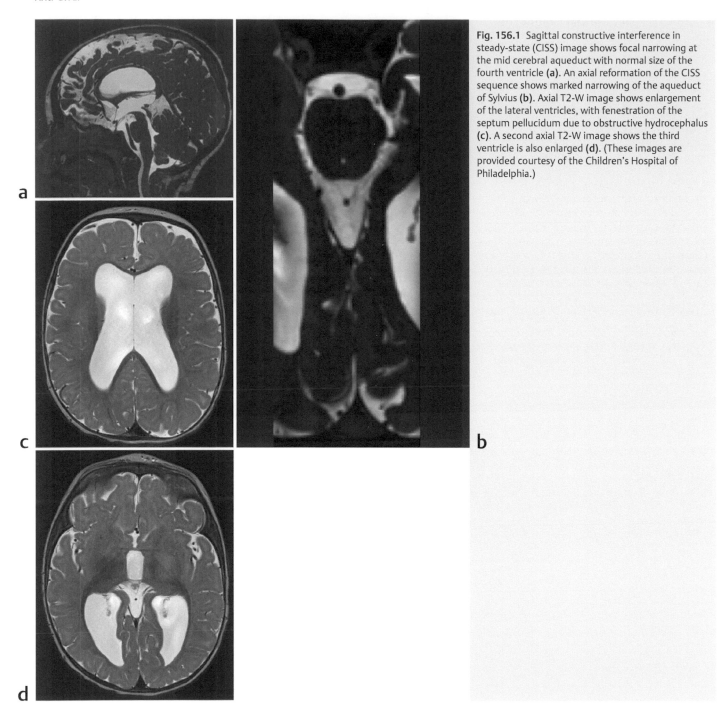

Fig. 156.1 Sagittal constructive interference in steady-state (CISS) image shows focal narrowing at the mid cerebral aqueduct with normal size of the fourth ventricle **(a)**. An axial reformation of the CISS sequence shows marked narrowing of the aqueduct of Sylvius **(b)**. Axial T2-W image shows enlargement of the lateral ventricles, with fenestration of the septum pellucidum due to obstructive hydrocephalus **(c)**. A second axial T2-W image shows the third ventricle is also enlarged **(d)**. (These images are provided courtesy of the Children's Hospital of Philadelphia.)

■ Clinical Presentation

A 9-month-old ex-preterm boy (▶Fig. 156.1).

■ Key Imaging Finding

Hydrocephalus.

■ Top Three Differential Diagnoses

- **Post-inflammatory hydrocephalus.** Intracranial hemorrhage or leptomeningeal infection may cause acquired hydrocephalus. Both entities often lead to ependymal inflammation. This—sometimes along with exudate or blood—may impair the flow or resorption of CSF, potentially resulting in communicating or, less often, noncommunicating hydrocephalus. In addition, chronic sequelae of inflammation sometimes cause fibrosis of the subarachnoid spaces, similarly impairing CSF flow and leading to delayed hydrocephalus. If only the lateral and third ventricles are enlarged, this would be considered acquired cerebral aqueductal stenosis.
- **Obstructive hydrocephalus.** A mass or cyst may obstruct the ventricular system anywhere. However, obstructive hydrocephalus most often occurs when the mass or cyst grows into the CSF outflow tracts, especially the aqueduct of Sylvius, the foramina of Monro, Magendie, and Luschka, and the third and fourth ventricles. CT depicts mass effect and may partly delineate the offending lesion. However, MRI is far superior and is essential for accurate diagnosis. Acute hydrocephalus may develop if mass effect causes acute obstruction, leading to a rapid increase in intracranial pressure. Patients present with headache, papilledema, poor feeding, irritability, nausea, and/or vomiting. Enlargement of the temporal horns of the lateral ventricles is the most sensitive indicator of acute obstructive hydrocephalus. In addition, there may be transependymal edema due to rapid increase in intraventricular pressure, appearing as periventricular T2 prolongation on MRI and hypodensity on CT. CSF spaces may be effaced. Severe acute hydrocephalus may cause brain herniation.

- **Congenital cerebral aqueductal stenosis.** Narrowing of the aqueduct of Sylvius may prevent outflow of CSF and lead to supratentorial obstructive hydrocephalus. To be considered congenital, there must be no causative lesion for such a mass or prior inflammation/hemorrhage. MRI is essential for excluding acquired causes of hydrocephalus and allowing definitive diagnosis of congenital aqueductal stenosis. MRI sequences should include thin section sagittal imaging through the midline. The superior portion of the aqueduct often appears funneled, and the narrowing may be focal or more extensive.

■ Diagnosis

Congenital cerebral aqueductal stenosis.

✓ Pearls

- Aqueductal stenosis shows dilatation of the lateral and third ventricles with a normal-sized fourth ventricle.
- Acute hydrocephalus may show transependymal fluid shift, and it is important to evaluate for evidence of herniation.

- Both hemorrhage and infection may cause post-inflammatory hydrocephalus.

Suggested Readings

Barkovich AJ, Raybaud C. Congenital malformations of the brain and skull. In Barkovich AJ, Raybaud C, eds. Pediatric Neuroimaging, 5th ed. Philadelphia, PA: Lippincott Williams & Wilkins; 2012:367–568

Medina LS, Frawley K, Zurakowski D, Buttros D, DeGrauw AJ, Crone KR. Children with macrocrania: clinical and imaging predictors of disorders requiring surgery. AJNR Am J Neuroradiol. 2001; 22(3):564–570

Case 157

Michael Doherty

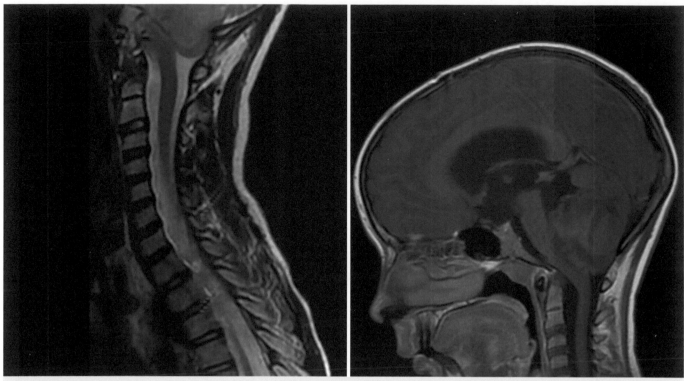

Fig. 157.1 Sagittal T2-W cervical spine MRI demonstrates inferior displacement of the cerebellar tonsils with posterior fossa crowding (displacement measured 10 mm) (**a**). Sagittal T1-W gadolinium-enhanced brain MRI shows the low-lying cerebellar tonsils, hydrocephalus, and enlargement of the cerebellum by a heterogeneous enhancing mass (**b**).

■ Clinical Presentation

An 8-year-old boy with ataxia (▶ Fig. 157.1).

■ Key Imaging Finding

Tonsillar herniation.

■ Top Three Differential Diagnoses

• **Chiari 1 malformation.** Most cases of Chiari 1 result from a small posterior fossa. This leads to a constellation of findings, including inferior displacement and elongation of the cerebellar tonsils, crowding of the posterior fossa, and compression of CSF spaces. Common symptoms include headache and neck pain, but up to 50% of patients are asymptomatic. On MRI, the cerebellar tonsils appear pointed and typically extend at least 5 mm below the foramen magnum (more than 6 mm is abnormal between ages 5 and 15 years). There is effacement of the foramen magnum. Cisterns are small or absent, and the fourth ventricle may appear elongated. Syringohydromyelia is common. Other associated abnormalities include basilar invagination and other osseous skull base anomalies, hydrocephalus, and fourth occipital sclerotome syndromes.

• **Chiari 2 malformation.** This complex hindbrain malformation occurs in the setting of neural tube closure defects. Folate deficiency and genetic predisposition (the methylene tetrahydrofolate reductase [MTHFR] mutation) combine to prevent neural tube closure at around estimated EGA 4 weeks. The open neural tube allows CSF to drain freely from the spine, and as a result mesenchyme does not develop normally. This leads to a small posterior fossa. There may also be absence of the corpus callosum and septum pellucidum, gray matter heterotopia, and dysmorphic posterior gyri. Characteristic findings on MRI include a crowded posterior fossa, tectal beaking, and inferior displacement of the medulla with cervicomedullary kinking. Supratentorial findings may include colpocephaly, hydrocephalus, fenestration of the falx with interdigitation of gyri, and absence of the corpus callosum. Classic features of the fetal brain include cerebellar compression (banana sign), frontal bone concavity (lemon sign), and ventriculomegaly.

• **Acute herniation.** The most common cause of acute brain herniation in children is a posterior fossa mass. Other etiologies include trauma, large infarcts, and inflammation. Acute herniation may be diagnosed with unenhanced CT. The cerebellar tonsils are pushed more than 5 mm inferiorly, impacted into the foramen magnum. The cisterna magna is obliterated, and hydrocephalus is common. MRI is usually needed to determine underlying etiology and assess for such complications as edema, hemorrhage, and infarcts. Other types of herniation include subfalcine, transalar, and transtentorial.

■ Diagnosis

Hydrocephalus and cerebellar tonsillar herniation secondary to medulloblastoma.

✓ Pearls

• Findings of Chiari 1 malformation include inferiorly displaced, elongated cerebellar tonsils, and a crowded posterior fossa; syringohydromyelia is common as well.

• Chiari 2 malformation is a complex hindbrain malformation that is virtually always associated with a neural tube defect.

• A posterior fossa mass is the most common cause of acute tonsillar herniation, resulting in obliteration of the cisterna magna and often secondary hydrocephalus and infarct.

Suggested Readings

Hussain SI, Cordero-Tumangday C, Goldenberg FD, Wollman R, Frank JI, Rosengart AJ. Brainstem ischemia in acute herniation syndrome. J Neurol Sci. 2008; 268(1–2):190–192

McVige JW, Leonardo J. Imaging of Chiari type I malformation and syringohydromyelia. Neurol Clin. 2014; 32(1):95–126

Case 158

Rebecca Stein-Wexler

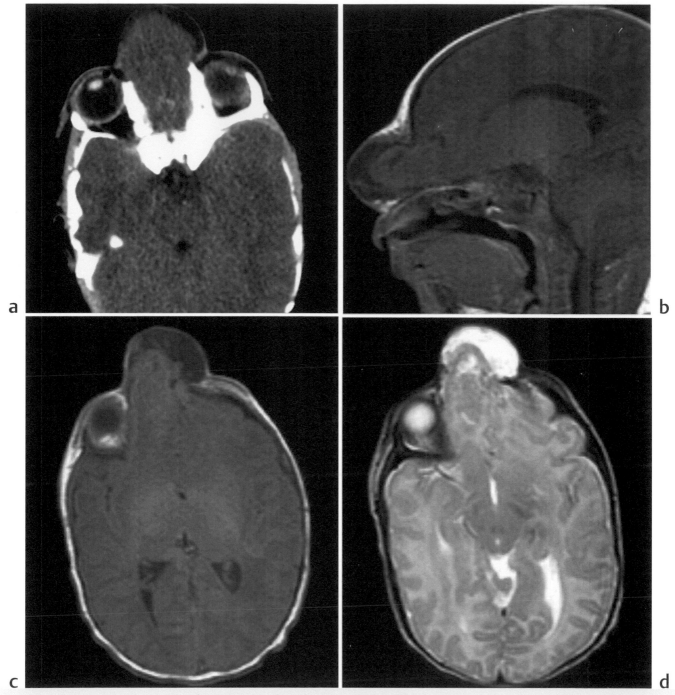

Fig. 158.1 Axial CT shows soft tissue extending anteriorly at the prefrontal region **(a)**. Sagittal T1-W image shows an osseous defect at the frontal midline, through which the frontal lobe protrudes **(b)**. Axial T1-W **(c)** and T2-W **(d)** images show dysplastic frontal lobes and a rim of CSF in the lesion.

■ **Clinical Presentation**

A newborn with a midline mass and nasal deformity (▶ Fig. 158.1).

■ Key Imaging Finding

Congenital midline nasal mass.

■ Top Three Differential Diagnoses

- **Dermoid/epidermoid.** These lesions present as a nasal mass, cyst, sinus, or draining fistula and are most common at the dorsum of the nose. They result from abnormal separation of dura and skin, which initially develop in close approximation. The dura should subsequently retract, and the foramen cecum should form a barrier between skin and dura. A nasal dermoid or epidermoid forms if the foramen does not close and/or if dural tissue does not retract. Dermoids are more common than epidermoids and are slightly more common in boys. They consist of both ectoderm and mesoderm, whereas epidermoids are ectoderm only. Dermoids may communicate with the CNS, whereas epidermoids typically do not. CT demonstrates an osseous defect. MRI depicts the defect as well as the lesion's contents. A dermoid has variable T1 and T2 signal, since it may contain fat as well as fluid. Fat suppression techniques are useful for diagnosing fat. Epidermoids contain simple fluid and—important for diagnosis—show restricted diffusion. The rims of both lesions may enhance. Since both dermoids and epidermoids are prone to infection—including, for dermoids, meningitis and cerebral abscess—complete resection of the cyst and potential tract is mandatory.
- **Nasofrontal encephalocele.** Formation of nasofrontal encephaloceles is similar to that of dermoids and epidermoids, but in addition the residual dura retains communication with the subarachnoid space. Only 15% of encephaloceles are anterior. Patients often also have anophthalmia, microphthalmia, microcephalus, hydrocephalus, dysgenesis of the corpus callosum, and/or cortical atrophy. Encephaloceles appear as soft, bluish masses that transilluminate and increase in size with Valsalva. They are located at the midline of the nose, glabella, or both. MRI shows a soft-tissue mass in continuity with the subarachnoid space, whose signal characteristics match those of the brain. CT demonstrates the osseous defect more clearly than does MRI. It is essential to image all nasal masses before biopsy, in order to exclude encephalocele.
- **Nasal cerebral heterotopia (aka glioma).** Development of these unusual masses is similar to that of dermoids. However, rests of sequestered glial tissue are retained, along with fibrovascular tissue. About 60% of these heterotopias are extranasal, and about 30% are intranasal; the rest span both regions. A few connect to the brain via a fibrous stalk that traverses the foramen cecum to end at the subarachnoid space, but most do not connect to neural tissue. Most patients present with a red or bluish, firm mass at the glabella, nasomaxillary suture, or within the nose. They uncommonly present with meningitis or CSF rhinorrhea. Nasal cerebral heterotopia appears as a soft-tissue mass at CT or MRI. Signal tends to be brighter than normal brain on T2, since the neural tissue is gliotic and dysplastic. It is important to differentiate nasal gliomas from encephaloceles.

■ Diagnosis

Nasofrontal encephalocele.

✓ Pearls

- Dermoids are the most common congenital nasal mass, may communicate with the CNS, and contain fluid, fat, skin, and/or bone.
- Epidermoids contain only fluid, do not communicate with the CNS, and demonstrate restricted diffusion.
- MRI of nasofrontal encephaloceles shows neural tissue in continuity with the frontal lobe.
- Nasal cerebral heterotopias may connect to the subarachnoid space; their T2 signal is brighter than that of brain.

Suggested Readings

Adil E, Huntley C, Choudhary A, Carr M. Congenital nasal obstruction: clinical and radiologic review. Eur J Pediatr. 2012; 171(4):641–650

Kadom N, Sze RW. Radiological reasoning: pediatric midline nasofrontal mass. AJR Am J Roentgenol. 2010; 194(3) Suppl:WS10–WS13

Saettele M, Alexander A, Markovich B, Morelli J, Lowe LH. Congenital midline nasofrontal masses. Pediatr Radiol. 2012; 42(9):1119–1125

Case 159

Rebecca Stein-Wexler

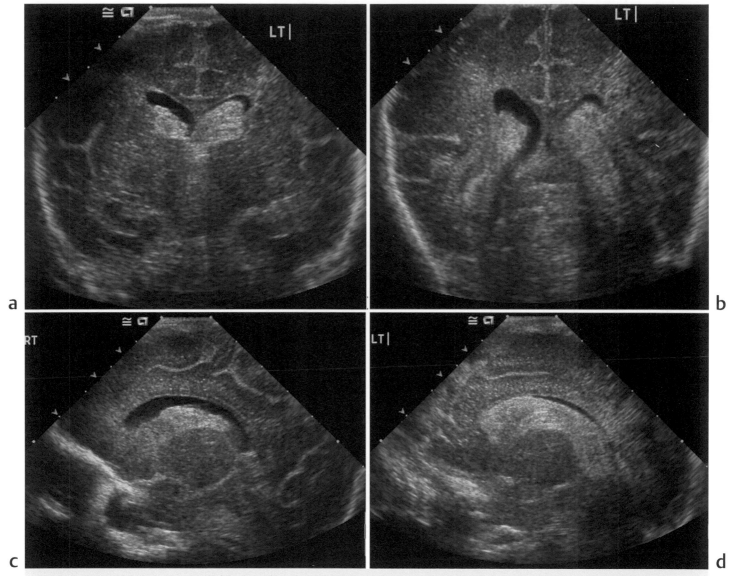

Fig. 159.1 Coronal head US at the level of the frontal horns shows echogenic material at both germinal matrices, extending into both frontal horns; the left is almost filled with echogenic material **(a)**. Coronal US at the posterior parietal/occipital regions shows echogenic material fills the left and partly fills the right lateral ventricles; both are mildly dilated **(b)**. Sagittal US to the right of midline shows the caudothalamic groove filled with hemorrhage that extends into the right lateral ventricle **(c)**. Sagittal US to the left of midline shows the left lateral ventricle is dilated and filled with echogenic material **(d)**.

■ Clinical Presentation

A 3-day-old premature newborn (▶Fig. 159.1).

■ **Key Imaging Finding**

Periventricular/intraventricular hemorrhage in a premature infant.

■ **Top Three Differential Diagnoses**

- **Grade 1 germinal matrix hemorrhage (GMH).** GMH accounts for about three-fourths of intracranial hemorrhage in preterm infants. It develops in about half of those who are very preterm. The germinal matrix (GM) is subependymal in location, initially located along the entire length of the lateral ventricles. By EGA 35 weeks, it is limited to the caudothalamic groove. Glial and neural cells develop in and migrate from this highly vascular area. Fragile vessels in the GM may rupture due to fluctuating blood flow in premature infants who lack cerebral autoregulation. GMH initially appears echogenic, bulging into the floor of the lateral ventricle. The hemorrhage retracts, becomes cystic, and eventually disappears. Clinical sequelae are uncommon.
- **Grade 2 IVH.** Grade 2 IVH develops when GMH perforates the ependyma and spills into the ventricular system. The ventricles may be dilated, but they are only partly filled with echogenic blood. Blood may pool in the occipital horns.

IVH is often isoechoic to choroid plexus, and the two may be confused. However, echogenic material in the frontal horns indicates IVH, as choroid plexus does not extend this far forward. As IVH evolves, the clot becomes hypoechoic and eventually contracts. If chemical ependymitis develops, the ventricular lining becomes echogenic. Hydrocephalus may develop if clot obstructs the foramina of Monro, the cerebral aqueduct, or—less often—the fourth ventricular outflow tracts. In the absence of hydrocephalus, clinical sequelae are unlikely.

- **Grade 3 IVH.** In this case, the hemorrhage fills at least 50% of the ventricle(s). The affected ventricles are dilated, and the hemorrhage forms an echogenic cast of the ventricular contour. As with grade 2 IVH, clot may block CSF pathways and lead to further ventricular enlargement. About 50% of patients with grade 3 IVH will develop cerebral palsy and/or developmental delay.

■ **Additional Differential Diagnoses**

- **Grade 4 periventricular hemorrhage (PVH).** Mass effect from GMH or severe ventricular enlargement may lead to blockage of parenchymal draining veins with subsequent venous ischemia. This may progress to arterial hemorrhage and hemorrhagic infarction. With venous ischemia, US shows a large GMH and extensive increased periventricular echogenicity. With hemorrhagic conversion, the hemorrhage

appears more masslike. It may lead to cystic encephalomalacia and porencephaly, with resultant cerebral palsy and/or developmental delay. PVH accounts for 5% of intracranial hemorrhage.
- **Choroid plexus hemorrhage.** Full-term infants may develop hemorrhage in their highly vascular choroid plexus. They may also develop thalamic and cerebellar hemorrhage.

■ **Diagnosis**

Bilateral germinal matrix hemorrhage (grade 1) with hemorrhage extending into the right lateral ventricle (grade 2) and filling the dilated left lateral ventricle (grade 3).

✓ **Pearls**

- Grade 1 germinal matrix hemorrhage is at the subependymal caudothalamic groove and bulges into the lateral ventricle floor.
- With grade 2 IVH, germinal matrix hemorrhage extends into the lateral ventricle, and blood partly fills the ventricle.

- Grade 3 intraventricular hemorrhage is complicated by ventricular enlargement, and blood mostly fills and forms a cast of the ventricle.
- Grade 4 periventricular hemorrhage develops when germinal matrix hemorrhage or hydrocephalus leads to obstruction of parenchymal veins with subsequent hemorrhagic ischemia.

Suggested Readings

Fritz J, Polansky SM, O'Connor SC. Neonatal neurosonography. Semin Ultrasound CT MR. 2014; 35(4):349–364

Orman G, Benson JE, Kweldam CF, et al. Neonatal head ultrasonography today: a powerful imaging tool! J Neuroimaging. 2015; 25(1):31–55

Riccabona M. Neonatal neurosonography. Eur J Radiol. 2014; 83(9):1495–1506

Case 160

Rebecca Stein-Wexler

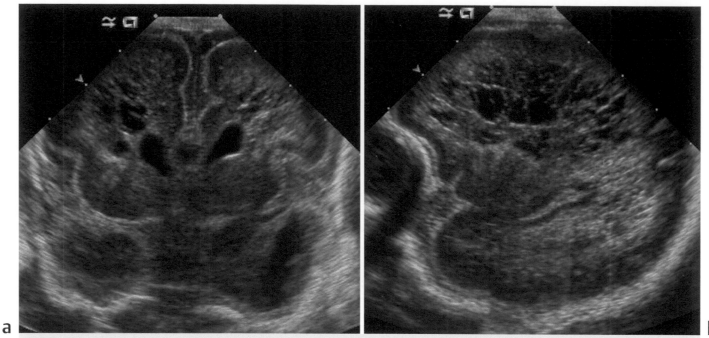

a

b

Fig. 160.1 Coronal US shows numerous irregular cystic lesions in the bilateral periventricular frontal lobes, more pronounced on the right **(a)**. Sagittal image through the right centrum semiovale shows multiple cystic spaces radiating within the periventricular white matter **(b)**.

■ **Clinical Presentation**

A 4-week-old ex-26-week premature infant with apnea and bradycardia (▶Fig. 160.1).

■ Key Imaging Finding

Periventricular cysts.

■ Top Three Differential Diagnoses

- **Connatal cysts (aka frontal horn cysts, coarctation of the lateral ventricles).** These cysts probably represent normal variants that develop if the ependymal lining on apposing sides of the lateral ventricle abuts. They form at or just below the superolateral angle of the frontal horn or, less commonly, adjacent to the anterior body of the lateral ventricle. Most are anterior to the foramina of Monro.
- **Subependymal cysts.** Most subependymal cysts are located below the external angle of the lateral ventricle, posterior to the foramina of Monro. These cystic cavities may be seen in the general population. Some result from prenatal hemorrhage, ischemia, or infection (cytomegalovirus/rubella). Those located at the caudothalamic notch are usually seen in premature infants and represent evolving germinal matrix hemorrhage.

- **Periventricular leukomalacia (PVL).** PVL develops in premature infants who have suffered perinatal hypoxia. Most cases occur in children born at less than 32 weeks EGA and weighing less than 1.5 kg. PVL forms in the periventricular white matter, which is the watershed zone. Most PVL develops in the peritrigonal area and anterolateral to the frontal horns, especially in the centrum semiovale and the optic and acoustic radiations. Screening US may initially demonstrate periventricular increased echogenicity that evolves to periventricular cysts by around age 2 weeks, but US may be normal. At this time, MRI may show periventricular necrosis and cavitation. MRI of toddlers with developmental delay may demonstrate undiagnosed PVL: loss of white matter volume, sulci extending close to enlarged lateral ventricles, and a correspondingly thin corpus callosum. White matter signal is increased on T2 and FLAIR due to gliosis.

■ Additional Differential Diagnosis

- **Mucopolysaccharidosis.** Deficiency of lysosomal enzymes leads to mucopolysaccharide deposition in many tissues, including in the perivascular spaces of the brain. This may lead to development of cysts in the white matter, basal ganglia, and corpus callosum. In addition, the deep white matter is usually hypodense on CT, hypointense on T1, and hyperintense on T2, perhaps due to accumulation of glycosaminoglycans and gan-

gliosides. Periventricular white matter is most often affected, but all parts of the cerebrum may be involved. Delayed myelination, hydrocephalus, and brain atrophy may be evident as well. Hurler syndrome is the most common mucopolysaccharidosis. Zellweger and oculocerebrorenal syndromes are other leukodystrophies that may develop deep periventricular white matter cysts.

■ Diagnosis

Periventricular leukomalacia.

✓ Pearls

- Connatal cysts usually form at or just below the superolateral angle of the lateral ventricle frontal horn.
- Subependymal cysts form posterior to the foramen of Monro, below the external angle of the lateral ventricle.

- Periventricular leukomalacia is usually seen in the peritrigonal area or anterolateral to the frontal horns, in the centrum semiovale.
- Perivascular mucopolysaccharide deposition may lead to white matter, basal ganglia, and corpus callosum cysts in patients with mucopolysaccharidosis.

Suggested Readings

Epelman M, Daneman A, Blaser SI, et al. Differential diagnosis of intracranial cystic lesions at head US: correlation with CT and MR imaging. Radiographics. 2006; 26(1):173–196

Phelan JA, Lowe LH, Glasier CM. Pediatric neurodegenerative white matter processes: leukodystrophies and beyond. Pediatr Radiol. 2008; 38(7):729–749

Simbrunner J, Riccabona M. Imaging of the neonatal CNS. Eur J Radiol. 2006; 60(2):133–151

Zafeiriou DI, Batzios SP. Brain and spinal MR imaging findings in mucopolysaccharidoses: a review. AJNR Am J Neuroradiol. 2013; 34(1):5–13

Case 161

Rebecca Stein-Wexler

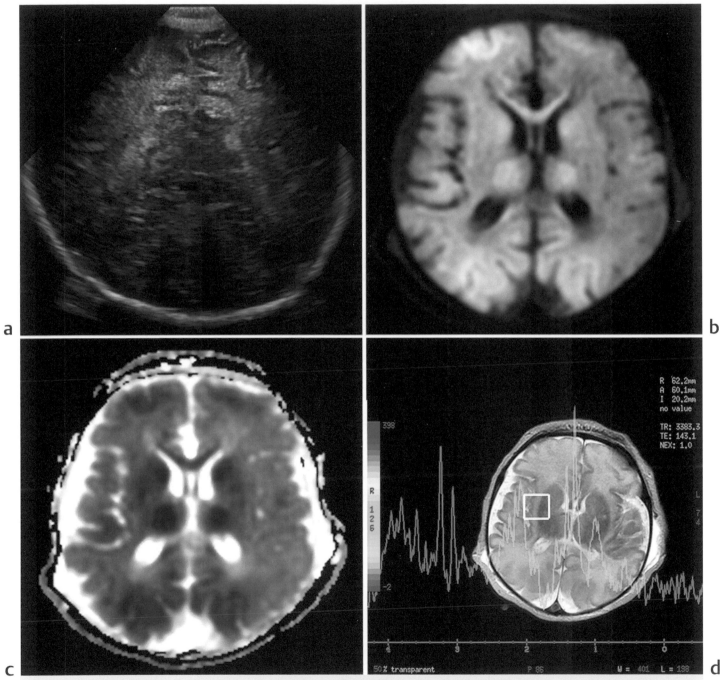

Fig. 161.1 Coronal head US shows diffuse increased echogenicity and a hypoechoic subcortical ribbon (**a**). Five days later, axial DWI shows restricted diffusion in the basal ganglia, thalami, and frontal and occipital watershed areas (**b**). Apparent diffusion coefficient (ADC) map shows corresponding hypointensity (**c**). MR spectroscopy shows a prominent lactate peak and reduced N-acetylaspartate peak (**d**).

■ **Clinical Presentation**

Term newborn with cardiopulmonary failure (▶Fig. 161.1).

■ **Key Imaging Finding**

Restricted diffusion.

■ **Top Three Differential Diagnoses**

• **Diffuse hypoxic-ischemic encephalopathy (HIE).** HIE can develop in a variety of settings. In the perinatal period, it often results from hypoperfusion due to failure of autoregulation. In the setting of nonaccidental trauma (NAT), it may result from strangulation or direct trauma to the brainstem respiratory center. Near drowning and other circulatory arrest may cause HIE in older children. Depending on patient age and insult severity, ischemia may be global or limited to the watershed areas and/or basal ganglia. Profound hypotension predominantly damages the most metabolically active and mature regions of the developing brain: in neonates, the brainstem, thalami, basal ganglia, and sensorimotor cortex. Milder hypotension damages the periventricular and deep white matter in premature infants and the watershed portions of the cerebral cortex (and adjacent white matter) in term infants. In older children, the basal ganglia and cerebral cortex are most vulnerable to profound hypotension, whereas milder hypotension causes watershed injury. In its early phase, the cytotoxic edema of HIE is best seen with DWI. DWI offers quantitative information about water motion and the microstructure of tissue. Diffusion is reduced immediately after traumatic, metabolic, or toxic brain injury. Restricted diffusion appears bright, whereas it appears dark on correlative ADC mapping, remaining abnormal for about 6 days. T2-W imaging becomes abnormal within about 24 hours; T1 takes longer. The presence of subdural hematoma, retinal hemorrhages, and suspicious fractures suggests NAT as etiology.

• **Localized infarction.** Stroke is one of the top 10 causes of death in children. Half the cases occur before age 1 year, and of these half occur in neonates. Metabolic abnormalities and coagulopathies cause some strokes, but at least half are idiopathic. Clinical signs and imaging manifestations vary with patient age. Prognosis is generally better for very young children, since the plastic pediatric brain can assume functions of damaged areas. US depicts perinatal strokes as ill-defined areas of moderately increased echogenicity. MRI is more useful, especially in older children. An acute infarct follows vascular territory and appears bright on DWI within hours. T2-W images become positive within 24 hours. The appearance of pediatric stroke resembles that of adults, except in infants whose high brain water content makes identification of stroke more difficult, especially on FLAIR.

• **Infection.** DWI depicts early cell necrosis in the setting of neonatal herpes encephalitis, which may cause multifocal destruction or predominantly affect the temporal lobes, deep gray matter, watershed areas, or occasionally the brainstem and cerebellum. Subtle T2 hyperintensity follows, with subsequent mild meningeal enhancement. Water diffusion is also decreased in brain abscesses, and this helps differentiate these lesions from cystic or necrotic tumors, in which diffusion is not restricted. Late cerebritis also demonstrates restricted water diffusion. Progressive normalization of diffusion indicates treatment is successful. If DWI remains bright, alternative therapies should be considered.

■ **Diagnosis**

Hypoxic ischemic encephalopathy in a term newborn.

✓ **Pearls**

• The pattern of diffuse hypoxic ischemic encephalopathy reflects the severity of hypotension and the maturity of the brain.
• DWI becomes abnormal within a few hours and normalizes within about 6 days.

• The high water content of the infant brain makes it difficult to identify stroke, especially on FLAIR.
• Water diffusion is restricted in abscess but not in tumor, making DWI useful for differentiation.

Suggested Readings

Badve CA, Khanna PC, Ishak GE. Neonatal ischemic brain injury: what every radiologist needs to know. Pediatr Radiol. 2012; 42(5):606–619

Parmar H, Ibrahim M. Pediatric intracranial infections. Neuroimaging Clin N Am. 2012; 22(4):707–725

Schwartz ES, Barkovich AJ. Brain and spine injuries in infancy and childhood. In Barkovich AJ, Raybaud C, eds. Pediatric Neuroimaging, 5th ed. Philadelphia, PA: Lippincott Williams & Wilkins; 2012:240–366

Case 162

Rebecca Stein-Wexler

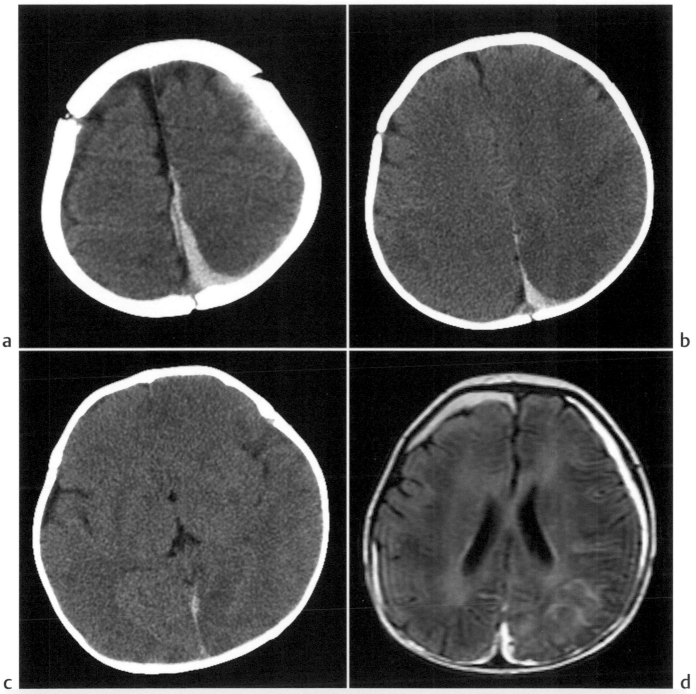

a

b

c

d

Fig. 162.1 Axial CT of the brain **(a–c)** shows dense fluid tracking along the falx and also along the left frontoparietal region **(a)**. There is patchy decreased density in the posterior parietal and occipital regions, and sulci are effaced **(b,c)**. Six days later, FLAIR MRI shows hyperintense extra-axial fluid, now present bilaterally, as well as heterogeneous areas of mixed signal, predominantly in the posterior parietal and occipital regions **(d)**.

■ **Clinical Presentation**

A 9-month-old girl with seizures (▶Fig. 162.1).

■ Key Imaging Finding

Subdural hemorrhage in an infant.

■ Top Three Differential Diagnoses

- **Spontaneous neonatal subdural hemorrhage (SDH).** Asymptomatic SDH is common in the neonatal period. Although usually seen with instrumented vaginal delivery, it may follow any type of delivery. SDH occurs most often in the posterior fossa but may also be found along the posterior falx and over the high convexities, locations that are also common with nonaccidental trauma (NAT)-induced SDH. These SDHs resolve in about 4 weeks and do not progress to chronic SDH. They have no clinical significance.
- **Posttraumatic SDH.** Accidental SDH results from motor vehicle collisions, falls greater than 3 feet, and other significant trauma. History facilitates diagnosis.

- **Nonaccidental trauma (NAT).** Multifocal SDH is a common manifestation of NAT. SDH is most common at the posterior interhemispheric fissure, along the vertex (where there are fragile bridging veins), and in the posterior fossa. Although usually hyperdense on CT, SDH may be heterogeneous if clot forms rapidly, if there are two temporally different hemorrhagic events, or if bleeding develops within a collection of CSF. Disruption of bridging veins may lead to venous infarction, seen in about 10%. Signal intensity of SDH varies on MRI, depending on the stage of evolution.

■ Additional Differential Diagnoses

- **Coagulopathy.** Hemophilia and von Willebrand disease are the most common coagulation disorders. Children with these diseases may present with bruising and joint swelling. Subdural and retinal hemorrhages resemble findings in children subjected to NAT.
- **Metabolic disorders.** Infants with glutaric aciduria type I may develop both subdural and retinal hemorrhage with minimal trauma. Patients with this autosomal-recessive disease have excessive quantities of glutaric acid due to an enzyme deficiency. Macrocephaly with rapid increase in head size is typical, and infants manifest hypotonia, head lag, and other neurological abnormalities. In addition to enlarged CSF spaces, there is temporal lobe hypoplasia, delayed myelination, and

abnormal T2 signal in the globi pallidi. Menkes disease may also demonstrate SDH and other extra-axial fluid collections, along with atrophy and infarctions.
- **Benign extra-axial fluid of infancy.** These CSF collections may mimic resolving SDH but result from increased fluid in the subarachnoid space. The subarachnoid location of fluid is confirmed by visualization of vessels traversing the enlarged extra-axial space, best appreciated at US or MRI. Fluid is also increased in the ventricles and cisterns. Patients are neurologically normal, and there is usually macrocranium and sometimes also a family history of macrocranium. This condition resolves by age 1 year.

■ Diagnosis

Parafalcine subdural hemorrhage and brain edema due to non-accidental trauma.

✓ Pearls

- Spontaneous neonatal subdural hemorrhage mimics non-accidental trauma–associated subdural hemorrhage, but is often associated with an instrumented vaginal delivery.
- Falls from more than 3 feet may result in accidental subdural hemorrhage.

- Subdural hemorrhage in the setting of non-accidental trauma is usually along the posterior falx, vertex, and posterior fossa.
- Benign extra-axial fluid of infancy is located in the subarachnoid space.

Suggested Readings

Cakmakci H. Essentials of trauma: head and spine. Pediatr Radiol. 2009; 39 Suppl 3:391–405

Girard N, Brunel H, Dory-Lautrec P, Chabrol B. Neuroimaging differential diagnoses to abusive head trauma. Pediatr Radiol. 2016; 46(5):603–614

Case 163

Rebecca Stein-Wexler

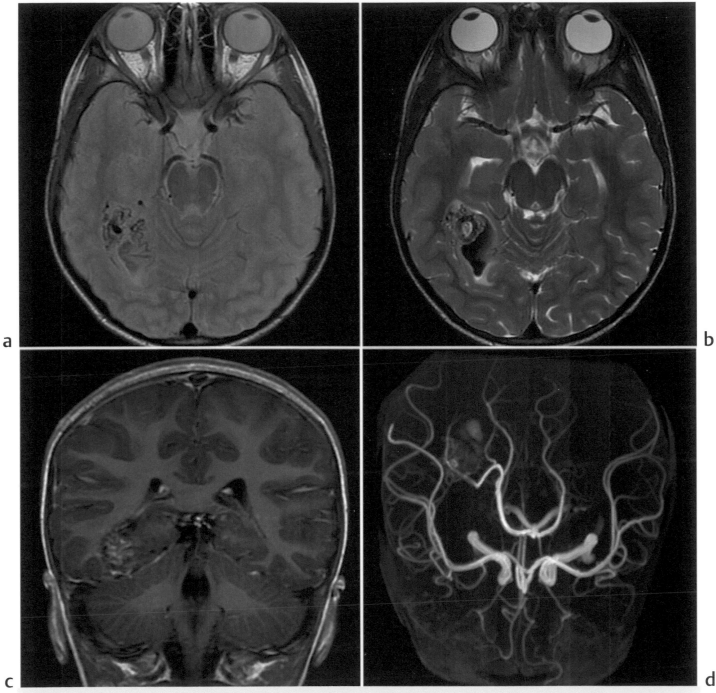

Fig. 163.1 Axial PD image shows serpiginous flow voids in the right temporal lobe (a). T2-W image also shows flow voids, along with susceptibility artifact secondary to hemorrhage (b). Coronal T1-FLAIR gadolinium-enhanced image shows flow voids along with contrast within serpiginous vessels (c). 3D time-of-flight MR angiography shows a temporal branch of the right posterior cerebral artery extending to the vascular nidus (d).

■ **Clinical Presentation**

A 5-year-old girl with seizure (▶Fig. 163.1).

■ Key Imaging Finding

Parenchymal hemorrhage.

■ Top Three Differential Diagnoses

- **Trauma.** This is the leading cause of parenchymal hemorrhage in children. History and evidence of trauma usually facilitate diagnosis. CT is often sufficient, but complex or questionable cases may proceed to MRI along with MR arteriography or MR venography. Appearance on T1 and T2 allows dating of parenchymal hematomas.
- **Vascular malformation (VM).** VM is the most common cause of spontaneous hemorrhage in children. Arteriovenous malformations (AVMs) are the most common VM to bleed. AVMs consist of a compact tangle of abnormal, thin-walled vessels (nidus) connecting arteries and veins and allowing rapid arteriovenous shunting. Most patients present with seizures, headache, and/or spontaneous hemorrhage. CT is useful for screening during the first 2 weeks after hemorrhage, but MRI provides much more information. The nidus appears as a serpiginous tangle of flow voids, with feeding arteries and draining veins. Hemosiderin from prior hemorrhage appears dark on T2/T2*. Catheter angiography delineates architecture and precedes possible microsurgery, radiation, or embolization. Developmental venous anomalies (DVAs) are the most common VM, but they never spontaneously bleed and are discovered incidentally. Rarely they may cause headache or seizures and—if the draining vein thromboses—intraparenchymal hemorrhage. DVAs are most common in the frontal lobes and posterior fossa. They consist of radially oriented dilated medullary or subcortical veins that drain into a single venous structure. MRI shows a uniformly enhancing tuft of radially arrayed small vessels. Vein of Galen malformations, another VM, rarely cause hemorrhage.
- **Hemorrhagic mass.** Ependymomas are the most common tumor to hemorrhage, but hemorrhage may also be seen with high-grade gliomas, primitive neuroectodermal tumors (PNETs), hemangioblastomas, and other neoplasms. MR angiography/venography help differentiate between hemorrhage due to tumor versus AVM or other VM.

■ Additional Differential Diagnoses

- **Hemorrhagic venous infarction.** Almost half of cases of dural venous occlusion (DVO) result in infarction, hemorrhagic in 70%. This causes some neonatal grade IV hemorrhage. US diagnoses DVO in young infants, but older patients require MRI. The affected sinus is enlarged and lacks signal void on fast spin echo (FSE) imaging. It contains clot, with signal intensity varying with thrombus stage (usually T1 bright when acute or subacute). Thrombus may also be seen in deep medullary veins. It is important to evaluate children with DVO for coagulation disorders. In infants, DVO often resolves without neurological sequelae.
- **Spontaneous intracranial hematoma in a newborn.** Most intracranial hematomas in newborns result from birth trauma, asphyxia, clotting disorder, or an underlying AVM. However, increased arterial and venous pressure and impaired autoregulation may cause spontaneous hematoma in otherwise normal infants.

■ Diagnosis

Arteriovenous malformation.

✓ Pearls

- Arteriovenous malformation is the most common cause of spontaneous parenchymal hemorrhage in children.
- Ependymomas, high-grade gliomas, PNETs, and hemangioblastomas are prone to hemorrhage.
- Venous infarction usually develops in the setting of thrombosis of the dural venous sinus.

Suggested Readings

Burch EA, Orbach DB. Pediatric central nervous system vascular malformations. Pediatr Radiol. 2015; 45 Suppl 3:S463–S472

Epelman M, Daneman A, Blaser SI, et al. Differential diagnosis of intracranial cystic lesions at head US: correlation with CT and MR imaging. Radiographics. 2006; 26(1):173–196

Case 164

Geoffrey D. McWilliams

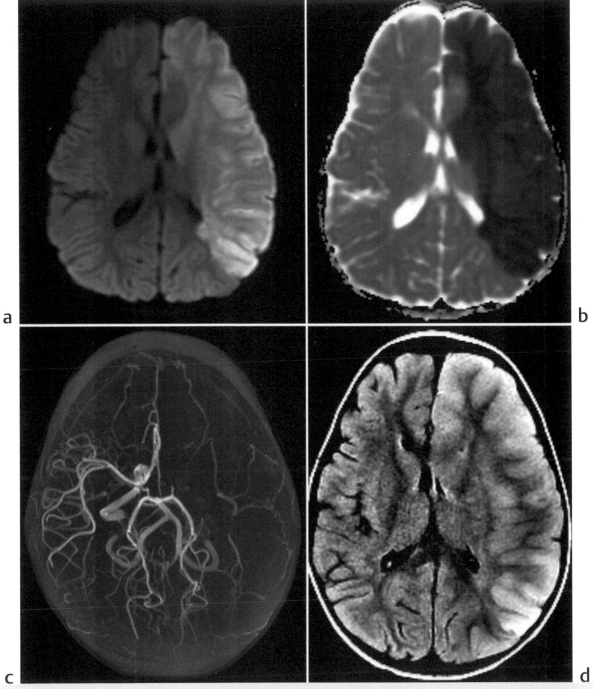

Fig. 164.1 Axial DWI image shows hyperintensity in the distribution of the left anterior and middle cerebral arteries, involving the frontal and parietal lobes as well as basal ganglia (a). This area is dark on ADC map (b). 3D time-of-flight MR angiography shows absent flow in the left internal carotid artery and left middle and anterior cerebral arteries (c). Axial FLAIR image 1 day later shows cortical edema and development of mild left to right midline shift (d).

■ Clinical Presentation

A 3-year-old with sudden onset of altered mental status
(▶Fig. 164.1).

■ Key Imaging Finding

Cerebral infarct.

■ Top Three Differential Diagnoses

- **Sickle cell disease.** Cerebral infarcts affect approximately 10% of children with sickle cell disease (an autosomal-recessive disorder of the hemoglobin β gene seen primarily in people of African descent). Red blood cells (RBCs) may become transiently misshapen and stiff, resulting in vascular occlusion or damage to the internal elastic lamina. This leads to ischemia, aneurysm formation, or vasculopathy. Infarcts are most common before age 5 years. They are usually ischemic but may be hemorrhagic in about 25%. In addition to acute infarction, vasculopathy may cause chronic arterial stenosis, often at the distal internal carotid artery or circle of Willis. Chronic occlusion results in development of lenticulostriate collaterals within the basal ganglia, leading to "moyamoya," or the "puff of smoke" appearance on cerebral angiography. Unenhanced CT in sickle cell patients often shows diffuse atrophy, prior infarcts, and occasionally intraventricular or intraparenchymal hemorrhage. Acute infarction is seen on MRI as diffusion restriction, evidenced by hyperintensity on DWI with corresponding low signal on ADC maps. Hyperintensity on T2 and FLAIR often manifests after 6 hours. Transcranial Doppler US is used to screen sickle cell patients for increased risk of cerebral infarction. Patients then receive prophylactic chronic transfusion therapy or hydroxyurea.

- **Vasculitis.** Vasculitis may also result in cerebral ischemia. The vasculitis may be primary or secondary to a variety of underlying systemic diseases. Though CT is often normal, there may be multifocal hypodensities in the deep gray or subcortical white matter, suggesting prior ischemia or infarction. MRI may show subcortical or deep gray matter FLAIR/T2 hyperintensities, with diffusion restriction if ischemia is acute. Rarely, hemorrhage may be evident on T2* gradient echo (GRE) sequences. Gadolinium-enhanced MRI may show patchy linear parenchymal enhancement. MR angiography is insensitive but may show concentric, smooth stenoses.

- **Posterior reversible encephalopathy syndrome (PRES), or acute hypertensive encephalopathy.** This is a disorder of cerebrovascular autoregulation related to acute or subacute hypertension, drug toxicity (immunosuppressants, chemotherapy), hematologic disease, or renal disease. Endothelial damage and resulting failure of autoregulation disrupt the blood–brain barrier, causing bilateral, symmetrical subcortical vasogenic edema, usually in a parietooccipital distribution—though any region of the brain may be involved. CT may show subtle bilateral, patchy, parietooccipital hypodense foci. MRI shows T2 and FLAIR hyperintensities. PRES rarely demonstrates restricted diffusion, hemorrhage, and patchy enhancement.

■ Diagnosis

Sickle cell disease–related acute left cerebral hemisphere infarction.

✓ Pearls

- Cerebral infarction shows high DWI and low ADC signal; FLAIR hyperintensity appears after 6 hours.
- Cerebral infarction affects about 10% of children with sickle cell disease; there may be "moyamoya" or "puff of smoke" appearance due to chronic occlusion and collateralization.

- Vasculitis is another common cause of pediatric cerebral infarct.
- Posterior reversible encephalopathy syndrome has a bilateral parietooccipital distribution and rarely demonstrates diffusion restriction.

Suggested Readings

Abdel Razek AA, Alvarez H, Bagg S, Refaat S, Castillo M. Imaging spectrum of CNS vasculitis. Radiographics. 2014; 34(4):873–894

Aviv RI, Benseler SM, Silverman ED, et al. MR Imaging and angiography of primary CNS vasculitis of childhood. AJNR Am J Neuroradiol. 2006; 27(1):192–199

Covarrubias DJ, Luetmer PH, Campeau NG. Posterior reversible encephalopathy syndrome: prognostic utility of quantitative diffusion-weighted MR images. AJNR Am J Neuroradiol. 2002; 23(6):1038–1048

Ohene-Frempong K, Weiner SJ, Sleeper LA, et al. Cerebrovascular accidents in sickle cell disease: rates and risk factors. Blood. 1998; 91(1):288–294

Case 165

Ethan Neufeld

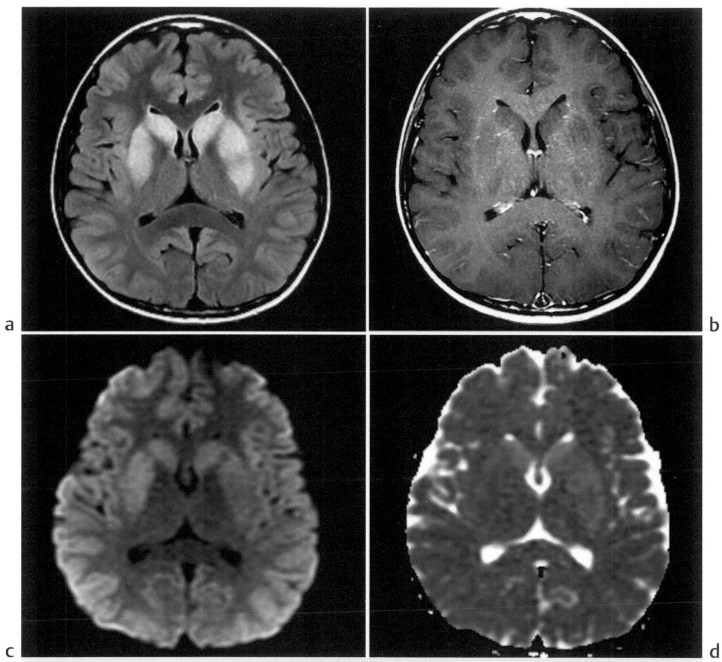

Fig. 165.1 Axial T2 FLAIR MRI shows symmetrical high signal in the bilateral caudate heads and putamina; the cortical gray and white matter is normal in signal and morphology (a). Axial gadolinium-enhanced T1-W image does not demonstrate abnormal parenchymal enhancement (b). On DWI the signal in the caudate heads and putamina is minimally increased (c). Axial ADC map also shows mildly increased signal in the caudate heads and putamina without appreciable signal loss, indicating that there is no restricted diffusion (d).

■ **Clinical Presentation**

A 7-year-old girl with seizures and motor dysfunction
(►Fig. 165.1).

■ Key Imaging Finding

Bilateral basal ganglia signal abnormality.

■ Top Three Differential Diagnoses

- **Hypoxic-ischemic injury.** Prolonged asphyxiation or near-drowning events may lead to profound neurological consequences with associated MRI findings. Injury occurs in the metabolically active gray matter, and thus the basal ganglia are preferentially affected, in addition to the cortex. High T2 signal is seen in the basal ganglia and thalami but may also be seen in the periphery, depending on the severity of injury. Sometimes white matter changes develop later in the process, indicating a poor prognosis.
- **Toxic exposure.** Various toxins cause encephalopathy with associated basal ganglia abnormalities. Carbon monoxide poisoning classically causes increased T2 signal in the globi pallidi, sometimes with increased T1 signal due to hemorrhagic

necrosis. There are often associated white matter lesions as well. Methanol poisoning causes increased T2 signal in the putamina, likewise with associated hemorrhage.
- **Thrombosis of deep cerebral veins.** Arterial occlusion is uncommon in children and would not be expected to cause bilateral pathology. However, venous occlusion can produce such findings. Venous occlusion may be seen in children with inherited coagulopathies or in those that are critically ill. Both internal cerebral veins are usually affected, associated with dural sinus thrombosis. The veins are hyperdense on CT. The thalami are affected, in addition to the globi pallidi and striatum, which can be a helpful distinguishing feature.

■ Additional Differential Diagnoses

- **Inherited metabolic disorder.** Several inherited metabolic disorders are characterized by abnormal basal ganglia and may not be suspected if family history is unknown or if the disorder is recessive. Leigh syndrome is an inherited mitochondrial disorder presenting in childhood with hypotonia and neurological regression. It features marked increased signal and swelling of the striatum, globi pallidi, and brainstem, along with characteristic lactate peaks on MR spectroscopy. Wilson disease is an autosomal-recessive disease that leads to copper accumulation; it sometimes presents in childhood.

MRI shows high signal in the striatum with predilection for the outer rim of the putamina.
- **Infectious encephalitis.** Several viruses produce encephalitis with deep gray matter involvement. Japanese encephalitis is caused by a flavivirus and is the most common infectious encephalitis in Asia. Asymmetrical, patchy high T2 signal is seen in the basal ganglia and thalami. There may be associated thalamic hemorrhage. Patients are typically febrile. The diagnosis is made by analysis of CSF.

■ Diagnosis

Hypoxic-ischemic injury.

✓ Pearls

- Bilateral basal ganglia signal abnormalities should prompt the search for a global process such as hypoxia/ischemia, toxic exposure, metabolic syndrome, or possibly infection.
- Characteristic patterns of toxicity include bilateral globi pallidi involvement for carbon monoxide poisoning and bilateral putaminal involvement for methanol toxicity.

- Venous thrombosis should be considered if the thalamus is involved; this should prompt CT venography or MR venography.

Suggested Readings

Beppu T. The role of MR imaging in assessment of brain damage from carbon monoxide poisoning: a review of the literature. AJNR Am J Neuroradiol. 2014; 35(4):625–631

Bonneville F. Imaging of cerebral venous thrombosis. Diagn Interv Imaging. 2014; 95(12):1145–1150

Hegde AN, Mohan S, Lath N, Lim CC. Differential diagnosis for bilateral abnormalities of the basal ganglia and thalamus. Radiographics. 2011; 31(1):5–30

Case 166

Rebecca Stein-Wexler

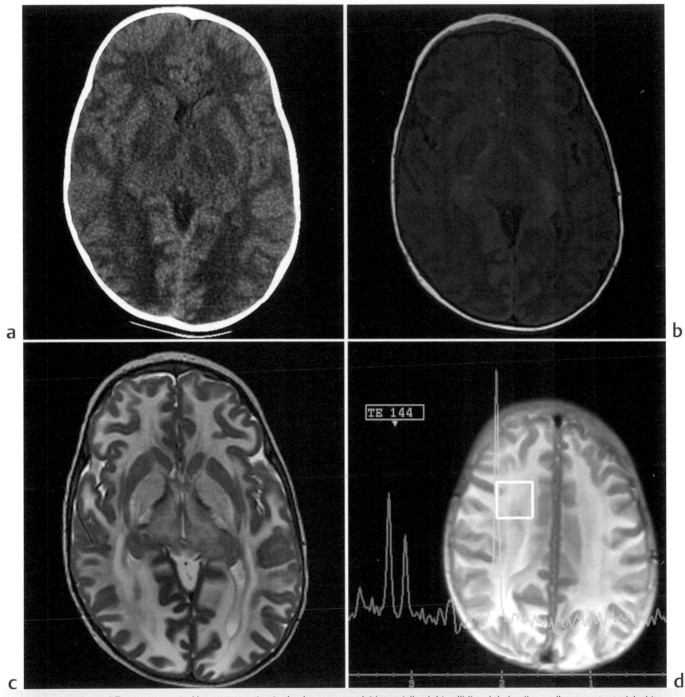

Fig. 166.1 CT shows diffuse, symmetrical hypoattenuation in the deep gray nuclei (especially globi pallidi and thalami) as well as supratentorial white matter (a). T1-W MRI shows profound corresponding T1 hypointensity (b). T2-W MRI shows these areas are T2 hyperintense (c). MR spectroscopy of the frontal lobe shows marked elevation of the N-acetylaspartate (NAA) concentration and increased NAA/Cre ratio (d).

■ Clinical Presentation

A 7-month-old with vomiting and nystagmus (▶ Fig. 166.1).

■ Key Imaging Finding

Symmetrical white matter abnormalities.

■ Top Three Differential Diagnoses

- **Periventricular leukomalacia.** Perinatal hypoxic injury to the premature brain may damage the watershed periventricular white matter. This is most likely in infants born at less than 32 weeks EGA and under 1.5 kg. Children who are not diagnosed early may present at age 1 to 2 years with developmental delay, motor impairment, and/or seizures. At this time, MRI will show often-symmetrical deep white matter loss. There may also be high-T1 and FLAIR periventricular signal due to gliosis, along with thinning of the associated portion of the corpus callosum and ex vacuo ventricular dilatation.
- **Adrenoleukodystrophy (ALD).** X-linked childhood cerebral ALD results from accumulation of very long chain fatty acids in the brain, adrenal glands, and testicles due to peroxisomal enzyme failure. Almost all patients are male. Patients are normal until age 4 to 10 years, when they develop behavioral changes and then sensory and motor deterioration. ALD is one of several white matter diseases that preferentially involve the periventricular white matter, sparing the cortex and subcortical U fibers (others include Tay–Sachs and Krabbe's diseases). Brain findings include extensive, contiguous demyelination in the periventricular white matter (especially parietooccipital), lymphocyte infiltration in the perivascular spaces, and

cavitation. MRI most often shows symmetrical findings in the deep parietooccipital white matter and in the splenium of the corpus callosum. The visual and acoustic pathways, posterior fossa, corticospinal tracts, frontal lobes, and other areas may also be affected. Three zones are seen on MRI. Gliosis and scarring cause the central zone to be T1 dark and T2 bright. The intermediate zone of active demyelination enhances. Finally, the peripheral demyelination zone is T1 bright and does not enhance. Chromosomal analysis and tissue/RBC assay confirm the diagnosis. Treatment with dietary manipulation and bone marrow transplantation may delay eventual atrophy.
- **Canavan disease.** This spongiform leukodystrophy, like Alexander disease, involves the subcortical white matter and leads to macrocephaly. Canavan disease is autosomal recessive and most common in Ashkenazi Jews. It results from deficiency of aspartoacylase, causing N-acetylaspartate (NAA) to accumulate and probably damage myelin. Patients present during the first month of life with head lag and hypotonia, soon followed by seizures and spasticity, with death by about age 3 years. MRI shows T1-dark and T2-bright globi pallidi and thalami, gradually extending to the cerebral cortex. A markedly elevated NAA peak at MR spectroscopy is diagnostic.

■ Diagnosis

Canavan disease.

✓ Pearls

- Periventricular leukomalacia, usually seen in ex-premature infants, demonstrates periventricular high-T1 and high-FLAIR signal, with associated ventricular dilatation and corpus callosum thinning.
- Adrenal leukodystrophy presents at age 4 to 10 years and shows periventricular white matter abnormalities that spare the cortex and subcortical U fibers.

- Adrenal leukodystrophy demonstrates classic zonal morphology on MRI, with enhancement only in the intermediate zone of active demyelination.
- Canavan disease involves the subcortical white matter, along with the globi pallidi and thalami; markedly increased N-acetylaspartate is diagnostic on MR spectroscopy.

Suggested Readings

Kim JH, Kim HJ. Childhood X-linked adrenoleukodystrophy: clinical-pathologic overview and MR imaging manifestations at initial evaluation and follow-up. Radiographics. 2005; 25(3):619–631

Phelan JA, Lowe LH, Glasier CM. Pediatric neurodegenerative white matter processes: leukodystrophies and beyond. Pediatr Radiol. 2008; 38(7):729–749

Case 167

Kriti Gwal

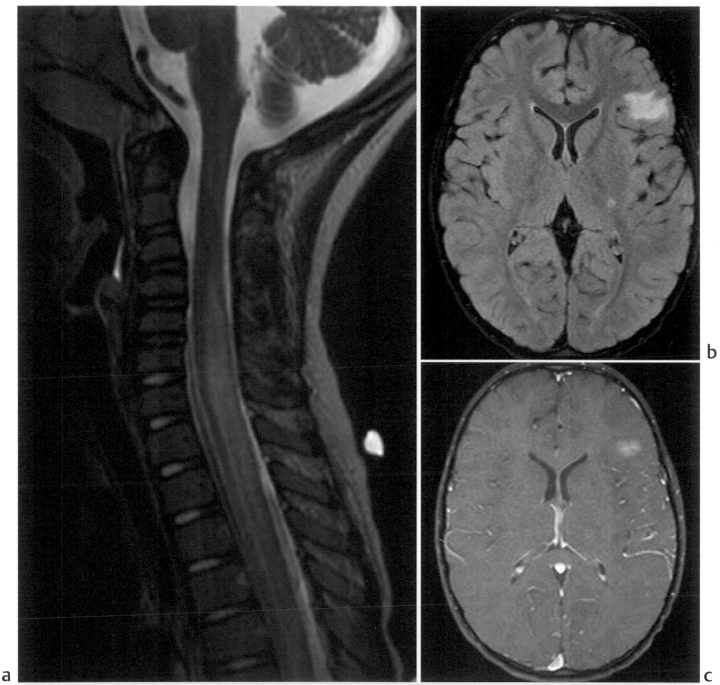

Fig. 167.1 Sagittal T2-W MRI **(a)** through the cervical spine demonstrates a T2-hyperintense focus in the midcervical spinal cord. Axial FLAIR image shows increased signal in the left frontal and capsular lesions **(b)**. T1-W gadolinium-enhanced image shows enhancement in the left frontal lesion **(c)**. (These images are provided courtesy of the Children's Hospital of Philadelphia.)

■ Clinical Presentation

A 5-year-old girl with lethargy and neurological defects (▶ Fig. 167.1).

■ **Key Imaging Finding**

Cerebral edema with asymmetrical white matter abnormalities.

■ **Top Three Differential Diagnoses**

• **Acute disseminated encephalomyelitis (ADEM).** This immune-mediated demyelinating disease affects gray and white matter, usually in multiple locations. The diagnosis requires a polyfocal acute neurological event with imaging findings of inflammatory demyelinating disease. The encephalopathy generally presents with headache, vomiting, seizures, and altered mental status after a viral infection or immunization. Symptoms usually resolve within 3 months, and most patients have few or no residual neurological abnormalities. However, ADEM is occasionally recurrent or multiphasic. Within 3 months of symptom onset, brain MRI should show diffuse, ill-defined, often asymmetrical lesions in the cerebral white matter, representing areas of demyelination. The corpus callosum and periventricular white matter are not usually involved. Lesions appear hypodense on CT, T1 hypointense, and T2 hyperintense. Gray matter may also be affected, including the central gray matter of the spinal cord. Cases of ADEM often show increased diffusion on DWI, differentiating ADEM from vasculitis, which shows restricted diffusion. Contrast enhancement is often minimal but may be diffuse, nodular, or ringlike.

• **Multiple sclerosis (MS).** This relapsing and usually progressive demyelinating disease can present in childhood with dramatic findings such as encephalopathy and altered mental status or with more focal neurological abnormalities such as optic neuritis or transverse myelitis. Knowledge of the clinical course is essential for diagnosis, since it is difficult to differentiate MS from ADEM based solely on imaging. Both MS and ADEM lesions are T1 dark and T2 bright, but periventricular white matter and the corpus callosum are more often involved with MS than with ADEM. MS is likely if at least two of the following are present: five or more lesions on T2-W MRI, two or more periventricular lesions, and/or at least one brainstem lesion. Active plaques may show central marked T2 hyperintensity, with peripheral intermediate hyperintensity. Plaques also enhance and may be DWI bright in the acute/early subacute phase. FLAIR demonstrates subtle lesions that might be missed on T2. Juxtacortical, deep white matter, and infratentorial lesions, along with tumefactive plaque (with an incomplete rim of enhancement) are more common in children than in adults.

• **Herpes encephalitis (HE).** Herpes virus is an important cause of encephalopathy in children. Patients often present with fever, headache, vomiting, seizures, altered mental status, or even coma, along with hyper-reflexia, focal neurological defects, and ataxia. DWI hyperintensity is the earliest finding. Affected brain parenchyma subsequently appears hypodense on CT, hypointense on T1, and hyperintense on T2, reflecting its high water content. In infants and newborns, HE results from primary CNS infection and causes multifocal abnormalities in the white matter and cerebral cortex. Disease begins in the temporal lobes, is often hemorrhagic, and may show enhancement and restricted diffusion. The findings may mimic infarction but do not follow vascular territories. In older patients, HE usually results from virus reactivation. In these patients, the limbic system is affected, specifically the medial frontotemporal lobes and the insula.

■ **Diagnosis**

Acute disseminated encephalomyelitis.

✓ **Pearls**

• Acute disseminated encephalomyelitis is triggered by infection or vaccination and usually resolves with few or no sequelae.
• Multiple sclerosis is likely if at least two of the following are present: five or more lesions on T2-W images, two or more periventricular lesions, and/or at least one brainstem lesion.

• Herpes encephalitis should be considered in patients with new-onset seizures and fevers and frontotemporal lesions on MRI.

Suggested Readings

Barkovich AJ, Patay Z. Metabolic, toxic, and inflammatory brain disorders. In Barkovich AJ, Raybaud C, eds. Pediatric Neuroimaging, 5th ed. Philadelphia, PA: Lippincott Williams & Wilkins; 2012:81–239

Tardieu M, Banwell B, Wolinsky JS, Pohl D, Krupp LB. Consensus definitions for pediatric MS and other demyelinating disorders in childhood. Neurology. 2016; 87(9) Suppl 2:S8–S11

Case 168

Kriti Gwal

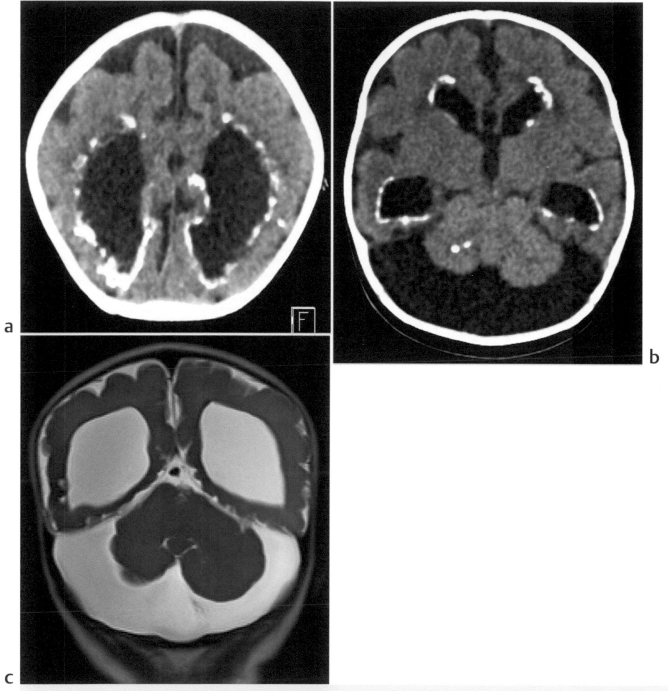

Fig. 168.1 Axial CT image shows coarse, predominantly periventricular calcifications, cerebral atrophy, and dilatation of the lateral ventricles (a). Another CT image shows there are also cerebellar hemisphere calcifications, with mildly asymmetrical cerebellar parenchymal atrophy (b). Coronal T2-W MRI shows the small cerebellum and the dilated ventricular system (c). (These images are provided courtesy of the Children's Hospital of Philadelphia.)

■ **Clinical Presentation**

A 3-month-old boy with seizures and hearing loss (►Fig. 168.1).

■ Key Imaging Finding

Scattered parenchymal calcifications.

■ Top Three Differential Diagnoses

- **Cytomegalovirus (CMV).** CMV is one of several important infections that are acquired transplacentally. Together, they are referred to as TORCH infections (toxoplasmosis, other [syphilis], rubella, CMV, and herpes). Many of these infections have similar clinical findings, and subtle differences in neuroimaging aid in diagnosis. CMV is the most common and affects many organ systems. Intracranial calcifications, which are one of the most common findings, are often central, in the periventricular regions and sometimes basal ganglia. Other findings include microcephaly (a poor prognostic sign), migrational anomalies (including lissencephaly), enlarged ventricles, and white matter disease. Germinal matrix, anterotemporal, and cerebellar cysts may also be seen. CNS infection has serious clinical consequences, such as sensorineural hearing loss, seizures, and developmental delay.

- **Toxoplasmosis.** This protozoa may lead to a number of neuroimaging findings, including calcifications in the basal ganglia, cerebral cortex, periventricular region, and subcortical white matter. Unlike congenital CMV infection, congenital toxoplasmosis often causes hydrocephalus. Head circumference should be obtained on every neonate undergoing imaging evaluation to aid in diagnosis. Neuronal migration anomalies are uncommon with toxoplasmosis, which also helps differentiate this from congenital CMV. Delayed myelination may be seen.
- **Rubella.** Congenital rubella infection demonstrates ventriculomegaly, cysts, and areas of hypodensity on CT throughout the white matter. These neonates may also have periventricular, cerebral cortex, and basal ganglia calcifications. Severe cases destroy brain parenchyma, resulting in microcephaly.

■ Additional Differential Diagnoses

- **Syphilis.** Congenital syphilis infection may cause leptomeningeal inflammation and resultant hydrocephalus. Other possible sequelae of the infection include infarction and pituitary dysfunction due to the inflammatory process. MRI shows leptomeningeal enhancement. Periventricular calcifications are not a frequent finding in syphilis, but the disease is mentioned here as it is one of the TORCH infections.
- **Tuberous sclerosis.** This systemic autosomal-dominant disorder is characterized by multiple hamartomas in the brain,

skin, kidneys, eyes, heart, and elsewhere. Seizures and developmental delay are common manifestations of CNS disease. Brain MRI may show subependymal hamartomas that appear nodular, and some may calcify. Additional findings include cortical lesions and linear transmantle dysplasias. Subependymal giant cell astrocytoma (SEGA) is an enlarging mass usually found near the foramen of Monro, potentially causing hydrocephalus. Serial growth differentiates SEGA from subependymal hamartoma.

■ Diagnosis

Congenital cytomegalovirus infection.

✓ Pearls

- Key imaging findings of cytomegalovirus include intracranial calcifications, microcephaly, neuronal migrational anomalies, ventriculomegaly, and cysts.
- Toxoplasmosis typically causes more scattered calcifications in the basal ganglia, cerebral cortex, periventricular region, and subcortical white matter, along with hydrocephalus.

- Features of tuberous sclerosis include subependymal hamartomas, cortical lesions, and occasionally subependymal giant cell astrocytoma.

Suggested Readings

Blaser S, Jay V, Becker L, et al. Neonatal brain infection. In Rutherford MA, ed. MRI of the Neonatal Brain, 4th ed. London, UK: Saunders; 2002

Fink KR, Thapa MM, Ishak GE, Pruthi S. Neuroimaging of pediatric central nervous system cytomegalovirus infection. Radiographics. 2010; 30(7):1779–1796

Hedlung G, Bale JF Jr, Barkovich AJ. Infections of the developing and mature nervous system. In Barkovich AJ, Raybaud C, eds. Pediatric Neuroimaging, 5th ed. Philadelphia, PA: Lippincott Williams & Wilkins; 2012:954–1050

Case 169

Ethan Neufeld

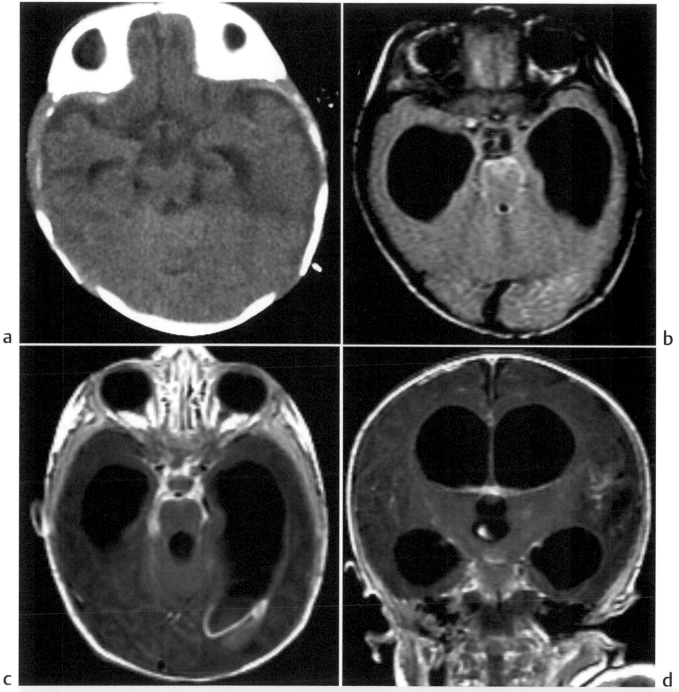

Fig. 169.1 Axial CT shows hydrocephalus, as evidenced by enlargement of the temporal horns of the lateral ventricles, along with ill-defined soft-tissue density material in the basal cisterns (**a**). Axial T2 FLAIR image obtained later in the clinical course shows marked worsening of the hydrocephalus, along with high signal in the basal cisterns (**b**). Axial gadolinium-enhanced T1-W MRI shows thickening and avid enhancement of the basilar meninges along with enhancement of the ependyma of the lateral ventricle (**c**). Coronal gadolinium-enhanced T1-W MRI shows similar findings without significant thickening or enhancement of the meninges along the cerebral convexities (**d**).

■ **Clinical Presentation**

Lethargy and fever (▶Fig. 169.1).

■ Key Imaging Finding

Basilar meningeal thickening and enhancement.

■ Top Three Differential Diagnoses

- **Tuberculous meningitis.** Meningitis is the most common intracranial manifestation of infection by *Mycobacterium tuberculosis*. The meninges are directly infected via hematogenous spread, and patients often have other infectious manifestations elsewhere in the body. Tuberculous meningitis is seen in all ages but has a peak incidence in younger children 0 to 4 years old. Risk factors include immunosuppression and underlying diabetes. The infection spreads along the leptomeninges within the basal cisterns, predominantly along the inferior frontal and anterior temporal lobes. It often involves the optic chiasm and suprasellar cistern but rarely if ever extends over the cerebral convexities. Affected areas feature irregular thickening of the leptomeninges, with florid enhancement. Complications include intraventricular extension as well as arteritis, possibly leading to infarction.
- **Fungal meningitis.** Many intracranial fungal infections can cause meningitis, namely coccidioidomycosis, histoplasmosis, blastomycosis, and candidiasis. Coccidioidomycosis is most associated with meningeal disease, which occurs in 30% of infected patients. Immunocompromised patients are prone to fungal infection. In general, the appearance resembles tuberculous meningitis, with thick, enhancing meninges in a basilar distribution. Parenchymal findings dominate the radiological picture, and ring enhancing lesions, arteritis, and basal ganglia involvement will be variably present depending on the specific pathogen.
- **Pyogenic meningitis.** Bacterial infection is a much more common cause of meningitis in children than is tuberculoid or fungal infection, but a predominantly basilar distribution is atypical. The most common agents in children are *Streptococcus pneumoniae* and *Neisseria meningitidis*. Meningeal thickening tends to be smoother than with tuberculoid or fungal infections and commonly extends over the cerebral convexities.

■ Additional Differential Diagnosis

- **Leptomeningeal carcinomatosis.** Medulloblastoma and leukemia (especially acute lymphocytic) may present with metastatic disease along the meninges. Children with medulloblastoma are distinguished by their primary site of disease in the posterior fossa, but those with leukemia may have a similar imaging appearance to infectious/granulomatous meningitis. The involved areas will demonstrate diffuse, nodular thickening. Spread along the cranial nerves is characteristic. Patients are usually diagnosed clinically by lack of infectious manifestations and also by cytology on serial lumbar punctures.

■ Diagnosis

Tuberculous meningitis.

✓ Pearls

- Tuberculous meningitis is characterized by thick, enhancing basilar meninges without extension over the cerebral convexities.
- Fungal meningitis may have an identical appearance to tuberculous meningitis and similarly affects the immunocompromised.

- Leptomeningeal metastases, especially from leukemia, should be considered in patients without clinical evidence of infection and can be diagnosed via lumbar puncture.

Suggested Readings

Maclean KA, Becker AK, Chang SD, Harris AC. Extrapulmonary tuberculosis: imaging features beyond the chest. Can Assoc Radiol J. 2013; 64(4):319–324

Porto L, Kieslich M, Bartels M, Schwabe D, Zanella FE, Du Mesnil R. Leptomeningeal metastases in pediatrics: magnetic resonance image manifestations and correlation with cerebral spinal fluid cytology. Pediatr Int. 2010; 52(4):541–546

Smirniotopoulos JG, Murphy FM, Rushing EJ, Rees JH, Schroeder JW. Patterns of contrast enhancement in the brain and meninges. Radiographics. 2007; 27(2):525–551

Case 170

Geoffrey D. McWilliams

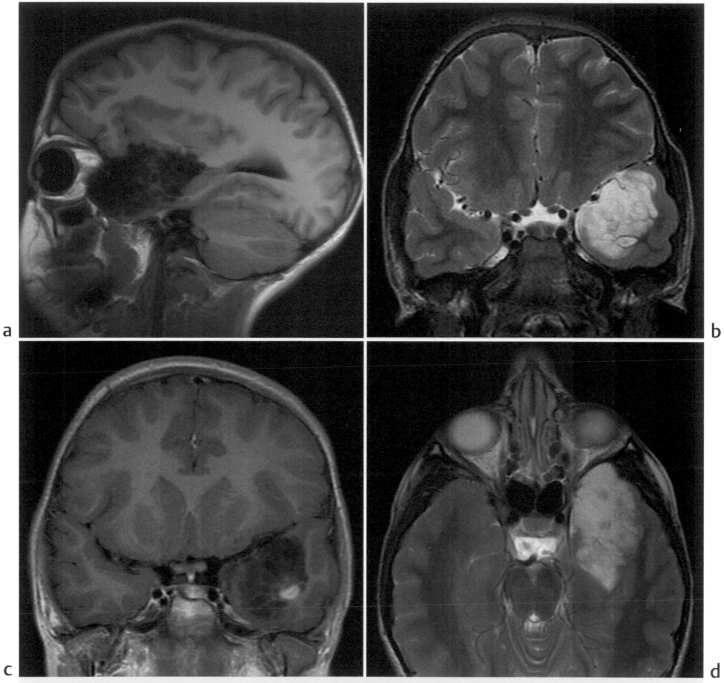

a

b

c

d

Fig. 170.1 Sagittal T1-W MRI shows a multicystic, well-circumscribed temporal lobe mass **(a)**. Coronal T2-W image shows the mass is well circumscribed, and there is no surrounding edema **(b)**. Coronal T1-W gadolinium-enhanced image shows that most of the mass does not enhance, but there is a small enhancing nodule **(c)**. Axial T2-W image demonstrates mass effect on and remodeling of the anterior wall of the middle cranial fossa **(d)**.

■ **Clinical Presentation**

An 11-year-old girl with facial droop and seizures (▶Fig. 170.1).

■ Key Imaging Finding

Well-circumscribed supratentorial mass.

■ Top Three Differential Diagnoses

- **Low-grade astrocytoma.** Pleomorphic xanthroastrocytoma (PXA) and juvenile pilocytic astrocytoma (JPCA) are both low-grade astrocytomas. PXA is considered a grade 2 World Health Organization (WHO) tumor, since although usually benign it may recur and undergo malignant transformation, whereas JPCA is WHO grade 1. PXA appears as a peripheral or cortical, well-defined, partly cystic mass, most often seen in the temporal lobe. JPCA is the most common primary brain tumor in children, but supratentorial lesions are rarely parenchymal (usually occurring in the optic chiasm or thalamus). It classically presents as a cystic mass with an enhancing nodule, although it may appear solid. With both PXA and JPCA, the cystic component follows CSF signal on T1 and T2. The solid component is isointense or hypointense to gray matter on T1 and hyperintense to gray matter on T2/FLAIR. The solid component of PXA enhances heterogeneously, whereas with JPCA enhancement is more uniformly intense. There may be meningeal thickening and enhancement adjacent to PXA.
- **Ganglioglioma (GG).** GG is a low-grade glioneuronal WHO grade 1 to 2 tumor with rare aggressive WHO grade 3 to 4 variants. It is a frequent cause of temporal lobe epilepsy. GG commonly appears as a cortically based cystic and solid mass within the temporal lobe, occasionally in the frontal or parietal lobe. However, it may occur anywhere within the CNS.

Surgical resection is usually curative. On CT, GG appears as a cystic or cystic/solid mass, with the solid component isodense or rarely hyperdense to brain parenchyma. The degree of calcification varies. Scalloping of the inner table of the skull results from osseous remodeling if the lesion is expansile. On MRI, the mass is T1 hypointense or isointense (relative to gray matter) and T2/FLAIR hyperintense. Susceptibility artifact may be seen with calcifications. The enhancement pattern is typically heterogeneous, but a minority of GGs do not enhance at all.
- **Dysembryoplastic neuroepithelial tumor (DNET).** This low-grade glioneuronal WHO grade 1 tumor is similar to ganglioglioma. DNET typically occurs in the temporal lobe, though it may be seen in other supratentorial locations. The tumor is a common cause of temporal lobe epilepsy. Like GG, DNET is often cortically based, may cause bony remodeling, and is usually cured by surgical resection. Unlike GG, DNET is multicystic or lobulated, with low T1 signal, high T2 signal, and a variable appearance on FLAIR. It has little to no edema and causes no mass effect. Enhancement is uncommon, but small enhancing nodules may be seen. Diffusion is not restricted. There are rare reports of hemorrhage, calcification, and tumor recurrence after resection. DNET is the most common brain tumor in patients with Noonan syndrome.

■ Diagnosis

Dysembryoplastic neuroepithelial tumor.

✓ Pearls

- Pleomorphic xanthroastrocytoma is a low-grade tumor that usually appears as a partly cystic, well-defined, peripheral or cortical temporal lobe mass.
- Gangliogliomas are low-grade, cortically based, mixed cystic/solid tumors frequently associated with temporal lobe epilepsy; they usually enhance and may be calcified.

- Dysembryoplastic neuroepithelial tumor is also a low-grade, cortically based tumor frequently associated with temporal lobe epilepsy, but unlike ganglioglioma it usually is multicystic/lobular, enhances little, and has little associated edema.

Suggested Readings

Adachi Y, Yagishita A. Gangliogliomas: Characteristic imaging findings and role in the temporal lobe epilepsy. Neuroradiology. 2008; 50(10).829–834

Borja MJ, Plaza MJ, Altman N, Saigal G. Conventional and advanced MRI features of pediatric intracranial tumors: supratentorial tumors. AJR Am J Roentgenol. 2013; 200(5):W483–W503

Collins VP, Jones DT, Giannini C. Pilocytic astrocytoma: pathology, molecular mechanisms and markers. Acta Neuropathol. 2015; 129(6):775–788

Daghistani R, Miller E, Kulkarni AV, Widjaja E. Atypical characteristics and behavior of dysembryoplastic neuroepithelial tumors. Neuroradiology. 2013; 55(2):217–224

Case 171

Rebecca Stein-Wexler

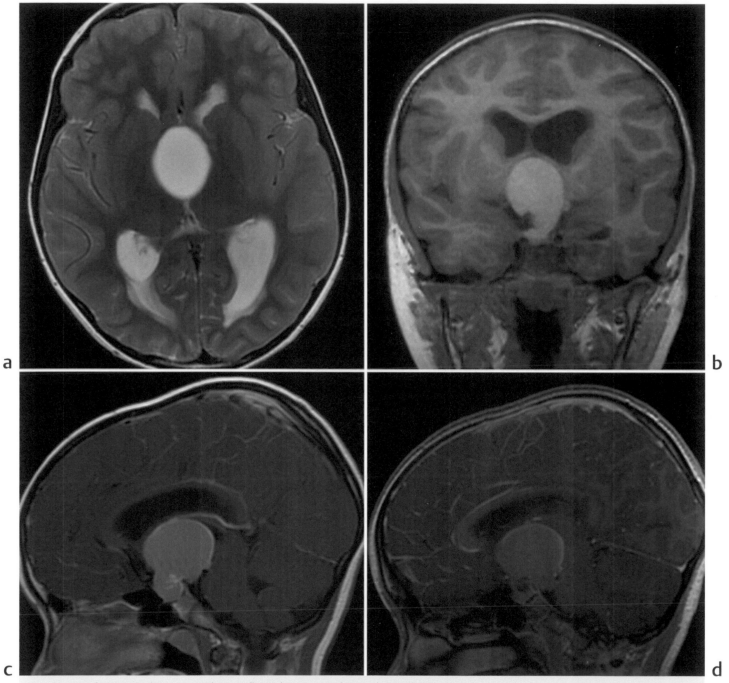

Fig. 171.1 Axial T2-W MRI shows an ovoid suprasellar T2-hyperintense lesion, along with hydrocephalus and transependymal fluid shift **(a)**. Coronal T1-W image shows the lesion is lobulated and has an intrasellar component; it is T1 hyperintense **(b)**. Midline sagittal T1-W gadolinium-enhanced image shows there is peripheral enhancement along with a small enhancing nodule **(c)**. Sagittal 3D-SPGR gadolinium-enhanced image also shows dark susceptibility artifact in an area of calcification **(d)**.

■ Clinical Presentation

A 7-year-old boy who has been awakened at night with head-ache and vomiting (▶Fig. 171.1).

■ Key Imaging Finding

Suprasellar mass.

■ Top Three Differential Diagnoses

- **Craniopharyngioma.** Ten percent of primary pediatric brain tumors arise in the sella and in the suprasellar region. In children, most are adamantinomatous. Almost all are suprasellar as well as intrasellar, and one-third extend into the anterior and middle cranial fossae. Mass effect causes clinical symptoms, including headaches, visual disturbance, and endocrine abnormalities. Adamantinomatous tumors appear cystic with lobulated contours, and almost all have calcifications. Cyst contents are often T1 bright and heterogeneous on T2. Solid components enhance, becoming brighter than the cyst contents. The less common papillary squamous tumors are isolated to the suprasellar region and are predominantly solid. Metastases are rare. The position of the tumor relative to the optic chiasm is important to surgical planning.

- **Germ cell tumor (GCT).** GCTs in girls are most common in the suprasellar region, whereas in boys they are usually pineal in location. Small lesions are confined to the pituitary stalk, but larger lesions often extend into the basal ganglia. T1 and T2 appearance varies with tumor composition. Solid elements are usually similar to or darker than gray matter on T2-W imaging, which helps differentiate GCTs from T2-bright gliomas. Solid areas usually enhance. Cysts are common.

- **Rathke cleft cyst.** This non-neoplastic congenital lesion develops from residua of Rathke cleft. It arises within but may extend above the sella. Curvilinear wall calcification may be seen in up to 15%, and many lesions have an intracystic nodule. Cyst fluid signal varies on MRI; those with mucin are bright on T1.

■ Additional Differential Diagnoses

- **Hypothalamic and optic chiasm glioma.** Hypothalamic and optic chiasm tumors in children are most often low-grade gliomas. Incidence is increased in children with neurofibromatosis type 1 (NF1), and in these children essentially all such tumors are juvenile pilocytic astrocytomas. Their tumors involve the optic nerve, are often bilateral, and often extend to the chiasm. In patients without NF1, the chiasm/hypothalamus is principally involved, and the tumors are larger and more masslike.

- **Pituitary adenoma.** Most children with pituitary adenomas (usually macroadenomas) are in their teens. Prolactinomas

are most common, followed by adrenocorticotropin and growth hormone tumors. Macroadenomas are solid masses in the anterior pituitary that are larger than 10 mm. They may have hemorrhagic or cystic foci. Microadenomas are smaller and show delayed enhancement.

- **Langerhans cell histiocytosis (LCH).** About one-fifth of patients with multicentric LCH have hypothalamic and pituitary infundibular involvement. The cerebellum is often affected as well, and gray and white matter lesions (including demyelination), extraparenchymal lesions, partial empty sella, and atrophy may be seen.

■ Diagnosis

Craniopharyngioma.

✓ Pearls

- Adamantinomatous craniopharyngiomas are usually cystic, lobulated, and T1 bright, often with calcification.
- Germ cell tumors may be confined to the pituitary stalk, or they may extend into the basil ganglia.

- Prolactinoma is the most common pituitary adenoma in children.
- Solid portions of hypothalamic/optic chiasm gliomas are bright on T2, whereas solid portions of germ cell tumor are dark on T2.

Suggested Readings

Poussaint TY, Panigrahy A, Huisman TA. Pediatric brain tumors. Pediatr Radiol. 2015; 45 Suppl 3:S443–S453

Schroeder JW, Vezina LG. Pediatric sellar and suprasellar lesions. Pediatr Radiol. 2011; 41(3):287–298, quiz 404–405

Case 172

Rebecca Stein-Wexler

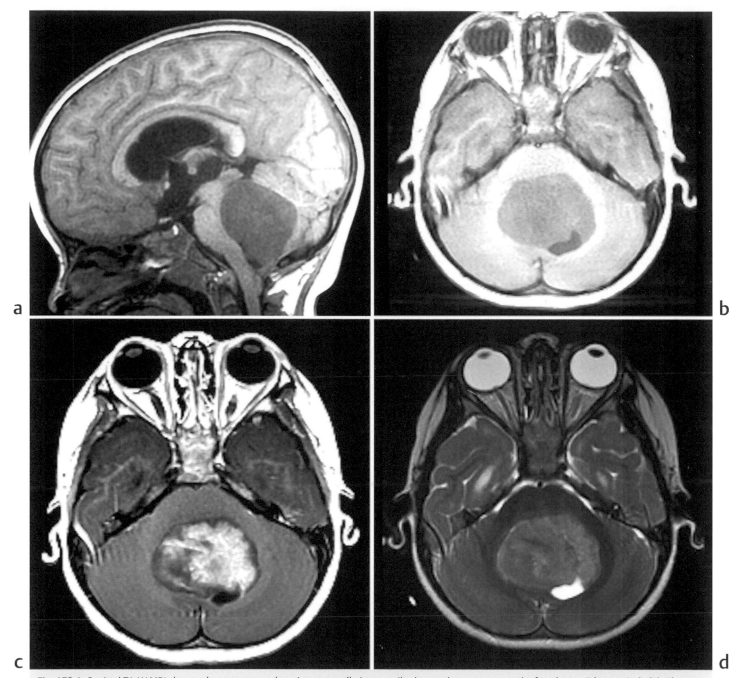

Fig. 172.1 Sagittal T1-W MRI shows a homogeneous, hypointense, well-circumscribed mass that compresses the fourth ventricle anteriorly **(a)**. The axial T1-W image shows there is a small, posterior, markedly hypointense element **(b)**. T1-W gadolinium-enhanced axial image shows heterogeneous enhancement **(c)**. T2-W axial image shows the mass is moderately heterogeneous, with hyperintense signal in the posterior cyst **(d)**.

▪ Clinical Presentation

A 3-year-old girl with ataxia and vomiting (▶Fig. 172.1).

■ Key Imaging Finding

Solid posterior fossa mass.

■ Top Three Differential Diagnoses

- **Medulloblastoma.** Medulloblastoma is a high-grade tumor that classically arises from the roof of the fourth ventricle and is usually midline. Peak incidence is age 4 years. The tumor may be parenchymal and paramedian in teens, who sometimes develop the relatively rare desmoplastic subtype. Classic medulloblastoma is highly cellular, leading to differentiating features of increased density on CT and restricted diffusion with a low ADC. The tumor is iso- to hypointense to gray matter on T2, and T2-hyperintense cysts are present in almost two-thirds of cases. Hemorrhage is rare, but calcifications are not unusual (about 20%). Most tumors show variable enhancement. Midline sagittal imaging may allow differentiation from ependymoma, since medulloblastoma arises from the roof of the fourth ventricle and ependymoma from the floor. Spine MRI should be performed at diagnosis, since seeding of subarachnoid space is common.
- **Ependymoma.** This tumor is most common between birth and age 4 years. Most cases of ependymoma arise from ependymal cells that line the floor of the fourth ventricle and foramen of Luschka. The tumor grows slowly, and patients often have insidious onset of headache, nausea, and vomiting.

Ependymomas have abundant intracellular myxoid material and numerous cysts, causing them to be bright on T2 and FLAIR. Calcifications are seen in about half of tumors, and this along with hemorrhage may be T2 hypointense. A relatively soft tumor, ependymoma has a tendency to extend through the foramina of Magendie and the foramen of Luschka. It demonstrates no restricted diffusion on DWI, helping differentiate ependymoma from medulloblastoma. Incidence of spinal—but not brain—ependymoma is increased in patients with neurofibromatosis type 2.

- **Atypical teratoid–rhabdoid tumor (ATRT).** ATRT usually occurs in infants and is unusual after age 3 years. It shares many imaging features with medulloblastoma. However, ATRT tends to be located off midline, may have areas of hemorrhage, appears relatively aggressive, and may invade the skull—features that help distinguish it from more common posterior fossa tumors. Its histopathology is complex, and thus enhancement is usually heterogeneous. This aggressive tumor has a poor prognosis, and treatment involves more intensive chemotherapy than other posterior fossa tumors.

■ Diagnosis

Medulloblastoma.

✓ Pearls

- Medulloblastoma arises from the roof of the fourth ventricle, appears T2 heterogeneous, often has cysts, and may calcify.
- Ependymoma arises from the floor of the fourth ventricle, often calcifies, and tends to extend through the foramina of Magendie and Luschka.

- Atypical teratoid-rhabdoid tumor resembles medulloblastoma but is more likely to have hemorrhagic foci and be located off midline.
- Atypical teratoid-rhabdoid tumor is most common up to age 3 years, ependymoma up to age 4 years, and medulloblastoma in slightly older patients.

Suggested Readings

Plaza MJ, Borja MJ, Altman N, Saigal G. Conventional and advanced MRI features of pediatric intracranial tumors: posterior fossa and suprasellar tumors. AJR Am J Roentgenol. 2013; 200(5):1115–1124

Poussaint TY, Panigrahy A, Huisman TA. Pediatric brain tumors. Pediatr Radiol. 2015; 45 Suppl 3:S443–S453

Case 173

Rebecca Stein-Wexler

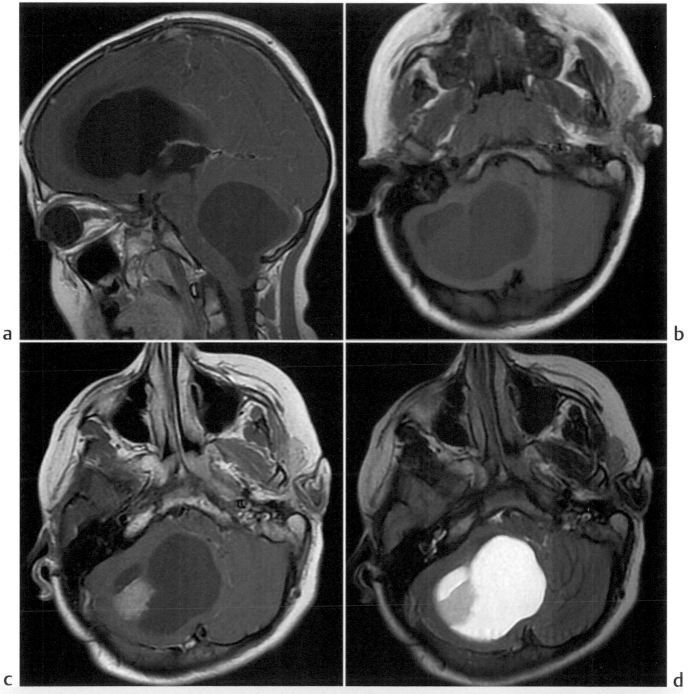

Fig. 173.1 Sagittal T1-W MRI shows a well-circumscribed cerebellar mass, which effaces the fourth ventricle and cerebral aqueduct, causing both hydrocephalus and cerebellar tonsillar herniation **(a)**. Axial T1-W image shows the mass is in the lateral cerebellar hemisphere **(b)**. T1-W gadolinium-enhanced image shows an enhancing mural nodule **(c)**. On T2, the cystic portion is very hyperintense and the mural nodule mildly hyperintense **(d)**.

■ Clinical Presentation

A 9-year-old boy with 1 month of headache and vomiting (►Fig. 173.1).

■ Key Imaging Finding

Cystic posterior fossa mass.

■ Top Three Differential Diagnoses

- **Juvenile pilocytic astrocytoma (JPCA).** Cerebellar astrocytoma is the most common posterior fossa tumor in children, with peak incidence between ages 5 and 13 years. Most cerebellar astrocytomas are the low-grade JPCA subtype, which is typically characterized by a large cyst with a solid mural nodule. The tumor is less often solid and/or necrotic. About half of posterior fossa JPCAs occur in the midline; the rest are in a cerebellar hemisphere. About two-fifths are supratentorial. Patients may complain of neck pain, headache, vomiting, and ataxia. On MRI, the cystic portion of the tumor shows fluid signal intensity. Since JPCAs are low grade, there is less surrounding vasogenic edema than with more aggressive tumors (such as medulloblastoma, ependymoma, and atypical rhabdoid tumor). The cyst lining and mural nodule usually enhance, and solid, non-necrotic portions enhance as well. Diffusion is not restricted. Gross total resection leads to a 10-year survival rate of around 90%. The incidence of JPCA is increased in patients with neurofibromatosis type 1 (NF1), but these tumors are usually located in the optic nerves or chiasm. Incidence is also increased with PHACES (posterior fossa malformations, hemangiomas, arterial anomalies, cardiac defects, eye abnormalities, sternal cleft, and supraumbilical raphe) syndrome, Turcot syndrome, and Ollier syndrome.
- **Hemangioblastoma.** Hemangioblastomas usually occur in adults. Multiple hemangioblastomas may be seen in children with von Hippel–Lindau syndrome (VHLS). Isolated lesions are usually encountered in otherwise normal patients. This tumor typically has a well-circumscribed cyst with a mural nodule and a rich vascular plexus. It is dark on T1 and bright on T2, and the mural nodule often enhances intensely. Calcifications are rare, but hemorrhage—manifested as T1 hyperintensity—is common. Hemangioblastoma somewhat resemble JPCA on MRI. However, hemangioblastoma typically demonstrates prominent serpiginous, enhancing vessels. In addition, perfusion MRI is useful for differentiation, since the relative cerebral blood volume is higher in hemangioblastoma than in JPCA.
- **Epidermoid.** Incomplete separation of neuroectoderm from cutaneous ectoderm results in formation of intracranial epidermoid cysts, which contain cholesterol and desquamated keratin. They are rare in children. The most common location is at the cerebellopontine angle, where they usually present with cranial neuropathy. Epidermoids are occasionally seen in the pineal and suprasellar regions, and in the middle cranial fossa. These lobulated masses are hypodense on CT. They are usually dark on T1 and bright on T2, although occasionally they will be T1 bright. The lesions neither calcify nor enhance. There may be internal linear heterogeneity. Epidermoids are typically slightly hyperintense on FLAIR.

■ Diagnosis

Juvenile pilocytic astrocytoma.

✓ Pearls

- Juvenile pilocytic astrocytoma usually has a large cyst with a solid, enhancing mural nodule with relatively little adjacent edema.
- Hemangioblastoma may be differentiated from juvenile pilocytic astrocytoma by the presence of prominent, serpiginous, enhancing vessels and a higher relative cerebral blood volume on perfusion MRI.
- Epidermoid tumors are usually located at the cerebellopontine angle; they are slightly hyperintense on FLAIR.

Suggested Readings

Plaza MJ, Borja MJ, Altman N, Saigal G. Conventional and advanced MRI features of pediatric intracranial tumors: posterior fossa and suprasellar tumors. AJR Am J Roentgenol. 2013; 200(5):1115–1124

Poretti A, Meoded A, Huisman TA. Neuroimaging of pediatric posterior fossa tumors including review of the literature. J Magn Reson Imaging. 2012; 35(1):32–47

Case 174

Rebecca Stein-Wexler

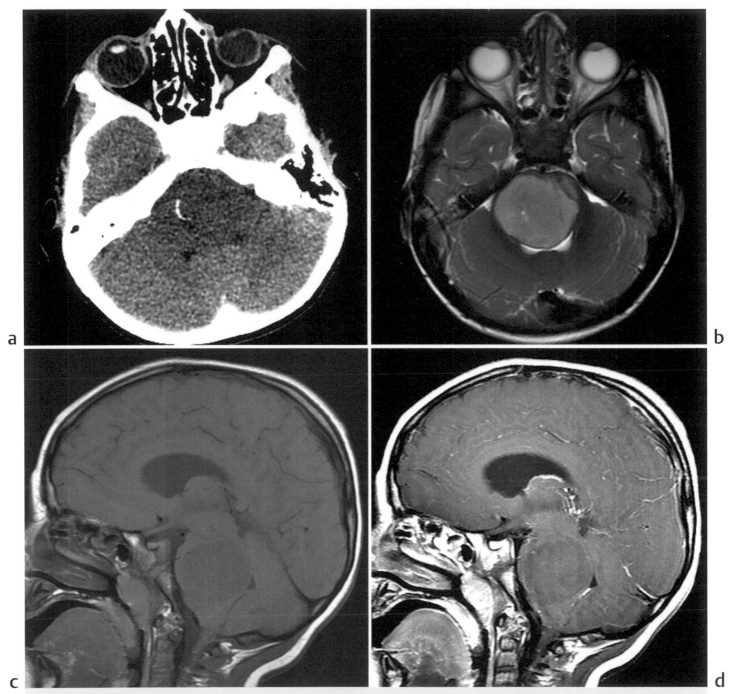

a   b   c   d

Fig. 174.1 Axial CT shows the brainstem is hypodense and swollen, effacing the fourth ventricle; there is a curvilinear calcification **(a)**. Axial T2-W MRI shows a mildly hyperintense lesion infiltrating the pons **(b)**. Sagittal T1-W image shows the lesion is slightly more hypointense than gray matter **(c)**. T1-W gadolinium-enhanced image shows that the lesion does not enhance **(d)**.

■ **Clinical Presentation**

A 3-year-old boy with a tremor and abnormal gait (▶Fig. 174.1).

■ Key Imaging Finding

Brainstem mass.

■ Top Three Differential Diagnoses

• **Brainstem glioma.** Most brainstem gliomas occur in children between 3 and 10 years old. Most are located in the pons (diffuse intrinsic pontine glioma [DIPG]). They are usually diffusely infiltrative, but they may be well circumscribed. Children often present with a long history of at least one of the following: long tract signs, cranial nerve deficits, and ataxia. Imaging shows diffuse enlargement of the pons. The tumors are usually T1 hypointense and T2 hyperintense compared with gray matter. Enhancement is unusual and, if present, is minimal and heterogeneous. The subset of focal midbrain tumors may, however, enhance intensely. Diffusion is usually not restricted, and ADC values are higher than with medulloblastoma. Most brainstem gliomas are low grade, but they may evolve into high-grade tumors. DWI, MR perfusion, and MR spectroscopy allow early assessment of disease progression. Patients with neurofibromatosis type 1 (NF1) have an increased risk of posterior fossa gliomas. Their tumors are usually located in the medulla instead of the pons, and they have a better prognosis. DIPG is treated with radiation therapy, with chemotherapy reserved for cases that continue to progress. Surgery does not play a role. Prognosis for DIPG is poor, with median survival around 9 months. However, the focal midbrain tumors have an excellent prognosis and are often followed on imaging without attempts at treatment.

• **Acute disseminated encephalomyelitis (ADEM).** This immune-mediated demyelinating disease affects gray and white matter, usually in multiple locations. Supratentorial disease is most common, but the brainstem, middle cerebellar peduncles, and cerebellar white matter are affected in about half of cases. One-third of patients also have spinal cord involvement. There is initially edema, demyelination, and macrophage infiltration, evolving to perivascular gliosis. ADEM usually follows several weeks after a viral or occasionally bacterial upper respiratory infection. Vaccination may also trigger the disease. Symptoms vary, have relatively rapid onset (unlike DIPG), and typically progress. Encephalopathy (altered behavior or consciousness) must be present for diagnosis of ADEM. Patients usually recover with steroid therapy. Demyelination causes lesions to appear hypodense on CT, slightly hypointense on T1, and hyperintense on T2 or FLAIR. The brainstem may appear swollen. However, lesions elsewhere in the brain do not typically cause mass effect. Unlike DIPG, ADEM rarely involves the entire pons. ADEM lesions rarely enhance. Tractography is useful for differentiating ADEM from brainstem glioma. ADEM truncates fibers, whereas gliomas deflect fiber tracts. If there is also multifocal supratentorial disease, multiple sclerosis becomes a consideration (CSF studies help differentiate).

• **Rhombencephalitis.** Rhombencephalitis describes an inflammatory disease affecting the brainstem, due to infection, autoimmune disease, or paraneoplastic syndromes. The condition is uncommon in children, but those affected are usually less than 5 years old. Appearance varies with etiology. Lesions are generally T2 bright.

■ Diagnosis

Diffuse intrinsic pontine glioma.

✓ Pearls

• Diffuse intrinsic pontine glioma is usually diffusely infiltrative but may be well circumscribed.
• Diffuse intrinsic pontine glioma is slightly T1 dark and slightly T2 bright; enhancement is uncommon.

• Acute disseminated encephalomyelitis usually follows a viral illness or vaccination; symptoms typically progress and then resolve.
• Acute disseminated encephalomyelitis resembles diffuse intrinsic pontine glioma but is often accompanied with supratentorial or spinal cord disease as well.

Suggested Readings

Plaza MJ, Borja MJ, Altman N, Saigal G. Conventional and advanced MRI features of pediatric intracranial tumors: posterior fossa and suprasellar tumors. AJR Am J Roentgenol. 2013; 200(5):1115–1124

Rossi A. Imaging of acute disseminated encephalomyelitis. Neuroimaging Clin N Am. 2008; 18(1):149–161, ix

Rossi A, Martinetti C, Morana G, Severino M, Tortora D. Neuroimaging of infectious and inflammatory diseases of the pediatric cerebellum and brainstem. Neuroimaging Clin N Am. 2016; 26(3):471–487

Case 175

Kriti Gwal

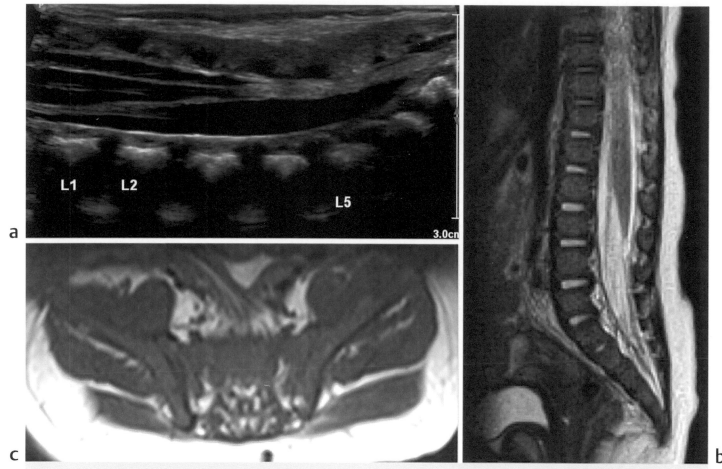

Fig. 175.1 Sagittal spine US shows the conus terminates at L3–L4 **(a)**. Axial T1-W MRI shows high signal in and thickening of the filum terminale **(b)**. Sagittal T2-W image also shows the elongated spinal cord **(c)**. (These images are provided courtesy of the Children's Hospital of Philadelphia.)

■ Clinical Presentation

Newborn with sacral dimple (▶Fig. 175.1).

■ Key Imaging Finding

Low position of the conus medullaris.

■ Top Three Differential Diagnoses

- **Tethered cord syndrome (TCS).** TCS is a clinical manifestation of spinal dysraphism. Although tethered spinal cord may occur in isolation, it often accompanies other forms of dysraphism, such as meningocele, myelomeningocele, split cord, and dermoid. Scarring may cause retethering after apparently successful detethering procedures. Patients may present with symptoms of TCS at any age. They typically have difficulty walking, abnormal reflexes, voiding dysfunction, and orthopedic issues. Tension on nerve roots is thought to cause these symptoms, since the filum terminale is often abnormally short or tight and the conus medullaris is therefore abnormally low. There may be fatty infiltration or fibrofatty proliferation within the filum terminale, either in addition to the low conus or as the only abnormality. In some patients with TCS, all imaging studies are normal, but surgical "detethering" may still relieve symptoms. The conus is considered borderline low if it terminates at the inferior endplate of L2 (slightly lower is acceptable in very young infants). Axial T1- and T2-W MRI are essential to evaluate for a fatty filum, which is considered pathological if the diameter exceeds 2 mm. A tethered cord may terminate in a lipoma along the caudal aspect of the spine or in a more complex malformation.
- **Dorsal dermal sinus.** The dorsal dermal sinus is a tract that extends from the skin surface to the spinal canal. It forms due to incomplete separation of the superficial cutaneous ectoderm and neural ectoderm. Since the neural tube closes from the middle out, the occipital and lumbar regions are most often affected. Most patients present with a midline dimple, tuft of hair, or hairy nevus that launches an investigation for underlying spinal anomalies. Since the dermal sinus tract extends from the spinal canal to the skin, patients are at high risk for infections, such as meningitis and intraspinal abscess. T1-W images without fat suppression depict the subcutaneous portions of the tract. Thin section T2-W images demonstrate the sinus tract within the spinal canal. Approximately 50% of dorsal dermal sinuses terminate in a dermoid or epidermoid cyst. However, most dermoids and epidermoids are not associated with a dermal sinus tract.
- **Lipomyelocele/lipomyelomeningocele.** These closed spinal dysraphisms develop when mesenchymal tissue enters the spinal canal via a dural defect. Both are always associated with tethered cord. Lipomyeloceles consist of fatty tissue at the dorsal neural placode extending through the dysraphic defect, contiguous with subcutaneous fat. Lipomyelomeningoceles consist of a mass containing fat, neural placode, and meninges that protrudes dorsally across the dysraphic defect into a skin-covered bulge. Patients often present with a lumbosacral mass and may have such neurological findings as lower extremity weakness, leg pain, bladder dysfunction, and sensory issues. MRI shows the bony defect and fatty tissue, as well as (for lipomyelomeningocele) neural placode, meninges, and bulging CSF.

■ Diagnosis

Tethered spinal cord with lipoma of the filum terminale.

✓ Pearls

- The tethered cord syndrome results from anomalies of the filum terminale, with the conus medullaris considered borderline low if it reaches the lower endplate of L2.
- Risk of meningitis and intraspinal abscess is considerably increased in patients with dorsal dermal sinus.

- Lipomeningocele consists of a lipoma affixed to a neural placode, extending through an area of closed spinal dysraphism into the subcutaneous tissues, with tethering of the cord at the level.

Suggested Readings

Raghavan N, Barkovich AJ, Edwards M, Norman D. MR imaging in the tethered spinal cord syndrome. AJR Am J Roentgenol. 1989; 152(4):843–852

Schwartz ES, Barkovich AJ. Congenital anomalies of the spine. In Barkovich AJ, Raybaud C, eds. Pediatric Neuroimaging, 5th ed. Philadelphia, PA: Lippincott Williams & Wilkins; 2012:857–922

Schwartz ES, Rossi A. Congenital spine anomalies: the closed spinal dysraphisms. Pediatr Radiol. 2015; 45 Suppl 3:S413–S419

Case 176

Rebecca Stein-Wexler

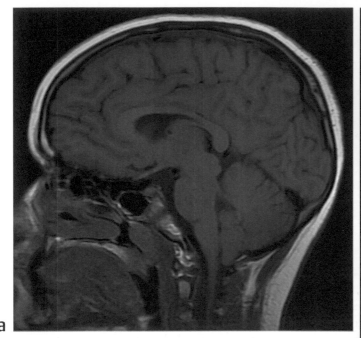

a

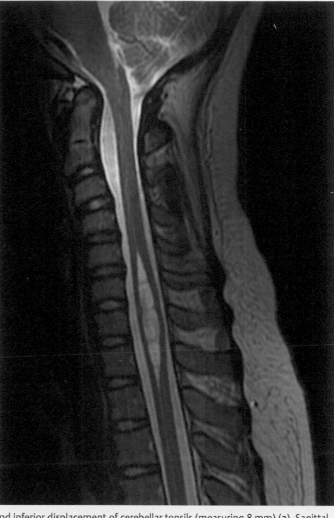

b

Fig. 176.1 Sagittal T1-W MRI demonstrates crowding of the posterior fossa and inferior displacement of cerebellar tonsils (measuring 8 mm) (a). Sagittal T2-W MRI shows the low-lying cerebellar tonsils as well as a septated collection of fluid within the central part of an expanded spinal cord (b).

■ Clinical Presentation

A 12-year-old girl with headache and ataxia (▶Fig. 176.1).

■ Key Imaging Finding

Syringohydromyelia.

■ Top Three Differential Diagnoses

- **Normal variant.** Focal, filiform enlargement of the central canal of the spinal cord may be seen in a small percentage of the general population. The fluid collection is typically slightly asymmetrical in the sagittal plane, within the ventral part of the low cervical or midthoracic cord. It is less common in the lumbar region, where it is central in location. If the dilatation exceeds 2 mm, follow-up MRI may be considered to exclude an early syrinx or neoplasm. This entity is distinct from the ventriculus terminalis, or "fifth ventricle," which is normal focal central dilatation of the proximal conus medullaris.
- **Chiari 1 malformation (C1M).** Most cases of C1M are due to underdevelopment of the occipital bone, which results in a small posterior fossa that leads to inferior displacement and elongation of the cerebellar tonsils, crowding of the posterior fossa, and compression of CSF spaces. Syringohydromyelia (SHM) is encountered in up to 70%. Children may complain of occipital headache and neck pain or symptoms related to brainstem compression, such as dysphagia, ataxia, and breathing abnormalities. Symptoms referable to SHM usually develop in older children or young adults and include paresis of the upper extremities and sensory deficits in the upper and lower extremities. About 30% of children with syrinx develop a progressive single curve levoconvex scoliosis, associated with neurological abnormalities on the left. However, many children with C1M are asymptomatic. On MRI, the cerebellar tonsils appear pointed and typically extend at least 5 mm below the foramen magnum. There is effacement of the foramen magnum and compression of the fourth ventricle and cisterns. SHM usually extends from the midcervical to the upper thoracic cord, though the entire cord length may be affected. MRI often shows multiple incomplete septations within the central fluid collection, resulting in a beaded appearance. There may be high T2 signal in the cord proximal and distal to the syrinx, due to microcysts or astrogliosis. However, there is no abnormal enhancement. Dynamic CSF flow studies show abnormal or absent flow across the foramen magnum. SHM may develop in patients with Chiari 2 malformation after surgical repair of meningomyeloceles.
- **Spinal cord tumor.** Ependymomas and astrocytomas are the most common intramedullary tumors of the spinal cord. They are commonly associated with both tumoral and nontumoral polar cysts. In addition, they are often accompanied with SHM. SHM may precede the development of tumor in patients with underlying conditions such as C1M. Alternatively, the SHM may form because the tumor obstructs normal CSF flow within the cord and subarachnoid space. Such tumoral SHM resolves after tumor resection. Intravenous (IV) contrast administration is important for excluding the presence of spinal cord tumor in patients with SHM.

■ Diagnosis

Syringohydromyelia along with inferior displacement of the cerebellar tonsils secondary to Chiari 1 malformation.

✓ Pearls

- Focal, filiform enlargement of the central canal up to 2 mm is a normal finding.
- The tight foramen magnum seen in patients with Chiari 1 malformation may disturb CSF flow, resulting in syringohydromyelia in up to 70% of patients.
- Progressive single curve levoscoliosis is seen in about one-third of patients with Chiari 1 malformation.
- IV contrast should be administered to patients with syringohydromyelia to exclude the presence of spinal cord tumor.

Suggested Readings

Koeller KK, Rosenblum RS, Morrison AL. Neoplasms of the spinal cord and filum terminale: radiologic-pathologic correlation. Radiographics. 2000; 20(6):1721–1749

Poretti A, Boltshauser E, Huisman TA. Chiari malformations and syringohydromyelia in children. Semin Ultrasound CT MR. 2016; 37(2):129–142

Schwartz ES, Barkovich AJ. Congenital anomalies of the spine. In Barkovich AJ, Raybaud C, eds. Pediatric Neuroimaging, 5th ed. Philadelphia, PA: Lippincott Williams & Wilkins; 2012:857–922

Case 177

Rebecca Stein-Wexler

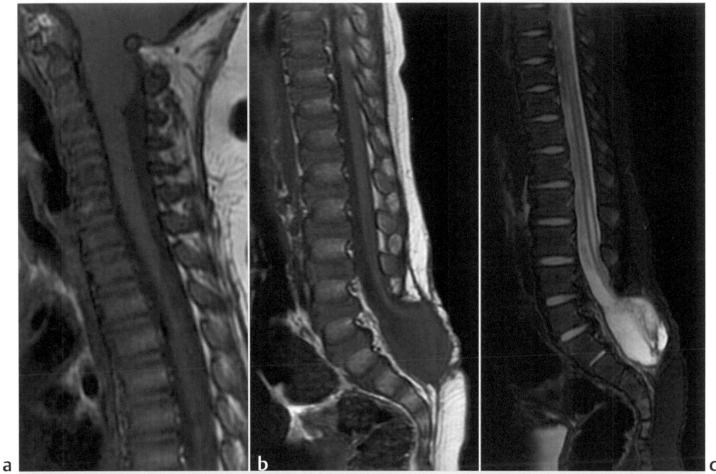

Fig. 177.1 Sagittal T1-W cervicothoracic spine MRI shows that the cerebellar tonsils extend down to C2–C3 and the foramen magnum appears tight **(a)**. Sagittal T1-W lumbosacral MRI shows there is low lumbar and upper sacral dysraphism and that the spinal cord appears elongated and stretched, terminating at a neural placode at L5/S1; the overlying skin appears irregular **(b)**. Sagittal T2-W image also shows focal dilatation of the lumbar spinal cord **(c)**.

◼ Clinical Presentation

A 10-month-old male infant with flaccid lower extremities
(▶Fig. 177.1).

■ Key Imaging Finding

Spinal dysraphism.

■ Top Three Differential Diagnoses

- **Myelocele/myelomeningocele (MC/MMC).** Open spinal dysraphism (aka "non-skin-covered dysraphism") develops when the neural tube fails to close in the midline and creates a neural placode instead of the distal spinal cord. Ectodermal elements, such as skin, and mesodermal elements, such as bone and muscle, fail to develop over this area. The neural placode is thus exposed to amniotic fluid in the womb and to outside air after birth. The bone- and skin-forming mesenchyme remains anterolateral to nervous tissue, so pedicles and lamina form abnormally and are splayed open. Vertebral segmentation abnormalities are common. With MMC, the meninges and cord protrude through the defect, whereas with MC only the cord protrudes. The neural tissue is flush with the skin with MC, but it protrudes posteriorly with MMC. MMC and MC are imaged postnatally only if neurological deficits progress after perinatal surgery. Diagnosis is usually made with prenatal US and imaged further with prenatal MRI, which shows neural tissue, CSF, and variably meninges extending through a dorsal bone/skin defect. The spinal cord terminates in an open neural placode, the unclosed neural tube. With lumbar or lumbosacral defects, the spinal cord is usually tethered and the conus low lying. Postsurgical imaging may show syringohydromyelia, other abnormal fluid collections, and persistent cord tethering. If fetal surgery is not performed, all patients also have Chiari 2 malformation, perhaps because CSF leaks through an open spinal defect, disturbing the pressure needed for normal posterior fossa and brain development.
- **Lipomyelomeningocele (LMM).** This closed spinal dysraphism (also termed "skin-covered dysraphism") develops when the neural tube fails to close after being covered with cutaneous ectoderm. Fat forms when the surrounding mesoderm comes in contact with ependymal cells that line the inner surface of the open neural tube. A mass consisting of fat, neural placode, and meninges protrudes dorsally across the dysraphic defect into a skin-covered bulge. LMM is recognized clinically by the presence of a fatty, subcutaneous mass above the gluteal cleft. With lipomyelocele, which is closely related, the neural/fatty mass does not protrude posteriorly. MRI shows the bony defect and fatty tissue as well as neural placode, meninges, and bulging CSF.
- **Meningocele.** This closed spinal dysraphism consists of meninges and CSF—but no neural tissue—herniating through an osseous defect. Posterior meningoceles are most common in the lumbosacral area, but may be occipital or cervical. Anterior meningoceles are usually presacral. Lateral meningoceles protrude through the intervertebral foramina and are a feature of neurofibromatosis type 1.

■ Diagnosis

Chiari 2 malformation with lumbosacral dysraphism, repaired lumbosacral MMC, syringohydromyelia, and low-lying conus.

✓ Pearls

- Myelomeningocele is an open spinal dysraphism that consists of a neural placode, meninges, and CSF extending through a dorsal osseous defect, with no overlying skin.
- Almost all patients with myelomeningocele also have Chiari 2 malformation, likely due to altered fluid dynamics.
- Lipomyelomeningocele is a closed spinal dysraphism consisting of a mass composed of fat, neural placode, and meninges protruding into a dorsal dysraphic defect, covered with skin.
- Meningoceles are usually posterior and are most common in the lumbosacral spine.

Suggested Readings

Poretti A, Boltshauser E, Huisman TA. Chiari malformations and syringohydromyelia in children. Semin Ultrasound CT MR. 2016; 37(2):129–142

Rufener SL, Ibrahim M, Raybaud CA, Parmar HA. Congenital spine and spinal cord malformations: pictorial review. AJR Am J Roentgenol. 2010; 194(3), Suppl:S26–S37

Schwartz ES, Barkovich AJ. Congenital anomalies of the spine. In Barkovich AJ, Raybaud C, eds. Pediatric Neuroimaging, 5th ed. Philadelphia, PA: Lippincott Williams & Wilkins; 2012:857–922

Taragin BH, Wootton-Gorges SL. The spine: congenital and developmental conditions. In Stein-Wexler R, Wootton-Gorges SL, Ozonoff MB, eds. Pediatric Orthopedic Imaging. Berlin/Heidelberg: Springer; 2015:43–105

Case 178

Rebecca Stein-Wexler

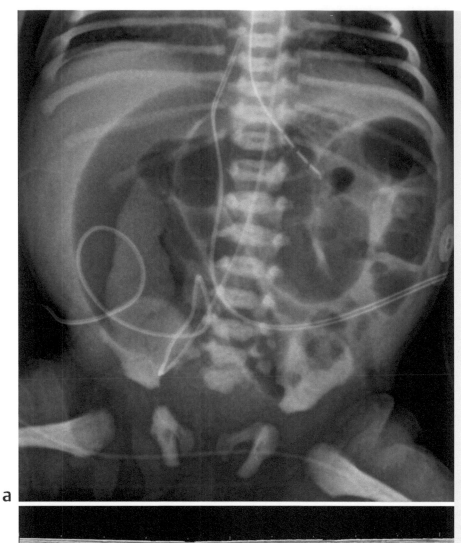

a

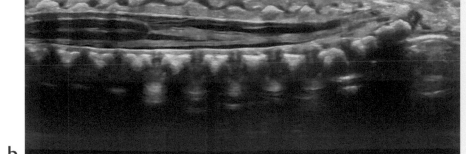

b

Fig. 178.1 Supine abdomen radiograph shows multiple very dilated bowel loops, with no gas in the rectum; there are only three ossified sacral segments, and S2 and S3 are dysmorphic **(a)**. Sagittal spine US shows the conus ends relatively high (L1) and has a blunt end that does not taper normally; the sacrum is deficient **(b)**.

■ Clinical Presentation

A newborn with failure to pass meconium at 24 hours (▶Fig. 178.1).

■ Key Imaging Finding

Lower spine deformity.

■ Top Three Differential Diagnoses

- **Spinal dysraphism.** Midline vertebral structures may fail to fuse, leading to closed (skin covered) or open (uncovered) dysraphism. Most open dysraphism is identified early, but covered defects may be diagnosed in older children presenting with constipation and urinary difficulties. The skin overlying closed defects may be abnormal (hairy patch, lipoma, hemangioma), and spinal cord abnormalities are common. Radiographs usually show structural defects in the vertebrae, such as abnormally wide neural arches, intersegmental fusion, vertebral scalloping, and diffuse enlargement of the spinal canal. US screening may be employed until age 3 months, after which MRI becomes necessary.
- **Caudal regression.** Abnormal regression of the mesoderm may lead to malformation of the lower spine. Most common in infants of diabetic mothers, caudal regression varies greatly in severity. In its most extreme form, the lower extremities are fused (sirenomelia), the sacrum is completely absent, and the iliac bones are fused in the midline. Lumbar vertebrae may be absent as well. Milder forms include partial absence of the sacrum (with S1 present), a hemisacrum, and absence of only the coccyx. Imperforate anus and other anorectal malformations are commonly associated, and patients with the milder forms of caudal regression may present simply with constipation. Neurogenic bladder is present in all patients who lack one or more sacral segments. Renal US is therefore essential to evaluate for hydronephrosis. Furthermore, caudal regression is associated with renal agenesis. The urethra may be abnormal (megalourethra or urethral valves). The spinal cord is often malformed. It may appear tethered or have an unusually high termination, in which case the conus medullaris often appears spade-shaped.
- **Currarino triad.** This condition consists of a scimitar-shaped sacrum, anorectal malformation, and presacral mass. A variety of neurological, genitourinary, and other abnormalities may be associated. A rectoperineal fistula is common. Alternatively, a fistula may extend to the bladder, urethra, or vagina. The presacral mass may consist of an anterior meningocele, teratoma, dermoid, rectal duplication, or a combination thereof. Tethered cord and lipoma commonly coexist, and therefore evaluation of the spine is essential. Hirschsprung disease and other dysganglionoses may also be present. Constipation is common and may be the only symptom. It is therefore especially important to carefully evaluate the sacrum on radiographs obtained to evaluate constipation. Duplex kidney/ureter, horseshoe kidney, renal dysplasia, and hypospadias may be seen. Currarino triad is also associated with trisomy 21. Currarino syndrome describes an autosomal-dominant form of Currarino triad.

■ Diagnosis

Imperforate anus with caudal regression syndrome and spade configuration of conus medullaris.

✓ Pearls

- Patients with low spine dysraphism or milder forms of caudal regression may present with constipation or bladder dysfunction, so it is important to always carefully evaluate the sacrum and lumbar spine.
- The Currarino triad consists of a scimitar-shaped sacrum, an anorectal malformation, and a presacral mass.
- Caudal regression varies greatly in severity and is most common in infants of diabetic mothers.
- The differential for a presacral mass in patients with Currarino triad includes anterior meningocele, teratoma, dermoid, and rectal duplication.

Suggested Readings

Kocaoglu M, Frush DP. Pediatric presacral masses. Radiographics. 2006; 26(3):833–857

Lynch SA, Wang Y, Strachan T, Burn J, Lindsay S. Autosomal dominant sacral agenesis: Currarino syndrome. J Med Genet. 2000; 37(8):561–566

Martucciello G, Torre M, Belloni E, et al. Currarino syndrome: proposal of a diagnostic and therapeutic protocol. J Pediatr Surg. 2004; 39(9):1305–1311

Tortori-Donati P, Rossi A, Cama A. Spinal dysraphism: a review of neuroradiological features with embryological correlations and proposal for a new classification. Neuroradiology. 2000; 42(7):471–491

Case 179

Rebecca Stein-Wexler

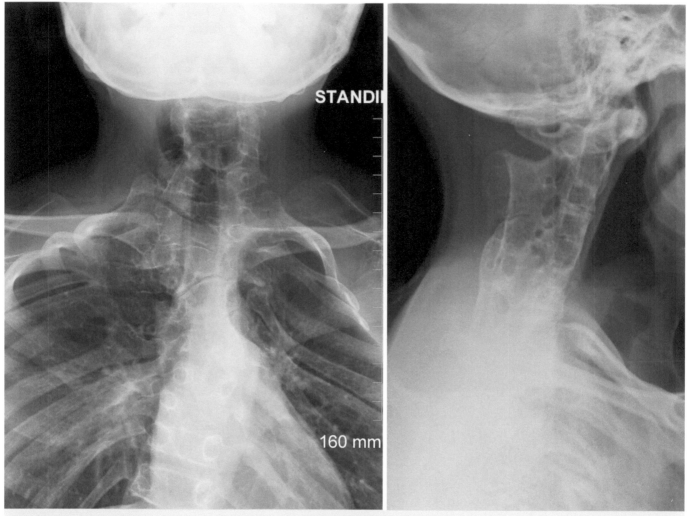

a

b

Fig. 179.1 Frontal view shows multiple hemivertebrae and other segmentation abnormalities, rib fusions, and an elevated and rotated left scapula (a). Lateral view shows multilevel block vertebra formation, with fusion of vertebral bodies as well as posterior elements (b).

■ Clinical Presentation

A 17-year-old with limited neck and shoulder mobility ▶Fig. 179.1).

■ Key Imaging Finding

Cervical spine fusion.

■ Top Three Differential Diagnoses

- **Klippel–Feil syndrome.** This condition describes partial or complete fusion of the cervical and upper thoracic spine, along with such vertebral anomalies as hemivertebrae, butterfly vertebrae, and wedge vertebrae. C2–C3 and C5–C6 are most often affected. Scoliosis is common, and ribs are often fused. The kidneys are abnormal in 50%. Unilateral agenesis is most common, but ectopia and horseshoe kidney are also seen. Increased mobility in unfused areas of the spine may lead to acute and/or chronic neurological damage. Spinal cord impingement is usually anterior, as a result of excess flexion, but hypertrophy of the ligamentum flavum may lead to dorsal impingement.
- **Juvenile idiopathic arthritis (JIA).** JIA is a clinical diagnosis with varied manifestations. It encompasses all arthritides of unknown origin that last more than 6 weeks in patients less than 16 years old. The disease is stratified based on the number of joints involved, along with the presence or absence of other clinical findings. If fewer than five joints are involved at diagnosis, the disease is termed oligoarticular, whereas with polyarticular disease five or more joints are involved. Fevers, rash, and hepatosplenomegaly suggest Still disease, a systemic and severe form of JIA. About 60% of patients with JIA develop cervical spine abnormalities, and this is especially common in those with polyarticular and systemic disease. Ankylosis may develop within 3 to 5 years of disease onset.

The upper cervical spine is most often affected, especially the apophyseal joints of C2–C3. Affected vertebrae appear unusually narrow, and intervertebral disks are narrowed and potentially entirely effaced. Synovial proliferation may erode the odontoid process, which combines with ligamentous laxity to cause spine instability.

- **Klippel–Feil syndrome along with Sprengel deformity.** Sprengel deformity, or undescended scapula, develops when the scapular anlage does not descend from the midcervical level to below T3. Sprengel deformity is seen in up to 50% of patients with Klippel–Feil syndrome, whereas up to 20% of patients with Sprengel deformity have Klippel–Feil syndrome. Patients with Sprengel deformity usually have a connection between the medial scapular border and the dorsal elements of a lower cervical vertebra or T1. In about half of patients, this connection is osseous (omovertebral bone). Radiographs show the scapula is tilted, lifted, and medially displaced. The number of ribs is often increased or decreased, and ribs may be fused or bifid. MRI and CT may demonstrate the omovertebral bone or its fibrocartilaginous anlage. Patients with Sprengel deformity have reduced shoulder mobility, along with fullness at the base of the neck. The condition is much more common in girls and is usually seen on the left. Genitourinary abnormalities are common.

■ Diagnosis

Klippel–Feil syndrome and Sprengel deformity.

✓ Pearls

- Klippel–Feil syndrome consists of fusion and segmentation abnormalities of the cervical spine, often resulting in scoliosis.
- Patients with juvenile idiopathic arthritis may develop cervical spine fusion, usually affecting the apophyseal joints of C2–C3.

- Affected vertebrae in juvenile idiopathic arthritis are usually tall and narrow, and intervertebral disks are at least partly effaced.
- Sprengel deformity, or undescended scapula, accompanies about 50% of cases of Klippel–Feil syndrome.

Suggested Readings

Azouz EM. CT demonstration of omovertebral bone. Pediatr Radiol. 2007; 37(4):404

Schwartz ES, Barkovich AJ. Congenital anomalies of the spine. In Barkovich AJ, Raybaud C, eds. Pediatric Neuroimaging, 5th ed. Philadelphia, PA: Lippincott Williams & Wilkins; 2012:857–922

Sheybani EF, Khanna G, White AJ, Demertzis JL. Imaging of juvenile idiopathic arthritis: a multimodality approach. Radiographics. 2013; 33(5):1253–1273

Case 180

Kriti Gwal

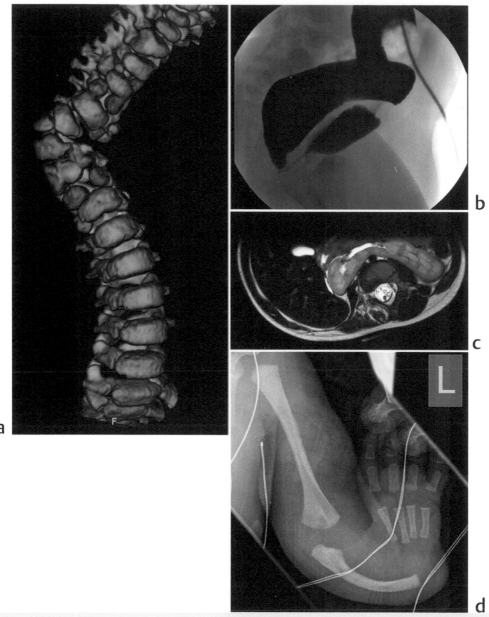

Fig. 180.1 3D-CT reconstruction of the spine demonstrates dextroscoliosis with a right hemivertebrae fused to the adjacent level, a butterfly vertebra, a right hemivertebrae with adjacent anomalous vertebrae, a wedge vertebra, and a second butterfly vertebra (listed cranial to caudal) (a). Fluoroscopic image obtained during a fistulogram after catheterization of a colostomy stoma shows a blind ending rectum with a fistulous connection to the bladder base and faint opacification of the normal prostatic urethra (different patient, newborn) (b). Axial T2-W image shows renal tissue fused in the midline; the filum terminale is thickened (c). Upper extremity radiograph shows the radius is absent, and the ulna foreshortened and bowed; the first ray is absent, and the hand is angled at 90 degrees to the forearm (d). (Images a, c, and d, all of the same patient at different ages, are provided courtesy of the Children's Hospital of Philadelphia.)

■ Clinical Presentation

Scoliosis and limb malformation (▶Fig. 180.1).

■ Key Imaging Finding

Vertebral segmentation abnormalities.

■ Top Three Differential Diagnoses

- **VACTERL association.** VACTERL or VATER describes the clinical association of multiple congenital anomalies that tend to occur together; it is not an actual syndrome. To qualify, the patient must have at least three of the following: **V**ertebral anomalies, **A**nal atresia, **C**ardiac defects, **T**racheo**E**sophageal fistula, **R**enal anomalies, with or without **L**imb malformations. Anal atresia (imperforate anus) is obvious at birth, and limb anomalies are usually apparent. Esophageal atresia with or without tracheoesophageal fistula is likewise diagnosed promptly when the neonate cannot tolerate feeds. The vertebral anomalies may be found on a radiograph evaluating scoliosis or obtained for other reasons. Vertebral anomalies include hemivertebrae, butterfly vertebrae, and wedge vertebrae, which, if unbalanced, often cause scoliosis. If any of the above criteria are identified, the other categories should be evaluated as well.
- **Alagille syndrome (aka arteriohepatic dysplasia).** Patients with Alagille syndrome may have butterfly vertebrae, cardiac anomalies such as tetralogy of Fallot, renal anomalies, and abnormal brain and spinal cord vessels. Intrahepatic bile duct abnormalities are common, mimicking biliary atresia and leading to cholestasis and liver damage in the newborn period. Identification of butterfly vertebrae suggesting Alagille syndrome is of critical importance, since the Kasai procedure does not help these patients and may cause symptoms to worsen. Patients often have characteristic facies with broad forehead and deep-set eyes.
- **Klippel–Feil syndrome.** This condition describes partial or complete fusion of the cervical and upper thoracic spine, along with such vertebral anomalies as hemivertebrae, butterfly vertebrae, and wedge vertebrae. C2–C3 and C5–C6 are most often affected, and scoliosis is common. Additional findings include decreased range of motion of the head and neck, short neck, and low posterior hairline. Associations include facial asymmetry, hearing and ocular abnormalities, and congenital cardiac and genitourinary problems. Sprengel deformity, congenital elevation of the scapula, is often present as well.

■ Diagnosis

VACTERL association with vertebral anomalies, anal atresia with fistula, horseshoe kidney, and longitudinal deficiency of the radius with radial clubhand.

✓ Pearls

- VACTERL or VATER association consists of at least three of the following: **V**ertebral anomalies, **A**nal atresia, **C**ardiac defects, **T**racheo**E**sophageal fistula, **R**enal anomalies, with or without **L**imb malformations.
- It is important to recognize butterfly vertebrae in patients with Alagille syndrome, since their biliary ductal abnormalities cannot be treated with the Kasai procedure.

- Klippel–Feil syndrome consists of cervical segmentation anomalies that cause decreased range of head/neck motion, short neck, and low posterior hairline.

Suggested Readings

Dilli A, Ayaz UY, Damar C, Ersan O, Hekimoglu B. Sprengel deformity: magnetic resonance imaging findings in two pediatric cases. J Clin Imaging Sci. 2011; 1:13

Saker E, Loukas M, Oskouian RJ, Tubbs RS. The intriguing history of vertebral fusion anomalies: the Klippel-Feil syndrome. Childs Nerv Syst. 2016; 32(9).1599–1602

Saleh M, Kamath BM, Chitayat D. Alagille syndrome: clinical perspectives. Appl Clin Genet. 2016; 9:75–82

Solomon BD. VACTERL/VATER Association. Orphanet J Rare Dis. 2011; 6:56

Case 181

Rebecca Stein-Wexler

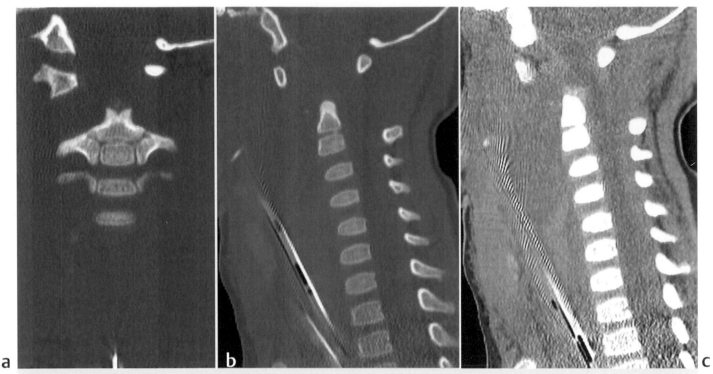

a b c

Fig. 181.1 Coronal reformatted CT shows wide separation between C1 and C2, slightly worse on the left (a). Sagittal reformatted CT shows extensive prevertebral soft tissue that displaces the esophageal catheter and endotracheal tube anteriorly, along with wide separation of C1 from C2, anterior displacement of the arch of C1, and a small fragment of bone anterior to the odontoid (b). Soft-tissue windows allow delineation of increased density anterior to the vertebral bodies and also in the dorsal aspect of the spinal canal (c).

■ Clinical Presentation

A 2-year-old girl who was hit by a car and required resuscitation en route to the emergency room (▶ Fig. 181.1).

■ Key Imaging Finding

Upper cervical spine fracture/dislocation.

■ Top Three Differential Diagnoses

• **Atlantoaxial joint disruption.** Young children are much more likely to injure the upper cervical spine than are older children and adults. This is due to a higher fulcrum of motion (C2–C3), ligamentous laxity, normal anterior vertebral body wedging, the configuration of the facet joints, and a relatively large head size. The mechanism of trauma in young children is usually related to motor vehicle, pedestrian, and bicycle accidents, whereas older children tend to have falls and sports injuries. In children, the normal gap between the posterior aspect of the anterior arch of C1 and the anterior cortex of the odontoid (atlanto-dens interval [ADI]) is up to 5 mm, larger than in adults. Injury to the transverse ligament allows the arch of C1 to slip forward, increasing the ADI. This is rarely an isolated injury in children and may be associated with rheumatoid disease or anatomical anomalies. Severe trauma may lead to extensive ligamentous injury and pronounced atlantoaxial disruption. Rotatory subluxation also occurs at this level.

• **Craniocervical separation (CCS).** Young children have relatively small occipital condyles and horizontal atlanto-occipital joints, predisposing them to this usually fatal injury. It results from sudden deceleration, causing ligamentous disruption. If the distance between the occipital condyles and the condylar surface of the atlas exceeds 5 mm, CCS may be present. The Wachenheim clivus line and the Powers ratio also assess CCS.

• **Jefferson fracture.** This results from axial load. Force transmitted through the occipital condyles to the lateral masses causes fractures through the anterior and posterior arches of C1. An open mouth odontoid view demonstrates asymmetry between the odontoid process and the lateral masses. Rupture of the transverse ligaments converts this from a stable to an unstable fracture, suggested if there is 6 mm or more between the lateral mass of C1 and the odontoid process. Decreased spinal canal width raises concern for cord injury.

■ Additional Differential Diagnoses

• **Hangman fracture.** Fractures of the pars interarticularis of C2 due to hyperextension injury result in traumatic spondylolisthesis of C2, the "hangman" fracture. This is less common than odontoid and C1 fractures. Evaluating the posterior cervical line (PCL), drawn along the anterior aspects of the spinous processes from C1 to C3, assesses alignment in this region. The spinous process of C2 should be within 1 mm of this line. If it is not, a hangman fracture may be present. Displacement of C2–C3 and to a lesser extent C3–C4 is usually physiological in young children.

• **Compression fracture.** This must be differentiated from the normal anterior wedging of up to 3 mm that is common in cervical vertebrae in children and which may be even more pronounced at C3. Wedge compression fractures are common but usually heal without sequelae if there are no retropulsed fragments.

■ Diagnosis

Severe atlantoaxial disruption with epidural hematoma.

✓ Pearls

• The upper cervical spine is injured most often in children.
• The Jefferson fracture of C1 is unstable if the distance between the lateral mass of C1 and the odontoid process is equal to or greater than 6 mm.

• Anterior cervical vertebral wedging of up to 3 mm is normal in children.

Suggested Readings

Egloff AM, Kadom N, Vezina G, Bulas D. Pediatric cervical spine trauma imaging: a practical approach. Pediatr Radiol. 2009; 39(5):447–456

Lustrin ES, Karakas SP, Ortiz AO, et al. Pediatric cervical spine: normal anatomy, variants, and trauma. Radiographics. 2003; 23(3):539–560

Case 182

Rebecca Stein-Wexler

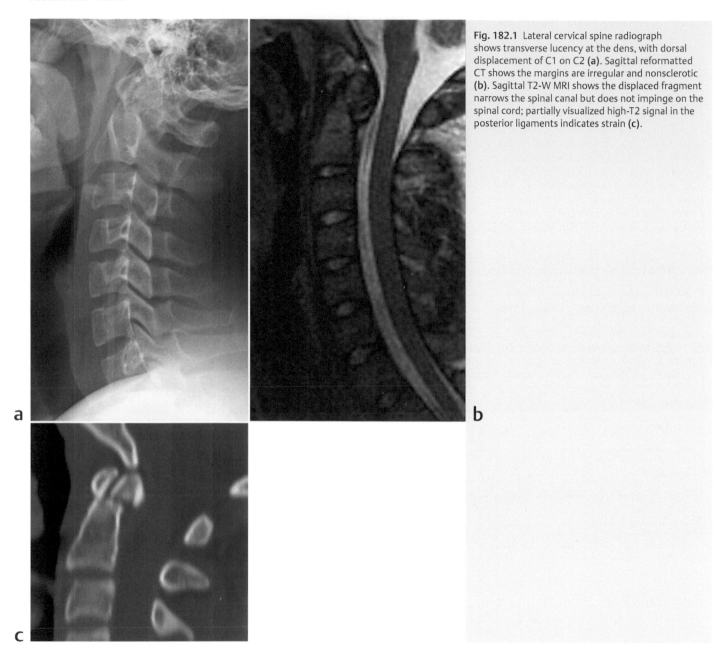

Fig. 182.1 Lateral cervical spine radiograph shows transverse lucency at the dens, with dorsal displacement of C1 on C2 **(a)**. Sagittal reformatted CT shows the margins are irregular and nonsclerotic **(b)**. Sagittal T2-W MRI shows the displaced fragment narrows the spinal canal but does not impinge on the spinal cord; partially visualized high-T2 signal in the posterior ligaments indicates strain **(c)**.

■ Clinical Presentation

A teen with neck pain after trauma (▶ Fig. 182.1).

■ Key Imaging Finding

Lucency in the odontoid process.

■ Top Three Differential Diagnoses

- **Ossiculum terminale.** Around age 3 to 6 years, the secondary ossification center at the top of the odontoid, the ossiculum terminale, begins to ossify. It usually fuses to the odontoid by about age 12 years, but in some patients it may never fuse. The ossiculum terminale is differentiated from fracture by its smooth, well-corticated margins.
- **C2/odontoid synchondrosis.** The odontoid fuses with the body of C2 around age 3 to 6 years, but the synchondrosis may remain evident on radiographs until adolescence and on MRI until early adulthood. Until fusion is complete, the synchondrosis may be confused with fracture. Margin contour helps differentiate.
- **Odontoid fracture.** This is the most common cervical spine fracture in children, especially in those younger than 7 years. It usually occurs through the synchondrosis (type 2 dens fracture) and heals without the complications that are common in adults. Radiographs show prevertebral swelling and anterior displacement with posterior tilt of the odontoid. The injury may be missed on axial CT, so sagittal and coronal reformatted images are essential. With type 3 dens fracture, which is the next most common, the fracture extends from the odontoid into the body of C2. The type 1 dens fracture is rare. It consists of an avulsion fracture of the tip of the odontoid at the insertion site of the alar ligament. It may be confused with an ossiculum terminale, but should be differentiated because of its sharp, nonsclerotic margins. Odontoid fractures in children usually respond well to immobilization in a halo, but internal fixation is often needed in adults, who have increased risk of nonunion.

■ Additional Differential Diagnosis

- **Os odontoideum.** This consists of a well-corticated bony density positioned above a relatively short odontoid. Congenital or residual from very early remote trauma, it is differentiated from an acute traumatic bone fragment by its smooth, well-corticated margins and its association with a relatively hypoplastic odontoid. There are two types of os odontoideum. The more common, orthotopic, type is positioned just above the superior margin of the dens. If it articulates with the posterior arch of C1, it may lead to atlanto-dens instability. The dystopic os is found in an unusual location, such as fused to the bottom of the clivus.

■ Diagnosis

Dorsally displaced type 2 odontoid fracture.

✓ Pearls

- The ossiculum terminale is a normal secondary ossification center, at the tip of the dens, which usually fuses around age 12 years.
- The synchondrosis at the base of the dens may persist into adulthood; it is differentiated from type 2 dens fracture by its smooth, well-corticated margins.
- Children with cervical spine fractures are likely to have injured their odontoid bone, either as a type 2 (base of dens) or type 3 (dens and body of C2) fracture.
- Either congenital or attributable to remote trauma, the os odontoideum is differentiated from ossiculum terminale by its association with a relatively short odontoid.

Suggested Readings

Egloff AM, Kadom N, Vezina G, Bulas D. Pediatric cervical spine trauma imaging: a practical approach. Pediatr Radiol. 2009; 39(5):447–456

Lustrin ES, Karakas SP, Ortiz AO, et al. Pediatric cervical spine: normal anatomy, variants, and trauma. Radiographics. 2003; 23(3):539–560

O'Brien WT Sr, Shen P, Lee P. The dens: Normal development, developmental variants and anomalies, and traumatic injuries. J Clin Imaging Sci. 2015; 5:38

Case 183

Ethan Neufeld

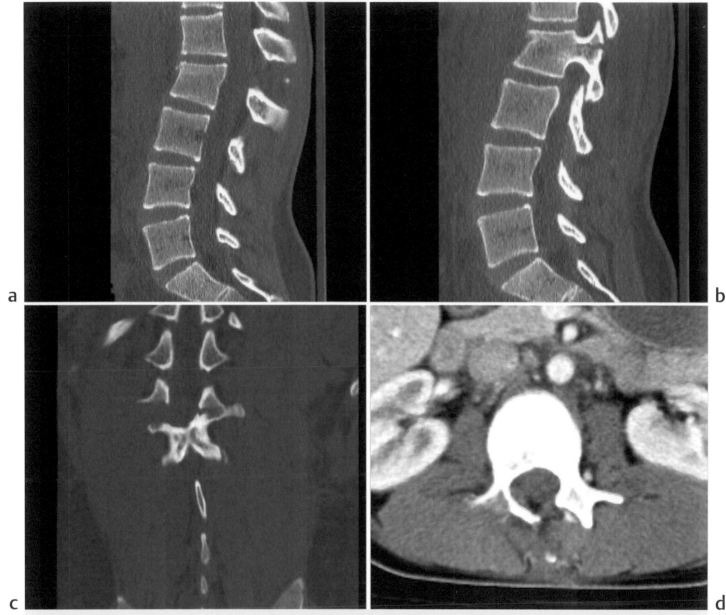

Fig. 183.1 Midline sagittal reformatted CT shows compression of the anterior aspect of the L2 vertebral body, along with superior endplate irregularity, distraction of the spinous processes of L1 and L2, and a bone fragment interposed between the spinous processes (a). Sagittal reformatted CT to the left of midline shows the fracture line extends through the left pedicle and superior articular process (b). Coronal reformatted CT better shows the posterior element extension (c). Axial CT in soft-tissue algorithm shows fat stranding in the prevertebral tissues at L2 as well as soft tissue surrounding the interspinous ligament posteriorly (d).

■ Clinical Presentation

A 15-year-old boy with back pain after motor vehicle collision
(▶Fig. 183.1).

■ Key Imaging Finding

Thoracolumbar spine traumatic injury.

■ Top Three Differential Diagnoses

- **Chance/seatbelt fracture.** Chance fractures are flexion–distraction injuries that are associated with motor vehicle collisions and tend to occur at the thoracolumbar junction and midlumbar spine. They involve all three spinal columns and are thus unstable. There is a strong association with intra-abdominal injuries in children, approaching 50%. The anterior aspect of the vertebral body demonstrates height loss and varying degrees of endplate irregularity. A horizontal fracture line extends through the pedicles and variably through the laminae, transverse processes, and articular processes. Attention should be paid to alignment of the spinous processes and facet joints, as ligamentous injury is very common.
- **Burst fracture.** Burst fractures are also characterized by vertebral body height loss, but they result from axial load, which in the thoracolumbar spine typically follows forceful landing from a significant height. The degree of height loss varies, but due to the compressive nature of injury there is a significant risk of retropulsion of osseous fragments into the spinal canal. There may be an associated fracture of the posterior elements, but the orientation will be vertical rather than horizontal as in Chance fractures. There is rarely if ever any malalignment of the posterior elements, as ligamentous injury is rare. Associated injuries are primarily musculoskeletal, with calcaneal fractures being especially common due to landing mechanism.
- **Hyperextension injury.** Pure hyperextension injuries are uncommon but are often associated with spinal cord injury. They occur at the lower thoracic spine and rarely in the lumbar and upper thoracic spine. The vertebral body heights are maintained, distinguishing this from Chance and burst fractures. The anterior disk space is widened due to disruption of the anterior longitudinal ligament, and there may be complex fractures of the posterior elements as they undergo compressive force.

■ Additional Differential Diagnosis

- **Pathological fracture.** If a complex fracture is out of proportion to the mechanism of injury, an underlying lesion should be suspected. Primary lesions like Ewing sarcoma should be considered, as should lesions associated with systemic processes such as Langerhans cell histiocytosis or leukemia. Findings that suggest an underlying pathological lesion include a background of abnormal bone marrow with a mottled appearance, an extensive soft-tissue component on CT/MRI, and any associated enhancement.

■ Diagnosis

Chance/seatbelt fracture (flexion–distraction injury).

✓ Pearls

- Chance fractures are characterized by anterior height loss, horizontal fracture lines through the posterior elements, and widening of the posterior articulations.
- Burst fractures are characterized by height loss with retropulsed fragments, vertical fracture lines through the posterior elements, and no significant ligamentous injury.
- The presence of an underlying lesion should be considered if the background bone is abnormal and/or the degree of injury is out of proportion to the mechanism of injury.

Suggested Readings

Bernstein MP, Mirvis SE, Shanmuganathan K. Chance-type fractures of the thoracolumbar spine: imaging analysis in 53 patients. AJR Am J Roentgenol. 2006; 187(4):859–868

Daniels AH, Sobel AD, Eberson CP. Pediatric thoracolumbar spine trauma. J Am Acad Orthop Surg. 2013; 21(12):707–716

Khurana B, Sheehan SE, Sodickson A, Bono CM, Harris MB. Traumatic thoracolumbar spine injuries: what the spine surgeon wants to know. Radiographics. 2013; 33(7):2031–2046

Case 184

Rebecca Stein-Wexler

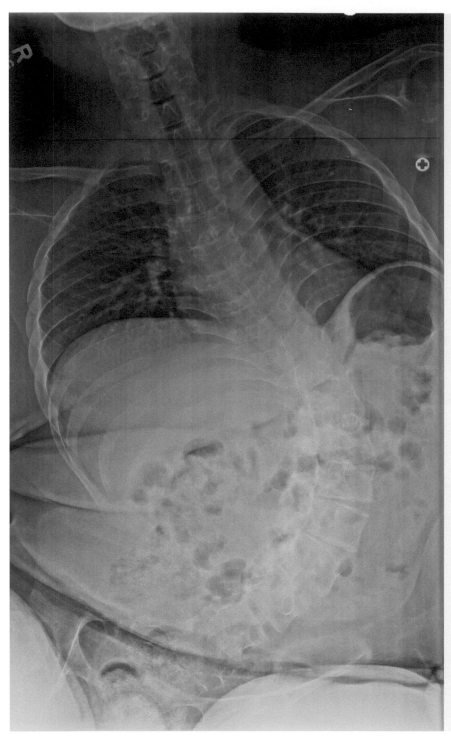

Fig. 184.1 Sitting anteroposterior view of the spine demonstrates long segment thoracolumbar levoscoliosis. Bones are osteopenic.

■ **Clinical Presentation**

A 16-year-old boy with deformity and profound weakness (▶ Fig. 184.1).

■ Key Imaging Finding

Scoliosis.

■ Top Three Differential Diagnoses

• **Idiopathic scoliosis (IS).** Adolescent IS presents after age 11, most often in girls, and usually with a primary thoracic dextroconvex curve and compensatory lumbar levoconvex curve. The primary curve does not correct with lateral bending, whereas the compensatory curve does. Curvature progresses most rapidly during growth spurts. Many centers employ the Cobb angle to measure curve progression. Juvenile IS has onset between ages 4 and 10 years, usually progresses, and, as in adolescents, has a dextroconvex primary curve. Infantile IS (age <4 years), by contrast, is levoconvex and usually resolves if treated before age 1 year.

• **Congenital scoliosis.** Segmentation abnormalities often cause scoliosis in young children. Hemivertebrae and wedge vertebrae may serve as the apex of a curve, whereas congenital bars restrict growth on the concave side of a curve. Symmetrical butterfly vertebrae and balanced hemivertebrae do not contribute to scoliosis. Curve progression is monitored on spine radiographs, but MRI is often performed to evaluate for associated tethered cord, syringohydromyelia, and split spinal cord malformation, present in up to 40%.

• **Neuromuscular scoliosis.** Neuromuscular scoliosis often presents in young patients, progresses rapidly, and continues to progress after skeletal maturity. Whether due to cerebral palsy, myelodysplasia, Duchenne muscular dystrophy, or spinal muscular atrophy, progressive trunk imbalance results from asymmetrical muscle forces. Neuromuscular scoliosis typically involves the entire spine in a single levoconvex C curve and also extends into the pelvis, causing pelvic obliquity. Bracing is the only nonoperative treatment, except for children with Duchenne muscular dystrophy, who may be treated with steroids.

■ Additional Differential Diagnoses

• **Bone and soft-tissue masses.** Osseous and paraspinal tumors may also cause scoliosis. Lesions to consider include neurofibroma, neural crest tumors, osteoid osteoma, aneurysmal bone cyst, osteoblastoma, Langerhans cell histiocytosis, lymphoma, and a variety of sarcomas.

• **Underlying spinal cord pathology.** A spinal cord tumor or syringohydromyelia often results in thoracic levoscoliosis. There may also be splaying and straightening of pedicles, due to long standing mass effect. Children may complain of back pain or neurological symptoms.

■ Diagnosis

Neuromuscular scoliosis due to Duchenne muscular dystrophy.

✓ Pearls

• Idiopathic adolescent scoliosis progresses most rapidly during growth spurts; it is usually dextroconvex in the thoracic spine and levoconvex in the lumbar spine.

• Hemivertebrae, wedge vertebrae, asymmetrical butterfly vertebrae, and congenital bars may cause congenital scoliosis.

• Neuromuscular scoliosis usually demonstrates a rapidly progressive long-segment thoracolumbar levoconvex curve.

• Patients with spinal cord tumor or syringohydromyelia may develop isolated thoracic levoscoliosis, along with remodeling of pedicles due to mass effect.

Suggested Readings

Schwartz ES, Barkovich AJ. Congenital anomalies of the spine. In Barkovich AJ, Raybaud C, eds. Pediatric Neuroimaging, 5th ed. Philadelphia, PA: Lippincott Williams & Wilkins; 2012:857–922

Taragin BH, Wootton-Gorges SL. The spine: congenital and developmental conditions. In Stein-Wexler R, Wootton-Gorges SL, Ozonoff MB, eds. Pediatric Orthopedic Imaging. Berlin/Heidelberg: Springer, 2015:43–105

Case 186

Geoffrey D. McWilliams

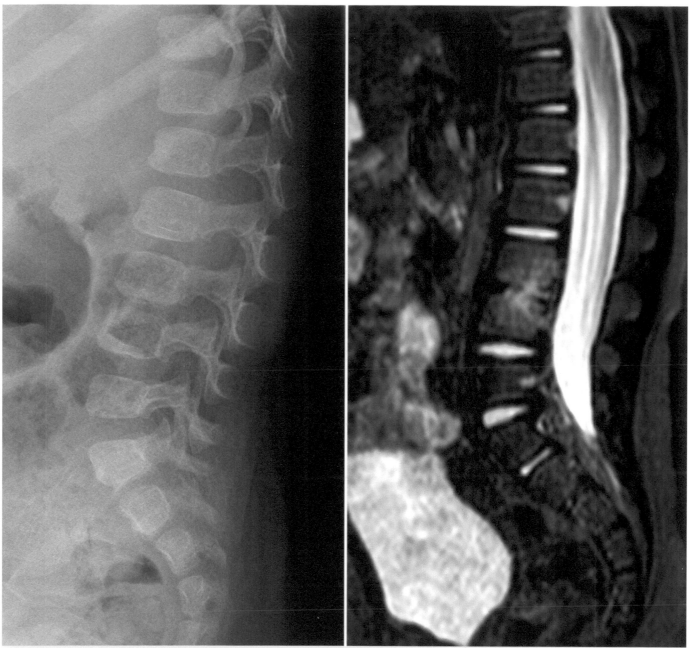

Fig. 186.1 Lateral lumbosacral spine radiograph shows mild narrowing of the intervertebral disk at L3–L4 with demineralization of the superior L4 endplate **(a)**. Two months later, T2-W sagittal MRI shows increased narrowing and T2 hyperintensity at the L3–L4 intervertebral disk, along with edema in the adjacent portions of the vertebral bodies **(b)**. (These images are provided courtesy of Hermann Kan.)

■ Clinical Presentation

A 2-year-old boy with a limp (▶ Fig. 186.1).

■ Key Imaging Finding

Vertebral body/disk inflammation.

■ Top Three Differential Diagnoses

- **Diskitis/osteomyelitis.** With pediatric diskitis/osteomyelitis, infection usually starts in the relatively vascular intervertebral disk and sometimes spreads to the vertebral body. Unlike in adults, primary bone infection is uncommon. Onset is insidious, and children often present with a limp or chronic back pain. Most cases occur before the age of 4 years, with a second peak at age 10 to 14 years. The disease typically involves the lumbar spine but may affect the thoracic and, less often, the cervical spine. Intervertebral disk height may be decreased, and end-plate cortical erosions are common. More advanced cases may show vertebral body collapse. Paraspinal or epidural abscesses or granulation tissue may lead to cord compression. X-rays may be normal for up to 2 months. In cases of diskitis, MRI shows low T1 disk signal with variably high T2 signal, diffuse enhancement of the disk, and indistinctness of adjacent endplates. Adjacent vertebral bodies often show mild reactive marrow edema (low on T1, high on STIR/T2) and enhancement, or there may be signs of more active infection. CT may show focal lytic and sclerotic changes at the vertebral endplate and enhancement of the intervertebral disk, marrow, and soft tissues.
- **Tuberculous spondylitis.** The spine is the most common site of osseous tuberculosis. Tuberculous spondylitis affects children more aggressively than adults. Thoracic spine involvement is most common in children, who usu-

ally develop contiguous infection of two or more vertebral bodies and resultant kyphotic deformity. Nearly all children also have a paraspinal or intraspinal soft-tissue mass, frequently abutting the spinal cord. Bone enhances, and the soft-tissue component shows variable rim enhancement. The disks between contiguous involved vertebral segments are destroyed, but those just above or below the affected region are usually intact.

- **Juvenile idiopathic arthritis (JIA).** JIA is a group of inflammatory arthropathies clinically defined by age and duration, occurring in children under 16 years with symptoms lasting longer than 6 weeks. Although any joint may be involved, large joints are most commonly affected. Many patients develop vertebral disease. Findings are most common in the cervical spine, but the thoracic spine is sometimes affected. X-rays show vertebral body growth anomalies such as intervertebral fusion and variable vertebral body size due to early fusion and overgrowth related to hyperemia. Erosive changes affect the odontoid, intervertebral, and costovertebral joints. Early degenerative disk disease may be seen. Multilevel subluxations are common and may affect the craniocervical junction. MRI may show cartilage erosion, periarticular pannus formation, joint effusions, and synovial thickening, while X-rays are still normal.

■ Diagnosis

Diskitis/osteomyelitis.

✓ Pearls

- Vertebral diskitis/osteomyelitis in children usually affects the lumbar spine, begins in the disk, and may not be apparent on radiographs for up to 8 weeks.
- Tuberculous spondylitis usually affects the thoracic spine and presents more aggressively than in adults, usually with kyphosis and a soft-tissue mass.

- Juvenile idiopathic arthritis usually affects the cervical spine and presents with growth disturbance, fusion, erosions, and subluxations.

Suggested Readings

Andronikou S, Jadwat S, Douis H. Patterns of disease on MRI in 53 children with tuberculous spondylitis and the role of gadolinium. Pediatr Radiol. 2002; 32(11):798–805

Elhai M, Wipff J, Bazeli R, et al. Radiological cervical spine involvement in young adults with polyarticular juvenile idiopathic arthritis. Rheumatology (Oxford). 2013; 52(2):267–275

Fucs PM, Meves R, Yamada HH. Spinal infections in children: a review. Int Orthop. 2012; 36(2):387–395

Case 188

Michael Doherty

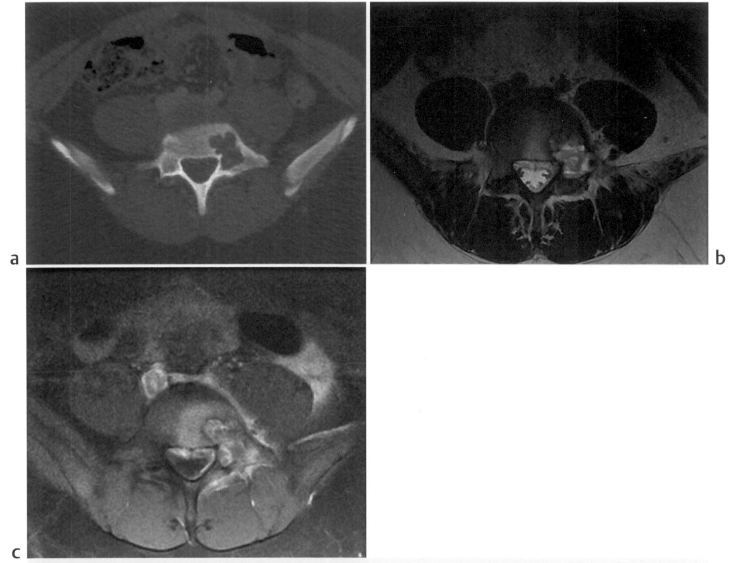

Fig. 188.1 Axial CT shows an expansile, lucent mass with a narrow zone of transition centered in the left L5 pedicle (**a**). T2-W MRI shows that the mass consists of cystic spaces of varying signal intensity with fluid–fluid levels and perilesional edema (**b**). Axial T1-W gadolinium-enhanced MRI shows septa enhance, and there is also perilesional enhancement (**c**).

■ **Clinical Presentation**

A 16-year-old with back pain (▶ Fig. 188.1).

■ **Key Imaging Finding**

Lytic mass in the posterior elements.

■ **Top Three Differential Diagnoses**

- **Aneurysmal bone cyst (ABC).** Up to one-third of ABCs occur in the spine, most often in the cervicothoracic region. Patients usually complain of insidious onset of back pain and neurological symptoms due to nerve root and/or spinal cord compression. The lesion has no malignant potential. ABC in the spine is usually subtle on X-rays, potentially showing expansion, lucency, and/or sclerosis of a posterior element. CT shows an expansile, lytic mass centered in the posterior element, with a narrow zone of transition and "eggshell" cortex. On MRI, there is a lobulated mass with a hypointense rim and perilesional edema. Cystic spaces contain fluid–fluid levels that vary in signal intensity. Cysts are separated by septa of varying thickness, which may enhance. Treatment options include surgical excision, injection with sclerosing agents, embolization, or radiation therapy. Giant cell tumor and telangiectatic osteosarcoma may contain areas of ABC.
- **Osteoblastoma.** About 40% of cases of this expansile, osteoid-forming benign tumor occur in the neural arch of the spine. Because of its large size at presentation (>1.5 cm), patients may present with pain or neurological deficits due to nerve root or spinal cord compression. X-rays may show expansion and/or sclerosis of the pedicle. On CT, osteoblastoma usually appears as a well-circumscribed expansile mass with a narrow zone of transition. Aggressive lesions may demonstrate cortical breakthrough. There is low to intermediate signal on T1 and low to high signal on T2/STIR as well as prominent peritumoral edema (flare phenomenon). The degree of enhancement varies.
- **Osteoid osteoma.** This tumor is differentiated from osteoblastoma by size less than 1.5 cm. Osteoid osteoma is much more common in the long bones. When it occurs in the spine, the posterior elements of the lumbar spine are most often affected. Patients typically present with painful scoliosis. CT shows a predominantly lucent central nidus with an associated dense reactive zone of sclerosis and variable periosteal reaction. The central nidus shows low signal intensity on T1 with low to high signal intensity on T2/STIR. It enhances intensely. The reactive zone is characterized by edema as well as enhancement that is delayed relative to the nidus.

■ **Additional Differential Diagnosis**

- **Metastatic disease.** Metastatic disease to the spine initially involves the vertebral body and may later spread to the pedicle. However, vertebral body involvement is relatively difficult to see, and posterior element lesions may be easier to recognize on X-rays. Spinal Langerhans cell histiocytosis usually presents with vertebra plana and uncommonly affects the posterior elements.

■ **Diagnosis**

Aneurysmal bone cyst.

✓ **Pearls**

- Spine aneurysmal bone cyst appears as an expansile mass centered in the posterior elements; MRI shows cystic spaces that contain fluid–fluid levels with enhancing septa.
- Osteoblastoma is an expansile, osteoid-forming benign tumor in the neural arch measuring greater than 1.5 cm, with prominent peritumoral edema.
- Osteoid osteoma is less than 1.5 cm and has a central lucent nidus with a reactive zone of sclerosis.

Suggested Readings

Doss VT, Weaver J, Didier S, et al. Serial endovascular embolization as stand-alone treatment of a sacral aneurysmal bone cyst. J Neurosurg Spine. 2014; 20:234–238

Zileli M, Isik HS, Ogut FE, et al. Aneurysmal bone cysts of the spine. Eur Spine J. 2013; 22:593–601

Index of Key Findings

Note: The index is ordered by case number within each section.